THE FIRST DECADE OF SAFE AND EFFECTIVE HIV VACCINES

THE FIRST DECADE OF SAFE AND EFFECTIVE HIV VACCINES

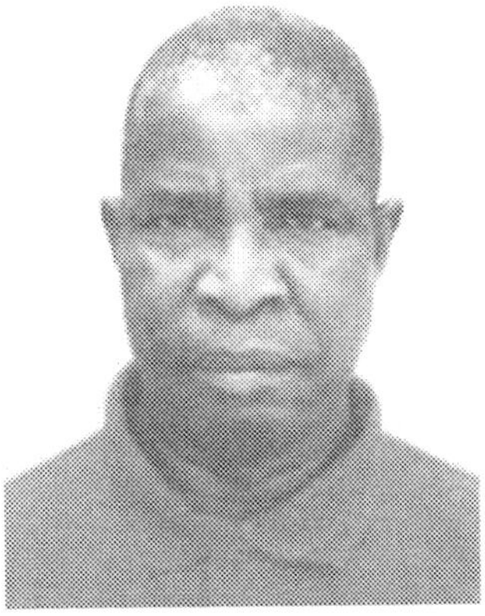

JEREMIAH O. A. ABALAKA

Nova Science Publishers, Inc.
New York

For permission to use material from this book please contact us:
Telephone 631-231-7269; Fax 631-231-8175
Web Site: http://www.novapublishers.com

Library of Congress Cataloging-in-Publication Data

Abalaka, Jeremiah O. A.
The first decade of safe and effective HIV vaccines / Jeremiah O.A. Abalaka.
p. ; cm.
Includes bibliographical references and index.
ISBN 978-1-60741-143-7 (hardcover)
1. AIDS vaccines. I. Title.
[DNLM: 1. AIDS Vaccines. 2. HIV Infections--prevention & control. WC 503.6 A117f 2009]
QR189.5.A33A23 2009
615'.372--dc22
2009002397

Published by Nova Science Publishers, Inc. ✦ New York

To mom Martha, brothers Tom and Akogu, daughter Irene, Frances Barre-Sinoussi, Jean-Claude Chermann, Luc Montagnier and the 9 others from the Pasteur Institut in Paris who first published the discovery of the AIDS virus in the Journal *Science* in May 1983, Robert Gallo and his team at the National Cancer Institutes in the US and all the other researchers that worked hard to facilitate the elucidation of the characteristics of the new virus,Frank Olize and the others in the Print and electronic media in Nigeria, Shareef Mohammed, Barrister Isaac Okpanachi, the staffs of Medicrest Specialist Hospital, the Editor of *Vaccine* Journal Professor Ray E. Spier, the many millions worldwide who are infected with HIV, the billions who are in dire need of a safe and effective preventive vaccine against the rampaging, dreaded and dreadful HIV and the memory of Professor Edington, daughter Amanda, wife Esther, dad Daniel, son Ronald, and the several millions that have callously been left to perish from HIV/AIDS by being victims of the sustained but false propaganda that safe and effective HIV vaccines do not exist.

Contents

Foreword

It is with great pleasure that I write the foreword to this book *"The First Decade of Safe and Effective HIV Vaccines"*. That a surgeon is writing on Human Immunodeficiency Virus (HIV) and vaccinology might sound absurd. But a young Dr. Jeremiah Ojonemi Alabi Abalaka did all the rotations in laboratory medicine, namely Haematology, Microbiology, Chemical Pathology and Histopathology. He finally settled for Histopathology. Later, he took a post-graduate certificate in immunology from Nigeria's premier University of Ibadan before suddenly abandoning laboratory medicine for surgery. Going through the book reveals that he is making good use of the knowledge and skills acquired in his earlier sojourn in the laboratory.

Dr. J. O. A. Abalaka is a person who also takes any work seriously. He is not afraid of voicing and/or doing what he believes even if people think otherwise. He has approached the issue of development of vaccines against HIV not exploiting modern sophisticated methods but rather believes other approaches including the so-called traditional or old-fashioned methods must not be thrown overboard when other approaches have not yielded the desired dividends.

The phrase "curative vaccine" may sound irritating to the ears of vaccinologists but this author uses it with ease to refer to any therapeutic vaccine that cures the infection. Others believe vaccines only prevent infection and that vaccines do not cure humans of already established infections.

The author is not afraid of controversies. Indeed controversies in science have proved, in the past, to be lubricants for more investigations sometimes leading to new discoveries. He has presented his views on HIV vaccine and other HIV-related issues in his characteristic bluntness, daring even the most internationally respected scientists on the subject of HIV/AIDS vaccines concept and development.

The author has presented in this book his experience in looking for HIV vaccines. He has discussed the immunological concepts he used vis-à-vis the futile international efforts made so far to develop safe and effective vaccines against HIV.

Since 1999, I have been conducting different tests on those who have been taking the author's HIV vaccines before and during treatment with the vaccines. Statistical analysis has shown that the vaccine has a highly significant positive effect on the CD4+ lymphocyte counts as well as a decrease in the HIV p24 antigen levels in the blood. The few who had an opportunity to do CD8+ lymphocyte counts outside Nigeria demonstrated a surge in this cell population at the onset of therapy with the vaccine. Quite a number have seroreverted, on repeated screening, to anti-HIV antibody negative for several months and even years. Whether one accepts or rejects that these developments mean a cure for HIV infection, the unavoidable conclusion is that these are remarkable achievements.

Personally, I was very sceptical at the beginning of 1999 when the author approached me about doing laboratory investigations for those taking his "innovative immunotherapy" for HIV infection. I know that the author does not shy away from any form of scientific investigation into his work. We have done all the tests that are within our capability to perform on the author's patients. The results so far are very exciting. Let those with the facilities and the expertise do more scientific investigations to their satisfaction to prove to the doubting Thomases either to confirm that Dr. Abalaka's HIV vaccine work and claims are fake and then celebrate it or recoil in shame that they have been proved wrong and that Dr. Abalaka's "Eureka" is real.

The author has also covered the politics and other extra and ultra scientific factors that have in one way or another influenced the yet to be successful international efforts at HIV vaccines development.

The HIV vaccines that Dr. Abalaka claims to have developed were marred by controversy both in Nigeria and abroad. This book also gives an insight into this controversy. This is a book that is a source of great encouragement for those genuinely interested in HIV vaccine development, scientific and extra/ultra scientific factors that influence it and a satisfying understanding of the author and his character.

This book is an invaluable and unique addition to all the futile efforts made so far for this generation to find a vaccine solution to this HIV/AIDS scourge that has afflicted mankind terribly and desperately. Desperate times may require that all possible solutions be pursued. This is true of Dr. Abalaka's efforts.

I strongly recommend this book not only to all scientific minds that are open or tend to be closed but also to all those who are genuinely interested in the beneficial science, politics and economics of HIV/AIDS vaccines.

Manason Rubainu
Chief Medical Laboratory Scientist
University of Abuja Teaching Hospital, Gwagwalada, Abuja.
and
National President
Association of Medical Laboratory Scientists of Nigeria.
GSM No.: +234 803 210 4412; +234 802 742 0925
Email: r_manason@yahoo.com

Preface

Dr. J. O. A. Abalaka has arranged this book *"The First Decade of Safe and Effective HIV Vaccines"* in a simple manner for ease of reading and understanding so that the reader will appreciate the complexities involved in developing a vaccine against the dreaded HIV in the third world.

The book is intended to capture the attention of the medical scientists of Nigeria, Africa, and the international community. Immunologists, HIV experts, vaccinologists and HIV vaccine developers will equally benefit from the immunological strategies described in this great work. All the 'soldiers' engaged in the battle against the dreaded common enemy—HIV/AIDS—stand to benefit immensely from reading this treatise.

It is a common saying that unusual situations require unusual approaches. With unusual intelligence, Dr Jeremiah Abalaka, the humble, unassuming medical practitioner and scientist from the middle belt of Nigeria, has unusually confronted the problem and developed potent, safe and acceptable vaccines against the unusual disease called HIV/AIDS. Of course, he did not use or follow the WHO or UNAIDS protocol for developing HIV vaccines, but the proof of the pudding (or the popular Nigerian food called *'moi moi'*) is in the eating. It is an effort that demonstrates the unusual dynamics, encourages research on the African continent and raises hope for the hopeless.

In this book, Dr Abalaka has made an in-depth analysis of his individual, self-sponsored efforts to produce safe and effective HIV vaccines, using modern scientific but unconventional and plausible approaches to achieve good results. His protocol is a radical departure from the generally accepted approaches known to and recognized by the medical scientific world, approaches that have yet to result in successful HIV vaccines.

Dr. Abalaka however has achieved remarkable breakthroughs in the fight against HIV/AIDS. I have used his HIV vaccines since 2000 and found them extremely safe and efficacious. His HIV vaccines relieve HIV-induced symptoms and signs rapidly. Many of my HIV-infected patients have been cured of HIV infection using Dr. Abalaka's HIV therapeutic vaccine; in other words, they have changed from HIV-antibody positive to a sustained HIV-antibody negative status with the doctor's HIV therapeutic vaccine. All those who have received his HIV preventive vaccine through me have remained HIV-antibody negative.

The emphasis in this book is that great scientific breakthroughs can occur in the hands of highly gifted medical scientists even if, as in Dr. Abalaka's case, they come from the Third World, with meagre resources and facilities at their disposal. Is this an HIV/AIDS saviour from Nazareth? Persecution and crucifixion have, and will come but resurrection is assured and world wide recognition is the deserved prize to be won.

Dr. Abalaka was my senior at the medical school in Ahmadu Bello University, Zaria. After graduation, both of us also worked together for some time at that University's Teaching Hospital in Zaria.

Born in Central Nigeria in 1948, Dr. Jeremiah Abalaka has had an outstanding and brilliant academic career throughout his education. Dr. Abalaka received his medical training at Nigeria's Ahmadu Bello University Zaria from where he graduated in 1972. He successfully studied Immunology at Nigeria's University of Ibadan in 1974 after which he attended a WHO-sponsored Immunopathological conference on Schistosomiasis in Geneva, Switzerland, in October 1974. In 1979 he obtained the Fellowship in General Surgery. He has been in continuous clinical medical practice since his graduation.

With the spreading menace of the HIV/AIDS in his country in the late 1980s and his constant professional vulnerability as a surgeon to the virus, he decided to fall back on his knowledge and training in Immunology to attempt to develop a prophylactic HIV vaccine in order to protect himself against the rampaging virus. His family's meagre resources were his only financial support for his HIV-vaccine adventure that began in early 1992.

Addressing his handicaps of lack of HIV viral cultures, modern approaches to vaccine development and experimental animals like chimpanzees for HIV-vaccine research, he decided eventually to work retrogradely by attempting to develop a safe and effective HIV therapeutic vaccine first.

After he had worked out how he would try and develop an HIV therapeutic vaccine, he used himself over a period of 21 months and established the safety of his approach. In October 1997, he started testing the efficacy of his approach on willing HIV-infected persons with their written and informed consent.

By December 1998, 4 of them had serodeconverted to HIV-antibody negative status. By March 1999, he developed his candidate HIV preventive vaccine that he took himself. After 3 months, he challenged his immune system with an intravenous dose of fresh whole HIV-infected blood from a confirmed HIV-positive person but he has remained protected against the virus, even after a total of 6 such challenges.

He then started giving normal persons the preventive vaccine with their written and informed consent but he did not challenge any of them with HIV as he had done to himself. He also made his HIV therapeutic vaccines available to his colleagues for their independent assessment of its efficacy and safety as they wished on their patients; they have all testified to the efficacy and safety of his HIV therapeutic vaccine.

As expected, his work triggered volleys of criticisms especially from far and near. Without assessing or verifying his claims, his own country's Government and its Ministry of Health announced at a press briefing on July 20, 2000 that President Olusegun Obasanjo had banned the author's HIV vaccines. The Vice-President Alhaji Atiku Abubakar then publicly declared that the author had been killing Nigerians with his illegal and untested HIV vaccines.

Dr. Abalaka has all along put me in the picture of what he had been going through because of his HIV vaccines work. I have visited and held discussions with him on countless occasions at his hospital and in court premises since I came to know about his HIV vaccine discoveries.

I know that a formidable team of opposition had assembled against him and his HIV vaccines, a team that includes but is not limited to the Nigerian Government, its Ministry of Health, the Medical and Dental Council of Nigeria, the Nigerian Academy of Science, the National Agency for Food and Drug Administration and Control, many eminent Nigerian scientists like the WHO recognized Virologist Professor Tam David-West, the UN, UNAIDS, WHO, UNICEF, the Western world and their powerful propaganda machinery, the recognized HIV experts and vaccine developers of our time such as Professor Robert Gallo of the American National Cancer Institutes, America's National Institutes of Allergy and Infectious Diseases (NIAID), its National Institutes of Health (NIH), and even the White House in Washington.

Dr. Abalaka has always been keen on an unbiased and proper scientific assessment or verification of his claims but such assessors are either unavailable or unwilling to perform such an exercise. He submitted his articles to a number of international and reputable medical scientific journals for publication, but one after the other turned it down.

He has treated over 4000 HIV/AIDS infected persons and over 400 normal persons with his vaccines. After critically looking into his data for several months, Professor Ray Spier, editor of the reputable journal *Vaccine* published a report in September 2004 about Dr. Abalaka's HIV vaccines work. Because he failed to find support from peer reviewers, the Professor wrote an editorial preceding the report, an editorial that answered the questions raised by the peer reviewers.

I know that Dr. Abalaka has been severely bruised and battered in the course of his constant battle with fires and infernos since 1999 that the public was informed about the HIV vaccines that he had developed. This book contains all the details that any reader would wish to have about Dr. Abalaka, his HIV vaccines and all the fires and infernos that emanated from his successful development of safe and effective HIV vaccines.

Many too have either stood solidly behind the author or come to his rescue as and when necessary. They include the Nigerian print and electronic media, the country's judiciary, his patients, some eminent scientists and doctors in his country, the Chief Medical Laboratory Scientist that performed the tests on his patients and me.

Read on.

ESamuel Tor-Agbidye, FWACP
M.D. / CEO
Family Practice Hospital
Makurdi, Nigeria
Email: *saminjeh@yahoo.com*
GSM +234 805 4516 307

Acknowledgments

Up till now, I would likely have been a stark illiterate in the rural community in which I found myself if I had not been lucky for my parentage especially my uneducated father who insisted on educating my elder brother Tom and me. In taking that decision, he went against the established culture and practice of his society. My parents and siblings have had a tremendous influence on my life and character. I thank them all.

In the course of my education, I was lucky to be influenced by honest, humane, dedicated and hardworking teachers who infected me with their qualities. In the medical school in Zaria, during training in basic immunology in Ibadan and during my surgical training both in Nigeria and in Liverpool in the UK, I continued to be influenced by teachers with these same qualities. I cannot find good enough words to convey the depth of my gratitude to all of them.

In my working career, the same luck continued to be my lot. I must express my appreciation to all of them, too.

Since the beginning of 1992 when I started my solo research into HIV vaccines, a new era opened in my life. I must sincerely thank all those who have contributed in one way or the other in the project. To list them all one by one would take so much space and time and at the end, I may not be able to list them all.

Some have made extraordinary contributions and sacrifices to my HIV vaccine work. I must start by thanking all my patients for their unyielding trust, confidence and support over the new remedies I developed against the HIV. I thank them all. I must not forget to also thank the members of my immediate and extended families, my siblings, Dr. Samson A. Shaibu, Mr. Manason Rubainu, Dr. Sam Tor-Agbidye, Mallam Shareef Mohammed, Barrister Isaac Okpanachi, Professor Jerry Gana, Professor Ray Spier, Dr. Aldar Bourinbaiar, Professor Nian Qing LU, Mr. Frank Olize and the other numerous practitioners of the Fourth Realm of the Estate (Print and electronic media), Nigerian University students, The Executive Governors and Governments of Nasarawa, Benue, Abia and Kogi States in Nigeria in 2000, Miss Nigeria 2000 Vien Bemigho Tetsola, the staffs of Medicrest Specialist Hospital and of Peak Medical Laboratories, The Nigerian Army, The Nigeria Police, all my professional colleagues that have used my HIV vaccines for their independent assessment of their safety and efficacy and all others that have made much sacrifice for the sake of my HIV vaccines. I am really very grateful to them all for their steadfast support, encouragement, sacrifice and advice.

I must express my sincere gratitude to all the Journals that received and processed my manuscripts for publication irrespective of whether they accepted the submission or not. I thank them all very sincerely. I must also not forget to thank all those who have offered constructive criticisms of my work for without such criticisms, science and other fields of human endeavour would make no meaningful progress.

I must not forget to thank Nova Publishers and its entire staff for all the initiative, encouragement, editorial expertise, guide and patience they have shown in the course of writing this book. I thank all of them very profoundly.

I accept full responsibility for, and offer sincere apologies for any typographical errors in this book and for any inconveniences that such errors may cause anybody, corporate or non-corporate.

Dr. J. O. A. Abalaka

Section I:
Infectious Diseases and *Some Human Vaccines*

Chapter I

Infectious Diseases and the Human Immune Responses

Abstract

In this chapter, we will discuss the rudiments of the normal human immune system from intrauterine days to independent existence after birth. Our immune system maintains our internal integrity by differentiating between self and nonself. The system also responds specifically to immunogens from infectious agents and their toxins. The responses are either cell-mediated (CMI) or humoral (antibody)-mediated or both. The antibodies involved in our immune response to viruses especially are generally beneficial in that their presence implies that the person has some degree of protection at least against the virus concerned; the higher the level of these antibodies, the better the protection they provide against the virus. Immunoglobulins (antibodies) from any person are not immunogenic when administered to another person; in other words, a normal person does not mount an immune response against immunoglobulins from another person. However, the normal person would produce specific and binding human immunoglobulins (antibodies) against, say, rabbit or monkey immunoglobulins. For this reason, the clinical use of immunoglobulins is limited, as much as possible, to human immunoglobulins.

Introduction

Though highly complex and still not completely understood, the normal human immune system maintains the integrity and individuality of the person by differentiating between self and nonself. In addition, our immune system detects foreign substances either as compounds (proteins and polysaccharides) or micro-organisms, and mounts specific immune responses (humoral and/or cell-mediated) against the immunogen it has detected. In this regard, antibodies are generally protective and beneficial. All our immune responses take place extracellularly.

Internal Surveillance of Own Cells

One of the key functions of our immune system is the internal surveillance of our own cells. The normal human immune system develops the ability to distinguish between self and nonself cells as early as the 8th–10th week of pregnancy. From then on, the normal human immune system ferociously destroys any cell, tissue or organ that it recognizes as nonself. This is one of the major problems facing tissue or organ transplants. The ferocity with which the normal human immune system destroys nonself cells, tissues or organs is amazing. It takes the normal human immune system just about 10–14 days to completely destroy a large organ like a transplanted but non-compatible liver or kidney from another human being.

The ABO, Rhesus D and major histocompatibility complex, MHC antigens elicit the most ferocious responses against non-compatible human cells, tissues or organs. As the author understands it, cellular immune responses, particularly the cytotoxic T lymphocytes (CTLs), otherwise called CD8+ lymphocytes are the effector cells responsible for cell, tissue or organ rejection.

Another interesting facet of our immune system's ability to recognize and differentiate self from nonself is the internal surveillance function of our immune system. Even from intra-uterine life, the normal human being literally develops many mutants from the uncountable numbers of mitotic divisions that take place throughout life. As a result of these divisions, many mutants appear. Our normal immune system usually detects or recognizes such abnormal mutants and destroys them. In this way, our internal integrity is maintained.

All of us must have developed many potential cancerous mutant cells since we came into existence. Such dangerous mutants however are destroyed by our immune cells carrying out their internal surveillance function. A person develops cancer when his immune system, for one reason or the other, fails to recognize as nonself the first mutant cancerous cell. Continued growth of the unrecognized cancerous cell, a wolf in sheep's clothing, eventually leads to the macroscopic tumour mass. Again, as the author understands it, cellular immune responses, particularly CTLs are responsible for this surveillance function.

Sometimes, for one reason or another, the immune system fails to recognize some self cells as self. As soon as that happens, the immune system begins to treat such cells as nonself and destroys them, resulting in a group of diseases called *'autoimmune diseases'*.

Infectious Agents

Infectious agents, viruses, rickettsiae, bacteria, protozoa, helminths, yeasts, molds and fungi abound in the environment in which we live. From conception, we must be protected against these potentially lethal agents. Until one develops his own competent immune system, he would need interim protection against these ubiquitous messengers of death. When a person is born, he is on his own in the unavoidable warfare against microbes.

Infections are caused by living organisms. Infectious diseases, like warfare, involve the following:

Parties:	Availability of both the person (host) and the hostile Infectious agent
Meeting:	The agent and the host meet or encounter each other
Entry:	The agent enters the host
Conflict:	The host's immune system recognises the invading agent as non-self and mounts a response against the invasion, but the hostile invader resists its elimination by the host
Spread:	The agent moves or spreads from the site of entry
Replication:	The agent multiplies or replicates in the host
Damage:	Damage to the host's tissues results from the host's response and/or the invading agent
Conflict resolution:	In this host-agent conflict, either the agent or the host emerges victorious or both compromise and agree to co-exist, a no victor no vanquished situation.

Immunity During Intrauterine Life

Conventionally, one's age starts counting from the day of his birth, as if his existence started then. In reality however, one's existence starts at conception and we all know that. During the nine months or so that we spend in our mothers' wombs, we normally live a completely aquatic life in a sterile environment, sheltered in the uterus where we lie cosily in the amniotic fluid within the tough amniotic membrane that also covers the foetal surface of the placenta. All these factors combine to very effectively shield us from the ubiquitous infectious agents that inhabit our external environment and planet.

The placental barrier is very efficient in preventing micro-organisms especially bacteria in the mother's circulation from passing across to the foetus. The placental capability however, like virtually everything else, is not 100 percent. Consequently, congenital infections like rubella (German measles), Japanese encephalitis virus (JEV), syphilis and CMV (cytomegalovirus) do occur; and when they occur in the first trimester of pregnancy, they really cause much morbidity and mortality to the offspring. These congenital infections are so terrible for the growing foetus because it lacks a competent immune system to powerfully resist the invaders and protect itself.

The sterile foetal environment in the uterus normally shields the foetus from infectious agents while it is developing its own immune system, but even then, the foetal immune system is not fully developed at birth. Most human beings encounter micro-organisms for the first time at birth. Anytime the author comes across the age or date of birth, DOB, he considers it as the date that person first came into contact with micro-organisms, that is to say, the beginning of a continuous and life-long battle against these disease-causing agents.

When a pathogenic micro-organism succeeds in getting entry into the host's tissues, it immediately comes into contact with the host's immune system, literally triggering a bitter war between the invader and the host. We will now look at this war more closely.

The Human Immune Responses

Our immunological responses are, broadly speaking, either humoral or cellular depending on either the use of plasma/serum (humors) or specific immune cells, even though both responses may occur together to varying degrees depending on the immunogen (antigen) that triggered the immune response. Both responses are generally highly specific.

While humoral immunity depends on the action of highly specific antibodies (gamma globulins), cellular immunity is mediated by direct cell-to-cell interaction of primed antigen-specific T lymphocytes that destroy infected cells. Both types of immune responses, triggered by the extracellular recognition of the immunogen by specific receptors on the cell membranes of the immune cells, also involve the secretion and action of soluble factors, cytokines. Both immune responses are extracellular, i.e. neither the specific antibodies nor specific effector cells of cell-mediated immunity (CMI) enter the cells during an immune response.

After our immune cells recognize an immunogen that would provoke the production of specific antibodies, it generally takes some weeks before detectable or significant quantities of such antibodies become detectable in the blood. This period represents the time it takes to prime the necessary cells and get them to produce the plasma cells that would pour out these specific antibodies. Generally, IgM antibodies are the first immunoglobulins to be produced in response to an antigen (the primary response); IgG antibodies are the predominant immunoglobulins in the secondary and other responses to the same antigen. Booster doses of most vaccines therefore provoke the outpouring of IgG antibodies. The catabolism of these IgG antibodies is a gradual process too. However, if there are small quantities of IgG antibodies in circulation and the appropriate immunogen is available, immune complexes consisting of the immunogen and the antibodies are rapidly formed and eliminated by our immune system, resulting in the rapid removal of such antibodies from the circulation.

These time frames are much faster for cell-mediated immune responses. Incompatible tissue or organ rejections, as we noted earlier on, take less than two weeks. Cell-mediated responses alone are largely responsible for such rejection. The two weeks interval is too short to involve any significant humoral (antibody) response in organ or tissue rejection especially when the ABO and MHC antigens are involved in the tissue or organ rejection.

Antibodies and Protective Immunity

Full-term neonates (babies), in particular, are born with substantial quantities of maternal IgG antibodies that pass across the placenta to the offspring during the last 4 weeks or so of pregnancy. Maternal antibodies in colostrum and in breast milk also pass to the offspring during breast feeding. These maternal antibodies help protect the offspring during the immediate months after birth. The normal child completely catabolizes (destroys) them before 18 months of age.

Premature neonates especially those born before the commencement of the ninth month of pregnancy have a hell of a time battling for survival against various infections because they were unlucky not to stay long enough in their mothers' wombs to passively receive their mothers IgG antibodies across the placenta before birth. Because such premature infants have not developed their sucking mechanism fully before birth, they are also unable without assistance to take in their mothers' colostrum from which they would have received some maternal IgG antibodies. The more premature a baby is, the greater the danger posed to it by the lack or paucity of its mother's protective IgG antibodies.

Accordingly, to imitate nature so to say, passive immunity using immunoglobulins is used clinically to prevent, delay or reduce the severity of some infections in exposed or high-risk cases, for example, human globulin administration for hepatitis B, and the use of human rabies immunoglobulin (HRIG), collected from immunized persons and given as soon as possible after rabies exposure especially rabid animal bites on the head and neck. Additionally, for those people who, for various reasons, cannot produce enough endogenous immunoglobulins, there is also the widespread intravenous use of human immunoglobulins especially in the developed countries, usually by weekly outpatient self-administration in a hospital's premises. Generally, the higher the level of these specific immunoglobulins, the better the degree of protection they provide against the virus involved. The reader would likely note that these human immunoglobulin remedies are human blood products /extracts.

Human immunoglobulins do not evoke an immune response when administered to another person; in other words, humans do not treat immunoglobulins from another human being as 'nonself'. This applies to human albumin and other plasma proteins, too. However, the normal human immune response would recognise immunoglobulins from other mammals such as the monkey or rabbit as 'nonself' and produce specific human anti-monkey or anti-rabbit immunoglobulins in response. Similarly, the normal monkey or rabbit immune system would recognise human immunoglobulins as nonself, and produce specific monkey or rabbit anti-human immunoglobulins in response.

Presently, vaccines for more than 20 diseases caused by infectious agents are in clinical use in human medicine. These vaccines include smallpox, rabies, diphtheria, tetanus, pertussis, polio, measles, chickenpox, mumps, influenza, rubella, hepatitis A and B, Haemophilus influenzae B, yellow fever and cholera vaccines. Virtually all these vaccines generate, or boost the production of large amounts of effective and highly specific antibodies against the causative organisms or their exotoxins, as the case may be.

Dating back to several decades ago, therefore, humanity has always regarded the presence of antibodies against disease-causing microbes in a person's blood as a very good and welcome prognostic parameter because it implies the person has some protection at least against the relevant microbe or its toxin. This is still not only generally true but it is apparently endorsed by nature, as described earlier!

Subconsciously therefore, we are all used to thinking of antimicrobial antibodies as not only beneficial but also inherently indispensable in protection against the diseases they cause. Like all generalizations, we should bear at least, in one corner of our mind that it is possible that this generalization may not apply to all infectious agents; there may be exceptions.

The Administration of Whole Human Blood or its Products

Experiments with blood transfusions, the transfer of blood or blood components into a person's blood stream, have been carried out for hundreds of years. Many patients died; it was not until 1901, when the Austrian Karl Landsteiner discovered human blood groups, that blood transfusions became safer.

Mixing blood from two individuals may result in agglutination that can cause serious toxic reactions that may be fatal. Karl Landsteiner discovered that the agglutination was an immunological reaction between the donor blood cells and antibodies in the recipient's blood against the donor blood cells.

Karl Landsteiner's work made it possible to determine blood types and thus paved the way for blood transfusions to be carried out safely. For this discovery he was awarded the Nobel Prize in 1930.

Phenotype	Genotype
A	AA or AO
B	BB or BO
AB	AB
O	OO

The ABO system is the most important blood group system in human blood transfusion. The associated anti-A and anti-B IgM antibodies are produced in the first years of life by sensitization to environmental substances such as food, bacteria and viruses.

The Rhesus system discovered in 1937 is the second most significant blood group system in human blood transfusion. The most significant Rhesus antigen is the RhD antigen because it is the most immunogenic of the five main rhesus antigens. Normally, RhD negative individuals do not to have any anti-RhD IgG or IgM antibodies, because anti-RhD antibodies are not usually produced by sensitization against environmental substances. However, on first exposure to RhD positive erythrocytes, RhD negative individuals can produce IgG anti-RhD antibodies following a sensitizing event such as a foetomaternal transfusion of RhD positive foetal blood cells from a fetus to its RhD negative mother in pregnancy or during parturition, or the transfusion of RhD positive red blood cells into an RhD negative recipient

Blood Group	A	B	AB	O
Antigens present on cells	A	B	A and B	None
Antibodies present in plasma	Anti-B	Anti-A	None	Anti-A and Anti-B

The International Society of Blood Transfusion (ISBT) currently recognizes 30 blood group systems (including the ABO and Rh systems). Thus, in addition to the ABO antigens and Rhesus antigens, many other antigens are expressed on the RBC surface membrane. For example, an individual can be AB RhD positive, and at the same time M and N positive (MNS system), K positive (Kell system), Le^a or Le^b negative (Lewis system), and so on, being positive or negative for each blood group system antigen. Many of the blood group systems were named after the patients in whom the corresponding antibodies were initially encountered [1, 2].

Conclusion

Our immune responses have the dual role of ensuring our internal security by differentiating self from non-self, and of protecting us from the constant threat throughout life of invasion, colonization and destruction by disease-causing agents. These highly specific immune responses are effected either through specifically primed immune cells that result in a cell-mediated immune response or through the production of highly specific antibodies (immunoglobulins) in a humoral immune response, or both. Both immune responses also involve the secretion of other soluble substances called cytokines and or chemokines. In almost all human viral infections especially, the presence of antibodies against the causative agent is good news because they imply some degree of protection against the infectious agent in the individual. Generally, too, the higher the level of these antibodies against an infectious agent, the higher the degree of protection against the agent involved. In the last few weeks of full-term pregnancy, the highly specific maternal IgG antibodies pass across the placenta to the offspring to protect the newborn baby against infectious agents during the early months of the baby's independent life after birth while its own immune system continues to develop and take over. By the time the baby is 18 months old, on average, it would have completely catabolised these maternal antibodies.

References

[1] http://nobelprize.org/educational_games/medicine/landsteiner/readmore.html
[2] http://en.wikipedia.org/wiki/Blood_type

Chapter II

Vaccines

Abstract

The acute infections of infancy and childhood result in much morbidity and mortality. Vaccines against the causative agents of these diseases have drastically reduced the incidence of these diseases. Vaccines are unlike orthodox drugs such as antibiotics that kill micro-organisms. Vaccines do not kill the micro-organisms at all. Instead, vaccines are teachers that specifically teach the immune system how to deal with the disease-causing agent whenever that agent should invade the body; vaccines prepare the body beforehand for the disease causing agent. Vaccines are produced by killing or inactivating the micro-organism, or weakening (attenuating) them so that they are no longer able to cause disease, or using a part of the micro-organism to provide protection against the causative agent of the disease, or rendering the toxins harmless (toxoids) that are then used to provide protection. Every effort is taken to ensure candidate vaccines are safe before and during trials for efficacy. Like all remedies, vaccines are not 100 percent efficacious. One must always weigh the potential benefits against the risks before prescribing any vaccine for a person. Generally, it takes on average at least 5 years to bring a vaccine into the market in the developed countries; that is the time it takes to go through the mandatory Phase I-III clinical trials. In the case of an emergency (an epidemic) for which no vaccine exists, however, it is natural that this time frame would be put on hold.

Introduction

Vaccines have literally transformed the landscape of medicine since Edward Jenner's cowpox vaccine for smallpox was developed around 1796. The vaccine eventually resulted in the global elimination of the smallpox disease whose last reported case was from Somalia in 1977.

In the US before the era of vaccines, for instance,

- Polio would paralyze 10,000 children every year;
- Rubella (German measles) would cause birth defects and mental retardation in as many as 20,000 newborns every year;

- Measles would infect about 4 million children, killing 3,000 every year;
- Diphtheria would be one of the most common causes of death in school-aged children every year;
- A bacterium called *Haemophilus influenzae* type b (Hib) would cause meningitis in 15,000 children, leaving many with permanent brain damage every year; and
- Pertussis (whooping cough) would kill thousands of infants every year [1].

Vaccines have greatly reduced and, in some cases, eliminated many diseases that killed or severely disabled people just a few generations before. For most people in the developed world today, vaccines are a routine part of healthcare. In the developing world, however, mortality and morbidity before the age of five are still very high partly because of poor immunization of the kids in these societies.

The disappearance of many childhood diseases in the developed world has led some parents to question whether vaccines are still necessary. Further, a growing number of parents are concerned that vaccines may actually be the cause of diseases such as autism, hyperactivity, developmental delay, attention deficit disorder, diabetes, multiple sclerosis, and sudden infant death syndrome (SIDS) among others. These concerns have caused some parents to delay vaccines or withhold them altogether from their children [1].

What Are Vaccines?

The author would define a vaccine as a suspension of attenuated or inactivated (killed) infectious agents, or portions of such infectious agents administered for the prevention, amelioration, or treatment of infectious diseases.

Broadly, there are two types of vaccine, the preventive vaccine and the therapeutic (treatment) vaccine. The former type is for preventing the infectious disease in those who, though their bodies have presently not been invaded by the infectious agent, stand the risk of being infected in the future; the preventive vaccine is to increase their resistance to the disease and reduce their chance of being infected, or if they do become infected, to make the disease milder. On the other hand, the therapeutic vaccine is for treating those people whose bodies have already been invaded by the infectious agent; a therapeutic or treatment vaccine that results in a cure of the infection is sometimes referred to as a curative vaccine.

In most circumstances in life, prevention is far better, cheaper, easier, wiser and more convenient than cure. Accordingly, for example, it is far better, cheaper, easier, wiser and more convenient to prevent any accident than to attempt to reverse or undo the effects of an accident that has already taken place. Generally therefore, it is the author's opinion that it is similarly far better, cheaper, easier, wiser and more convenient to prevent an infectious disease especially those caused by viruses by using a safe and effective (sae) preventive vaccine than it would be to try and cure such an infection by developing and using a sae-therapeutic vaccine.

Safety and Efficacy Only

Like all remedies in medicine, there are just two crucial requirements to be satisfied by any vaccine before it can be used clinically: safety first and foremost, and then, effectiveness or efficacy. *Any vaccine or other medical remedy that is both safe and effective qualifies immediately for use in patients that are willing to take it.*

Let us remember, however, that in practice, no medical remedy is absolutely safe and/or efficacious, like most other things in life. Whenever we discuss the issue of safety and/or efficacy of any medical remedy, we should bear in mind that what we are actually discussing is *relative* safety and/or efficacy of the remedy. Every medical remedy has a risk. Just to take a drink of clean safe water out of a sealed plastic bottle that has the approval of FDA or other similar regulatory body charged with that responsibility is not absolutely safe; it carries a risk indeed.

We all must have experienced, once in a while, the accidental inhalation of water or other drinks or food in the course of our taking drinks or food, and the invariably immediate punishment of very uncomfortable, painful, intense, violent and uncontrollable spasms of coughing mixed with profuse shedding of tears. That is one of the risks we take whenever we swallow not only food or drink but also our own saliva. The benefits of taking a drink or food, or of swallowing our saliva far outweigh this risk, and so we do not ever contemplate stopping to take drinks or food, or stopping to swallow our own saliva because of this risk. In fact, most people proceed to continue with the very drink that started the nasty experience even before the bout subsides completely.

Still on the issue of safety and efficacy of any vaccine or medical remedy, one should always imagine a weighing scale, put the risk posed to the person if he does not take the remedy on one side of the scale, and put the benefits to him if he takes the remedy on the other side of the imaginary balance. If the risks far outweigh the benefits, do not recommend or use the remedy. If on the other hand, the benefits far outweigh the risks, recommend the remedy to the patient. Of course, the final decision to take or refuse the remedy lies with the patient or his legal guardian.

Conventional Ways of Making Vaccines

The first safe and effective vaccine against any human diseases however was not developed until around 1796 A.D at a time that man did not even know about the existence of micro-organisms. Its development was empirical. And remember it was not 100 percent safe and efficacious. About 100 years further on, more vaccines were developed, again empirically. Among these vaccines were those effective against viruses, a group of micro-organisms completely unknown to humanity at the time the vaccines were developed against them. More vaccines were empirically developed especially in the 1950s and 1960s. Smallpox, rabies, diphtheria, tetanus, pertussis, polio, measles, chickenpox, mumps, rubella, hepatitis A and B, Haemophilus influenzae B, yellow fever and cholera vaccines were all developed empirically before cell-mediated immunity (CMI) was developed. In fact, the now vast fields of Immunology and Virology are recent specialties developed in the last half of the last century.

All the successful vaccines against the viruses that cause the acute infectious diseases of infancy and childhood employ either inactivated or live attenuated viruses.

Inactivation is achieved by heating, exposure to ultraviolet light or gamma radiation, treatment with inactivating agents such as formaldehyde or acetyl-ethylene-imine, or the use of denaturing agents such as urea or proteolytic enzymes. Live attenuated vaccines are usually developed in the laboratories by culturing the virus in laboratory animals, monkey or human cell culture lines, or chick embryos followed by purification.

Stabilizers, adjuvants and preservatives are usually added to both types of vaccines. Vaccines from inactivated viruses or bacteria are more likely to survive at ambient room temperatures below 20°C. Live vaccines however need to be stored refrigerated, frozen or freeze-dried [2].

Inactivated vaccines do not pose a risk of causing infection in the recipients because they do not contain infectious agents, but usually more doses are required to produce an immune response. Furthermore, inactivated vaccines can be safely given to those who are immunosuppressed from whatever cause.

Live attenuated vaccines, on the other hand, pose the risk of causing infection in the recipient especially those who are immunosuppressed because they contain live infectious agents. However, fewer doses are required to provide immunity. The immunity provided by live attenuated vaccine generally lasts longer than the one provided by killed micro-organisms.

Vaccines usually generate high titres of neutralizing antibodies to prevent infection upon exposure to the wild virus, and this is the way new vaccines are traditionally or conventionally tested. The vaccine doses and regimens are first tested in normal volunteers for their capacity to invoke high titres of neutralizing antibodies. Then, the vaccine and placebo are introduced into a population where the incidence of infection is high, and the frequencies of infections in the vaccinated group and in the placebo control group are compared.

This approach requires a reasonably high incidence of infection in the endogenous population, and a reasonable rate of infection, so that the trial can be conducted in a reasonable time frame. However, even under the best of circumstances, several thousand volunteers and several years are usually required to accumulate enough data for analysis to show whether the vaccine will work, and how well it works, i.e. whether it confers complete protection from infection, or only partially effective, affording protection for a fraction of recipients compared with the incidence in the placebo control group.

Therefore, vaccines are made in several ways. However, all vaccines have the same general goal: weaken the virus or bacteria in a way that allows the recipient to develop an immune response without developing any symptoms of infection. Vaccines are made using the same components that are found in the natural virus or bacteria.

Several basic strategies are used to make vaccines. The strengths and limitations of each approach are described below.

Weaken the Micro-Organism

Using this strategy, the infectious agents particularly viruses are weakened so that they reproduce themselves very poorly once inside the body. The measles, mumps, German measles (rubella) and chickenpox (varicella) vaccines are made this way. Viruses usually cause disease by reproducing themselves many times in the body. Whereas natural viruses reproduce themselves thousands of times, vaccine viruses usually reproduce themselves fewer than 20 times. Because vaccine viruses don't reproduce themselves very much, they don't cause disease, but vaccine viruses replicate well enough to induce "memory B cells" that protect against infection in the future.

The advantage of live, "weakened" vaccines is that one or two doses provide immunity that lasts for a long time. The limitation of this approach is that these vaccines usually cannot be given to people with weakened immune systems (like people with cancer or AIDS).

Inactivate or Kill the Micro-Organism

Using this strategy, the micro-organism is cultured in the laboratory before it is completely inactivated (or killed) usually with a chemical. By killing the infectious agent, it cannot possibly reproduce itself or cause disease. The inactivated polio, hepatitis A, influenza, and rabies vaccines are made this way. Because the killed or inactivated micro-organism is still recognized by the body's immune system as foreign, cells of the immune system that protect against disease are generated.

The strength of this approach is that the vaccine cannot possibly cause even a mild form of the disease that it prevents and can be given to people with weakened immune systems. The limitation of this approach is that several doses must be given to achieve immunity.

Use Part of the Micro-Organism

Using this strategy, just one part of the disease-causing micro-organism is removed or artificially produced in the lab by modern genetic engineering techniques, and used as a vaccine. The hepatitis B and HPV vaccines are made this way. The vaccine is composed of a protein that resides on the surface of the virus. This strategy can be used when an immune response to one part of the virus (or bacteria) is responsible for protection against disease.

The hepatitis B vaccine can be given even to people with weakened immunity and the vaccine appears to induce long-lived immunity after three doses.

Some bacteria cause disease by making a harmful protein called a toxin. Several vaccines are made by taking such toxins and inactivating them with a chemical (the toxin, once inactivated, is called a toxoid). By inactivating the toxin, it no longer causes disease. The diphtheria, tetanus and pertussis vaccines are made in this way.

Another strategy to make a vaccine is to use part of the sugar coating (or polysaccharide) of the micro-organism especially bacteria. Protection against infection by certain bacteria is based on immunity to this sugar coating (and not the whole bacteria). However, because young children don't make a very good immune response to the sugar coating alone, the coating is linked to a harmless protein (this is called a "conjugated polysaccharide" vaccine). The *Haemophilus influenzae* type B (or Hib), pneumococcal, and meningococcal vaccines are made in this way.

Just like for inactivated viral vaccines, bacterial vaccines can be given to people with weakened immune systems, but often require several doses to induce adequate immunity.

Ways of Making Vaccines in an Emergency

When discussing the making of vaccines, the author considers it as an emergency if there is an epidemic disease hitherto unknown to mankind, such as AIDS was unknown to mankind before 1981, or when mankind is under the scourge of serious epidemics caused by a disease previously known to man, such as polio epidemics, but in either situation, there are no extant vaccines for the prevention or treatment of such diseases. Accordingly, this situation applies to smallpox before Jennerian vaccination, polio before the Salk vaccine, etc. If there is an epidemic of a disease for which a vaccine exists, that would be a completely different scenario; all that is required is to produce the vaccine and apply it urgently in the affected area, and there would be no need of making a vaccine and bringing it to the market since that would have been done earlier after the development of the vaccine.

The author cannot find any documents anywhere for making vaccines in the emergency situation he has just defined. That is as it should be. If no vaccine exists for any disease, there cannot be a procedure, methodology or recipe for making it!

Conventional Procedure Before Bringing a Vaccine to the Market

Before a vaccine can be made, researchers are expected to spend time isolating and studying the virus or bacteria in question and learning how it causes disease. Researchers then begin studying how to protect someone from the disease. Sometimes researchers ask questions like: What is the best quantity of virus to give? Does one dose of the vaccine work? Do additional doses help even more? How long does protection last?

There are three phases of studies, called clinical trials that need to be done in people before the vaccine can be considered for the general population:

Phase I

Phase I studies are designed to answer two questions: Is the vaccine safe and does it induce an immune response? Of course, this presupposes that the induced immune response is of the type known to the researchers and must be of the type the researchers can evaluate. If the answer to either of these questions is "No", the vaccine cannot be developed further.

Roosevelt's former law partner, the first ball became a countrywide "celebration." What has been described as "the biggest radio network in history" was patched together so that Roosevelt could broadcast a live message from the White House. "I thank you but lack the words to tell you how deeply I appreciate what you have done," Roosevelt told the nation's revellers, "and I bid you good night on what is to me the happiest birthday I have ever known."

More than 4,000 communities staged balls that first year, raising a little over $1 million. Aside from Warm Springs, the money went to groups in towns that had held balls. Because health insurance was not yet common, city committees gave the money to polio victims. The Warm Springs Foundation, in turn, earmarked $100,000 to "stimulate and further the meritorious work being done in the field of infantile paralysis elsewhere," establishing the President's Birthday Ball Commission for Infantile Paralysis to distribute research grants. The next year, balls only took in $750,000, but $241,000 went to the new Commission for Infantile Paralysis.

Maurice Brodie of New York University in 1935 received the first massive grant from the commission, $65,000. Brodie, who reported that he had protected monkeys with a killed poliovirus vaccine, distributed the experimental vaccine to hospitals and health departments, which then inoculated more than 9,000 children. At around the same time, Temple University's John Kolmer, who had not received any Birthday Ball dollars, had cooked up a vaccine made from live but weakened poliovirus and, with the help of private physicians, had inoculated nearly 11,000 kids.

Allegations soon flew that the vaccines had paralyzed and even killed a few vaccinees, the Birthday Ball Commission taking the heat for both disasters. In retrospect, the live vaccine that Kolmer made probably was the more damaging of the two, though both were ineffective, if not dangerous. Officials publicly lambasted Kolmer and Brodie for rushing their vaccines into humans. Brodie died four years later; many have written that he killed himself, though his death certificate lists coronary thrombosis as the cause.

Stung by the vaccine failures, criticized by the chief surgeon at Warm Springs, charged with shamelessly politicizing polio, Roosevelt abandoned the birthday balls after the 1937 bash and announced the formation of a new group. Named the National Foundation for Infantile Paralysis and headquartered in O'Connor's New York law office, the group, announced Roosevelt, would "make every effort to ensure that every responsible research agency in the country is adequately financed to carry out investigations into the cause of infantile paralysis and the methods by which it may be prevented."

The first fund-raiser held by the National Foundation was a radio blitz, again coinciding with Roosevelt's birthday. Comedian Eddie Cantor supposedly hatched the idea of having radio stations donate time to ask for small contributions. "We could ask the people to send their dimes directly to the White House," Cantor enthused. "Think what a thrill people would get. . . . And we could call it the March of Dimes!" Two days after the appeal, only $17.50 had arrived at 1600 Pennsylvania Avenue. "You fellows have ruined the president," a White House aide groused.

A quarter of a million letters arrived during the following week stuffed with $1,823,045, including 2,680,000 dimes, all of which went to the National Foundation for Infantile

Paralysis/March of Dimes. For the first time, a serious war chest existed to research and develop a polio vaccine.

When man does not intervene, epidemic diseases rise and fall in waves; the number of impacted people crests over several years as the susceptibles become infected, and then steadily drops into a trough, allowing another population of susceptibles to build. That year, 1938, the United States recorded only 1,705 cases of polio, the deepest trough the country would enjoy until 23 years later, when the vaccine developed by Jonas Salk was in wide use.

Jonas Edward Salk was born October 28, 1914, and raised by his Russian immigrant parents in New York City. His father, Daniel, designed women's scarves and blouses. According to Jonas's younger brother Lee, their father "was something of a Willy Loman character from Death of a Salesman, beaten down in business but still believing that success would soon be his."

Jonas, who zealously shielded his private life over the years, once gave a speech to a group of educators in which he described the sway his mother, Dolly, had over him. When Jonas matriculated to the College of the City of New York as a precocious 15 year old, he registered as a prelaw student. "I had no notion of studying medicine ever," he told the educators. "Well, why did I suddenly make that change? Well, it was because my mother, who was a very powerful person [and] had enormous influence with me and everyone else with whom she was in contact, was able to put me into a state in which, when I had anything to say that was contrary to what seemed to be her wishes, I would stutter and stammer. And she didn't think I'd make a very good lawyer. She preferred that I become a teacher. . . . They got out of school in the midafternoon and they had long vacations, and she was one of those very overprotective mothers and didn't want her son to work very hard. And so, my form of protest was to study medicine. And that was the way I dropped out, so to speak. It was a discovery for me. But I didn't really want to study medicine. I decided that if I was going to do that then I'd do research."

In 1938–39, his final year of medical school at New York University, Salk met Thomas Francis Jr., chair of the Department of Bacteriology. Francis, a redoubtable influenza researcher, held the iconoclastic view that vaccines made from killed viruses had much to offer. Conventional wisdom held that only a live, attenuated vaccine could confer long-lasting immunity because it more closely mimicked a true infection. Salk, then 24, took an elective with Francis, who at the time was attempting to kill influenza virus with ultraviolet light. Salk, however modestly, helped isolate the virus from mice lungs and then irradiate it. The day after receiving his M.D., Salk married Donna Lindsay, a social worker. He stayed on with Francis until March 1940, whereupon he began an internship at Mount Sinai Hospital in New York.

In October 1941, Salk visited Francis at the University of Michigan in Ann Arbour, where Francis had moved a few months before to head the epidemiology department in the School of Public Health. Under contract with the Armed Forces Epidemiological Board, Francis was developing a killed-virus vaccine for influenza, which in the 1918–1919 epidemics had killed 43,000 doughboys—more than the number killed in combat during all of World War I. Salk wanted in on the project. Even though the work did not involve polio, Francis encouraged Salk to apply for a fellowship from the National Foundation for Infantile Paralysis, which groomed up-and-coming virologists. "My ultimate intentions are to do

investigative work in virus diseases," Salk wrote in a draft of his fellowship application. "At the present time, my chief interest lies in the fundamental aspects of this field relative to the problems of prophylactic immunization." Viruses. Vaccines. The 27-year-old Salk had charted his course.

The National Foundation awarded Salk the $2,100 fellowship, and he moved to Ann Arbour, beginning the yearlong project on April 12, 1942. Salk soon began publishing scientific papers, some of which revealed what his critics would call his essential flaw and his admirers would praise as his genius - his penchant for extrapolating from the data at hand. In Breakthrough: The Saga of Jonas Salk, a 1965 book by Richard Carter, Salk recounts how Francis once scolded him for attempting to publish a paper that was short on facts and long on inferences. "There may have been times when I made more of my data than might have been expected, but I was not functioning in the expected way," Salk said. "I was supplying immunological insights. I was attempting to elucidate the interaction of man and virus in a field which was accustomed to viewing the two separately. I engaged in extrapolation because I had always felt that it was a legitimate means of provoking scientific thought and discussion. I engaged in prediction because I felt it was the essence of scientific thought. The fact that neither extrapolation nor prediction was popular in virological circles seemed to me to be a shame."

Francis also grew impatient with Salk's independent streak. "Damn it, Salk," Francis chided his young assistant around that time, "why do you have to do things differently from other people?"

Salk rose through the ranks at Ann Arbour, becoming an assistant professor. But when the University of Pittsburgh approached Salk in 1947 and offered him his own viral research program, he eagerly made the move.

With a grant from the Armed Forces Epidemiological Board, Salk continued his work on killed-virus influenza vaccines, focusing on adjuvants. Adjuvants serve as a fuel additive to killed-virus vaccines, boosting potency and durability, and can make or break the effectiveness of a preparation. Though adjuvants have taken on something of an alchemical mystique, they work because they are made of substances so foreign to the human body that the immune system cannot help but take notice. At the time, Salk was interested in an adjuvant known as Incomplete Freund's, an emulsion of mineral oil and water with the gooey consistency of white glue. He began testing this killed influenza vaccine on thousands of soldiers stationed at Fort Dix, New Jersey.

Salk worked hard, and luck came his way in the form of Harry Weaver. Appointed as director of research at the National Foundation a few years before, Weaver, with the blessing of Basil O'Connor and the damnation of many, wanted to do just that—direct research. Until Weaver came on board, the National Foundation simply funded projects that independent researchers selected, maintaining the age-old stance that yoking the minds of scientists would leave fields fallow. The U.S. government also shied away from directing polio research, but for different reasons. The NIH, impressed with the polio research funded by the nongovernmental National Foundation, reserved most of its grant money for other scourges.

While researchers who are independent arguably unearth more truths about a disease, they often investigate questions that have little practical application. Soon after becoming research director at the National Foundation, Weaver began inviting leading polio researchers

to roundtable conferences in luxury hotels, where stenographers recorded their remarks, which the foundation then published as progress reports. He quickly concluded, as he wrote O'Connor, that "only an appalling few . . . were really trying to solve the problem of poliomyelitis in man." In a different reflective note to O'Connor, Weaver wrote, "It became evident that, if real progress were to be made, more exact methods of research would have to be instituted, objectives would have to be clearly defined, procedures and techniques would have to be developed to permit attaining these objectives, and individual groups of workers would have to sacrifice to some extent their inherent right to 'roam the field,' so to speak, and concentrate their energies on one or, at most, a few of the objectives."

At the behest of Weaver, the National Foundation spearheaded a research project in 1948 to identify strains of poliovirus, a critical step in the development of an effective vaccine. Researchers knew that there were at least three types of poliovirus, but no one knew how many existed. If a vaccine is not made from every type of the virus, people will remain susceptible to the disease. The National Foundation assembled an eminent advisory committee to lead the virus-typing project. Along with Thomas Francis Jr., Salk's old professor and boss, there was Albert Sabin from the Children's Hospital in Cincinnati. An M.D. who began studying poliovirus shortly after leaving Russia for the States in 1930, Sabin declared his interest in—though he had not yet begun devising—a weakened, live poliovirus vaccine.

The actual grunt work of typing viruses did not interest the members of the advisory committee, so Weaver went hunting for ambitious, younger researchers who had the necessary laboratory space. And that is what led Harry Weaver to Jonas Salk and Jonas Salk to polio research.

That year, 1948, Isabel Morgan of Johns Hopkins University in Baltimore successfully protected monkeys from one type of poliovirus with a killed-virus vaccine. Before the year was out, the United States recorded 27,726 new cases of polio. American polio cases surged to 42,033 in 1949. Public panic was building.

Science advances nanometre by nanometre, but in 1949, March of Dimes-funded research yielded a bona fide breakthrough: The lab of John Enders at Children's Hospital in Boston discovered a way to grow poliovirus in non-nervous tissue cultures, a feat that later earned a Nobel Prize. Not only did the culturing of virus in non-nervous tissue remove a safety concern; it also dramatically reduced the need for monkeys, as the testicles or kidneys of one animal provided enough tissue culture for 200 test tubes. One monkey, then, did what used to require 200. Anxious to apply this technique to making a vaccine, Salk had his own tissue-culturing system functioning by 1950, and by June of that year, revealed plans to make a killed-virus vaccine and test it in children. "My orientation at the moment is to see if we can develop a satisfactory procedure for the prevention of poliomyelitis by immunologic means," Salk wrote Weaver. "The approaches to the realization of this solution are obvious enough. The problem at hand is that of devising ways and means whereby it can be accomplished."

Problem. Solution. It was the language Weaver spoke, but he could not openly back the plan.

Developing a vaccine for humans clearly was the next step, but a cautious scientific mood prevailed, partly because the two vaccines in the 1930s had performed so pitifully. Scientific concerns and public ones, though, often differ greatly. The National Foundation

was a cross-breed, with both a scientific and a public lineage. Part of its soul belonged to the very researchers who found comfort in slow progress. Yet the National Foundation also worked for every person terrified by poliovirus: The mothers wearing paper hats, who had begun arming themselves with tin cans, marching door-to-door to collect dimes during January fund-raising drives. The girl in the iron lung who clenched a mallet in her teeth and played the xylophone for a March of Dimes newsreel. The crutched-up poster boy wearing a wide cowboy hat and a smile to match. And the Hollywood stars who gave generously to the cause. Weaver and Salk were the type of scientists who moved judiciously, but with a palpable sense of urgency, the very sense that the panicked public felt.

Weaver counselled Salk that if he wanted the National Foundation to help him make a vaccine, he could not speak of using children in experiments. And so it was that when Salk submitted his proposal for a 1951 National Foundation grant, which he got, he left out the idea of vaccinating children. Salk even sidestepped the controversial notion of pursuing a killed-virus vaccine, stating that a preparation containing live, but weakened poliovirus might be the way to go.

During the typing project, Salk found weakened strains of polio that intrigued him, but he never seriously considered making a live vaccine. Indeed, he would become the standard-bearer for the non-infectious killed vaccine and for a scientific principle that would open the door for a new era of vaccinology.

Back then, common wisdom held that the only way to develop long-lasting protection against a disease was by "convalescent immunity"—in other words, getting an infection and recovering. This, of course, was how people naturally became immune to polio. A vaccine could only hope to improve upon nature by creating a weak infection that could not lead to disease, but could create durable immunity. This is what the live, "attenuated" vaccines for smallpox, rabies, and yellow fever aimed to do. Salk found the common wisdom unwise. Since the time he was a medical student, he questioned why infection was needed for viral vaccines but not for the bacterial vaccines that worked so well against diphtheria and tetanus. "From my experience in chemistry, logic suggested that if one were possible then so should be the other," Salk once wrote.

Salk hardly thought up the idea of a killed-virus vaccine: the first was made in 1886 (for hog cholera), and France's Louis Pasteur had unwittingly made the first human one (for rabies) two years later. There also existed killed vaccines for human typhoid, cholera, plague, pertussis, and influenza before Salk began his polio work. Yet it was the diphtheria and tetanus vaccines that encouraged him to make a killed poliovirus vaccine. The bacteria responsible for diphtheria and tetanus cause disease by releasing toxins. In the mid-1920s, researchers found that chemically inactivating the toxins, creating what are now called "toxoids," made for effective vaccines. So then didn't it follow that infection and protection could be separated, that one was not necessary to create the other? That is a fundamental question Salk believed a killed poliovirus vaccine could answer. But the question tipped the dogma cart and, at least in the world of science, won him few friends and no shortage of detractors.

The National Foundation had competition in the vaccine search in 1950, most notably the New Jersey–based Ederle Pharmaceuticals. One of the hotshot researchers at Lederle was Hilary Koprowski. A Polish physician who studied piano at an Italian conservatory in 1939,

Koprowski sailed to Brazil once the war broke out and worked on an attenuated yellow fever vaccine. He came to Lederle in 1944 and by 1950 had developed a live vaccine that contained weakened virus, grown in the brains of cotton rats, to defeat one of what the typing project would later reveal were three main types of poliovirus. While a successful vaccine would need to be trivalent, this was an exciting start. In the spirit of self-experimentation, Koprowski and his boss ate their vaccine.

Koprowski subsequently inoculated 20 institutionalized children with his polio vaccine. The children developed antibodies to poliovirus without illness. Though their parents had put them up for the experiment, scientists branded Koprowski, two years Salk's junior, as brash and reckless. But as the first vaccine administered to humans since the fiascos of the thirties, it proved an important point. Humans, like monkeys and chimpanzees, responded to weakened poliovirus.

That year, 33,000 Americans got polio. One of them was Basil O'Connor's 30-year-old daughter. "When, in 1949, Dr. John Enders grew poliovirus, O'Connor sniffed victory," wrote science reporter Victor Cohn in the 1955 Minneapolis Morning Tribune, "and when in 1950 his daughter got polio, his quiet controlled frenzy was doubled. Now he wanted in on the kill."

Jonas Salk and Basil O'Connor became friends in 1951. Though they had met before, it was on the Queen Mary, carrying them home from the Second International Poliomyelitis Congress in Copenhagen, that their visions fused. Over the years, the friendship would draw charges of cronyism and, worse, that O'Connor exploited Salk or that Salk willingly let O'Connor exploit him. Time has rendered the once hot allegations inert. The robust Irish-American and the slightly built, reserved son of Jewish immigrants pushed each other higher than they might otherwise have risen and the world benefited. "We made a good team," Salk explained to me. "Whatever it was, he was hoping to succeed. That was his narrow outlook."

In 1951, 28,386 Americans got polio.

By the middle of 1952, Salk had developed a killed poliovirus vaccine designed to work against all three strains of the virus, had tested it in monkeys, and was ready to inject it into humans. In keeping with the trusting nature of the times, he did not have to clear this proposed human trial with a group of ethicists at his university, scientists at the Food and Drug Administration (which didn't exist), or even the scientific committee of the National Foundation. Rather, he just had to find people willing to participate, which he did at the D. T. Watson Home for Crippled Children, just outside of Pittsburgh.

Salk chose to test his vaccine on a few dozen sufferers of polio at the home, whose parents had agreed to let them participate in the trial. He chose this group for safety reasons: If something were dangerous about his vaccine—if, say, not all of the poliovirus was killed, as some critics of the approach feared—these kids would not contract polio anew. And his goal was simply to assess whether the vaccine could boost production of antibodies against the three distinct types of poliovirus. On July 2, Salk began vaccinating the children with three vaccines, each containing a different type of poliovirus that had been killed with the chemical Formalin, a formaldehyde solution. In all, 43 children received one of the three types of vaccines. Everyone involved swore to secrecy, and only the top brass at the National Foundation, which was funding the study, even knew of its existence.

The vaccine, just as Salk had hoped, goosed the immune system and led it to crank out antibodies that could "neutralize" the virus. Specifically, when Salk and his co-workers mixed fresh samples of the vaccinees' blood with poliovirus growing in tissue culture, the virus could no longer destroy the tissue. The vaccine, it seemed, worked. As Salk told writer Richard Carter, "It was the thrill of my life. Compared to the feeling I got seeing those results under the microscope, everything that followed was anticlimactic."

That year, 57,879 Americans got polio. The United States had never experienced a higher crest in the epidemiological wave—and never would again.

At a National Foundation Committee on Immunization meeting in January 1953, Salk presented his results from the Watson Home and from another institution where he had tested his experimental polio vaccines on humans, the Polk State School, a home for the retarded. Both trials indicated that the killed vaccines were safe and triggered a strong immune response, stronger even than the one caused by natural infection. Some committee members immediately called for a larger field trial. Others, most notably Sabin and John Enders, cautioned against an expanded trial.

The next month, the National Foundation gathered luminaries, none of whom were directly involved with polio research, from the Rockefeller Foundation, the American Medical Association, academia, and the U.S. government to toss about the idea of launching a large clinical trial of a killed-virus vaccine made by Salk. One of the attendees, Thomas Rivers of the Rockefeller Institute, had long been a key adviser to the National Foundation, having come aboard during the days of the Birthday Ball Commission. After Salk told the group his findings, Rivers explained how Salk would soon publish his data in the Journal of the American Medical Association (JAMA). "Dr. Salk is over a barrel," Rivers said. *"Terrific pressure is going to be put on him. Terrific pressure is going to be put on the foundation and there is always the danger of moving too fast. There is also the danger of going too slow, because if you have something that is good, the public should have it as soon as possible and at a safe time. That is the problem before the group this morning. . . .*

"Wouldn't it be silly to wait 50 years or to wait 10 years to develop the ideal vaccine when there is the possibility of a vaccine being developed very rapidly that will last, say, for two or three years with one injection perhaps? We don't know anything about that, but have we the right to wait until the ideal vaccine comes along?"

The attendees concurred that, as Salk wished, he should move ahead cautiously, and that Rivers should write a letter to JAMA explaining their decision. The intent of these formalities was to inform professionals about the vaccine Salk was developing, while keeping the public enthusiasm in check. All of these careful manoeuvres were undermined however; when a syndicated New York columnist ran a story headlined "New Polio Vaccine! Big Hopes Seen." Insiders have speculated that someone at the National Foundation, anxious to march more dimes into the coffers, leaked the story.

Salk, worried that the attention would slow him down and make him seem a publicity hound, forged a deal with O'Connor that he would speak directly to the public in a radio address the evening before the JAMA article came out. "I knew goddamn well the next day they [the media] would be exaggerating," Salk told me. "I wanted to modulate."

Entitled "The Scientist Speaks for Himself" and broadcast over CBS radio, the speech Salk gave, which followed a brief introduction by O'Connor, stressed patience and the fact

that he was but one of many polio researchers. "We want to reach our goal as quickly as possible," Salk told listeners across the country, "and I am certain that you will understand that the actual accomplishment of our purposes cannot be achieved in a day."

Salk had to duck behind this door and that over the next few weeks to avoid the torrent of press. It would be this way, off and on, for the rest of his life. Whether by design or default, Salk had walked into a hall that few scientists ever enter. The bold, tall letters of the daily press had spelled out his name. Sonorous announcers had repeated it over the wireless, on television and newsreels. The kind-faced, soft-spoken Dr. Jonas Edward Salk was famous.

Whatever the effect on Salk's personal life, the radio speech bridled any hopes the public had for a large-scale trial in 1953. With help from a paediatrician at the Watson Home and more than 500 volunteers, Salk and his little viral research lab spent the summer improving his vaccine.

During the summer of 1953, Harry Weaver left the National Foundation, in part because of a clash over the design of a large-scale field trial. The Foundation also lost the support of several high-powered members of its Committee on Immunization, including Albert Sabin, when it indelicately sprung the news at an October meeting that plans were far along for a large-scale test of Salk's killed-virus vaccine.

As one committee member later wrote, "Decks had been cleared for action on a vaccine, and if in the process some individuals had been hurt and some wrong decisions had been made, that was just too bad."

That year, 35,592 Americans got polio.

In 1954, the National Foundation's polio field trials mobilized the country. One writer, looking back, compared organizing the experiment to teaching a large troupe of elephants to do the mambo. Trial officials, true to the gee-whiz fifties, compiled the largely meaningless but otherwise staggering tally of how many people pitched in: 20,000 doctors and public health officials, 40,000 registered nurses, 14,000 school principals, 50,000 teachers, and 200,000 lay volunteers.

The one figure that was anything but meaningless was 1,830,000 - the number of first-, second-, and third-grade children in 44 states who participated. They were the patients, though the National Foundation, fearful of having them labelled guinea pigs, dubbed them "Polio Pioneers."

An illustration of Salk appeared on the cover of Time magazine a month before the trial began, further lionizing him. The March 29, 1954, article itself, though, did not glorify Salk, recounting the contributions of many polio researchers and even quoting unnamed colleagues criticizing the young researcher. One particularly harsh complaint was that Salk had not published much of his data. Wrote Time, "A cautious Yankee with long years of experiences with viruses and vaccines objects: 'We want Salk to show us, not tell us.' "

From the outset of the trial, which formally began on April 26, 1954, Basil O'Connor foresaw that if the vaccine worked, there would be a stampede of parents demanding it for their children. So that summer, O'Connor decided to pay six pharmaceutical houses a total of $9 million to produce the vaccine. If the vaccine proved effective, warehoused vials would be at the ready. The only thing standing in the way would be the government licensing authority.

That year, 38,476 Americans got polio.

In February 1955, Salk appeared on See It Now, the popular television interview program hosted by Edward R. Murrow. Salk had a strong distaste for journalists. (He once described a press conference to me as "feeding the animals in the zoo.") But the no-nonsense Murrow, the exemplar of broadcast journalists who made his name dispatching clear-eyed radio reports while Nazi bombs crashed around him in London, much impressed Salk.

Salk discussed the colossal trial underway; the criticism pelting him, and the contributions others made to the development of what he wished was not being called the "Salk vaccine." "You must remember that nothing happens quite by chance," he told Murrow, intonating in the high style that was his wont. "It's a question of the accretion of information and experience. You must see - it should be obvious that there is an enormous heritage into which I was born, so to speak, and it's just chance that I happen to be here at this particular time when there was available and at my disposal the great experience of all the investigators who plodded along for a number of years. And essentially that's what we've been doing ourselves, but acknowledging fully that which has been contributed by everyone else. . . . So what I am really saying is that the . . . science of immunology is not a new one, and it's one that has been contributed to by many investigators ever since the time of Pasteur."

On April 12, 1955, Thomas Francis Jr., who oversaw data analysis of the trial, revealed the results. The announcement fittingly was made in Ann Arbour on the campus of the University of Michigan, 13 years to the day after Salk first arrived there to work with Francis. The 150 journalists who attended acted something like zoo animals being fed, climbing atop tables, fighting for copies of the report, elbowing each other as they rushed to phone in their copy. Having assembled and analyzed 144,000,000 separate pieces of data, Francis stated that the vaccine worked at least 60% of the time, and had not caused any significant harm to a single child.

Two hours later, the Department of Health, Education, and Welfare licensed the vaccine.

The country—the world—exploded with joy, dancing and singing and hugging, and blasting, ringing, and clinking anything that would make noise. Page 1 of the New York Times had a photo of Salk and Francis with this ebullient headline above it: SALK POLIO VACCINE PROVES SUCCESS; MILLIONS WILL BE IMMUNIZED SOON. Boxes filled with vaccine, RUSH printed on their sides, were whisked out of the warehouses.

That night, Salk and Francis appeared on See It Now with Murrow, live from the University of Michigan. "Who owns the patent on the vaccine?" Murrow asked Salk at one point.

"Well," said Salk, "the people I would say. There is no patent. Could you patent the sun?"

During the next few weeks, letters, telegrams, phone calls, and in-the-flesh well-wishers descended on Salk. Elated folks suggested Salk make vaccines for cancer, multiple sclerosis, colds, Lou Gehrig's disease, Parkinson's, diabetes, herpes, colitis, and even anti-Semitism. There was no end to the awards, honorary degrees, and donations. It was a train of elation, with ever more cars hooking on [4].

From this account, it is clear that the US Government was deeply involved in the events that led to the development of the Salk polio vaccine – it provided funds, arranged the mass

immunization with the unregistered Salk vaccine, collected, collated, analyzed and announced the data from the mass trials, etc.

The lesson from the polio experience in the US is that extant procedures and regulations are, of necessity, waived in the face of major epidemics wrecking much morbidity and mortality. Readers may wish to note that the new polio cases and mortality rates from polio in the US in the days before the Salk vaccine are relatively insignificant when compared with the figures for the HIV/AIDS pandemic that has been ravaging the world since 1981, especially in sub-Saharan Africa that harbours about 70 per cent of the HIV/AIDS cases in the world

With the deadly HIV/AIDS pandemic on the rampage since 1981, the lengthy procedure involved in the conventional approach to bring a vaccine to the market leaves the scourge to cause the death of tens of millions of people and tens of millions of new cases of the infection. Is it proper and ethical then to spend, say 10 years to develop and evaluate a vaccine when in those 10 years, the disease kills tens of millions of people with tens of millions of new cases of the infection that has no cure? In the recent case of Merck's V520 HIV vaccine that took 10 years and several billion dollars to develop and evaluate, the vaccine failed to deliver on its promise even though the scientific community had all placed high hopes on the vaccine, describing it as 'the vaccine of vaccines'.

Let us imagine that the V520 HIV preventive vaccine had been partly effective in preventing HIV infection after 10 years of research, development and evaluation. How many new cases of HIV occurred worldwide in those 10 years? We all know the answer - tens of millions. The V520 cannot do anything to help those victims of the infection. In other words, a mediocre but safe HIV preventive vaccine that, let us say, is only 10 per cent efficacious, if introduced today, would be far more helpful to mankind than a fantastic HIV preventive vaccine introduced 10 years hence. It would be more prudent and pragmatic, in the author's view, to introduce and use such a mediocre HIV vaccine today and change to better ones as better ones are developed.

Conclusion

We have looked at what vaccines are, as well as the conventional ways of making them and bringing them to the market. As one would expect, there cannot be any laid down procedures either for making any vaccine that has never been developed before or for bringing such a vaccine to the market. The development of a new vaccine is the result of an open field with different researchers working hard to develop a safe and effective vaccine against the disease.

The conventional ways of making vaccines that have been described cannot be exhaustive. New methods of making safe and effective vaccines may be developed in the future. Since 1981, man has been facing a new disease, AIDS, hitherto unknown to man. It became clear within a few years that the disease was turning out to be a global epidemic. In 1983/84, the causative agent, a virus, was discovered, first by the French and independently a year later by the Americans, but the latter were the first to announce it to the world in April 1984. The causative agent of AIDS was eventually called HIV. Since 1984, the HIV/AIDS

scourge has become a major pandemic unlike any known to man. Several millions have died from the scourge, and several millions are infected with the deadly and 'incurable' virus every year. The search for its vaccine has been on since 1984, but the world claims there is none yet. As happened to the polio epidemics in the US before the Salk vaccine in 1954, there cannot be a procedure either for making an HIV vaccine or for bringing it the market. The problem that has been facing humanity since 1984 is the development of safe and effective HIV vaccines.

References

[1] http://www.chop.edu/consumer/jsp/microsite/microsite.jsp?id=75918

[2] Plotkin S.A, Orenstein W.A., Editors (2003). *Vaccines* (4th Edition), Elsevier Books, Oxford.

[3] http://www.chop.edu/consumer/jsp/division/generic.jsp?id=75749

[4] Cohen J (2001). Chapter 2 'The Next Breakthrough' in *Shots in the dark: the wayward search for an AIDS vaccine.* W.W. Norton and Company, New York. The quotations are from the author's copy that he kindly emailed to the author in September 2004 after *Vaccine* published a report on the author's HIV vaccines effort.

Chapter III

Plague

Abstract

In days past, plague was a terror to mankind. Mighty armies were sometimes devastated by it. This chapter recalls, again from history, man's response to this infectious and highly contagious and infectious disease in order for us to learn lessons from it. The bubonic form of plague is the commonest and is highly contagious. The pneumonic form is extremely infectious and highly lethal. The septicaemic form arises from time to time in bubonic cases. All forms of the disease have a short incubation period of a few hours to just 3 or 4 days. An attack of plague left the victim immune from another attack if he survived it. Unfortunately, there is still no effective and safe vaccine against this bacterial disease.

Introduction

Plague is among the more virulent infectious diseases. Its association with humans is an ancient one. The disease is caused by a bacterium, *Yersinia pestis* (Lehman and Neumann). The pathogen is transmitted by fleas, particularly the oriental rat flea, *Xenopsylla cheopis* (Rothschild), but it also can be transmitted from human to human in its pneumonic form (a lung infection).

Plague primarily is a disease of rodents. Under certain circumstances, however, plague can be introduced to humans, where it is devastating. Fleas that have fed on plague-infected rats or other rodent species become infected. Plague bacilli multiply in the gut of the flea, and, if humans are in close association with infected rats, the fleas may attempt to feed on them. During feeding, the plague bacilli are introduced into the victim. In humans, after the bacteria are introduced, the onset of the disease usually occurs in three to four days [1].

Clinically, there are three forms of the disease, bubonic, pneumonic and septicaemic. Following a short incubation period of less than a week, there follows an acute illness with death within a few days or in the septicaemic form of the disease, within hours.

Historically, plague destroyed entire civilizations. In the 1300s, the "*Black Death*," as it was called, killed approximately one-third (20 to 30 million) of Europe's population. In the

mid-1800s, it killed 12 million people in China. Today, thanks to better living conditions, antibiotics, and improved sanitation, current World Health Organization statistics show there were only 2,118 cases in 2003 worldwide.

Approximately 10 to 20 people in the United States develop plague each year from flea or rodent bites—primarily from infected prairie dogs—in rural areas of the south-western United States. About 1 in 7 of those infected die from the disease. There has not been a case of person-to-person infection in the United States since 1924.

Worldwide, there have been small plague outbreaks in Asia, Africa, and South America [2].

The Black Death in the 14th Century A.D.

In the 14th Century, Europe found itself at the mercy of the Black Death. Historians have left this account for us:

The Black Death, 1348

Coming out of the East, the Black Death reached the shores of Italy in the spring of 1348 unleashing a rampage of death across Europe unprecedented in recorded history. By the time the epidemic played itself out three years later, anywhere between 25% and 50% of Europe's population had fallen victim to the pestilence.

The plague presented itself in three interrelated forms. The bubonic variant (the most common) derives its name from the swellings or buboes that appeared on a victim's neck, armpits or groin. These tumours could range in size from that of an egg to that of an apple.

Although some survived the painful ordeal, the manifestation of these lesions usually signalled the victim had a life expectancy of up to a week. Infected fleas that attached themselves to rats and then to humans spread this bubonic type of the plague. A second variation—pneumonic plague—attacked the respiratory system and was spread by merely breathing the exhaled air of a victim. It was much more virulent than its bubonic cousin—life expectancy was measured in one or two days. Finally, the septicaemic version of the disease attacked the blood system.

Having no defence and no understanding of the cause of the pestilence, the men, women and children caught in its onslaught were bewildered, panicked, and finally devastated.

The Italian writer Giovanni Boccaccio lived through the plague as it ravaged the city of Florence in 1348. The experience inspired him to write The Decameron, *a story of seven men and three women who escape the disease by fleeing to a villa outside the city. In his introduction to the fictional portion of his book, Boccaccio gives a graphic description of the effects of the epidemic on his city [3].*

The Signs of Impending Death

"The symptoms were not the same as in the East, where a gush of blood from the nose was the plain sign of inevitable death; but it began both in men and women with certain swellings in the groin or under the armpit. They grew to the size of a small apple or an egg, more or less, and were vulgarly called tumours. In a short space of time these tumours spread from the two parts named to all over the body. Soon after this the symptoms changed and black or purple spots appeared on the arms or thighs or any other part of the body, sometimes a few large ones, sometimes many little ones. These spots were a certain sign of death, just as the original tumour had been and still remained.

No doctor's advice, no medicine could overcome or alleviate this disease, an enormous number of ignorant men and women set up as doctors in addition to those who were trained. Either the disease was such that no treatment was possible or the doctors were so ignorant that they did not know what caused it, and consequently could not administer the proper remedy. In any case very few recovered; most people died within about three days of the appearance of the tumours described above, most of them without any fever or other symptoms.

The violence of this disease was such that the sick communicated it to the healthy who came near them, just as a fire catches anything dry or oily near it. And it even went further. To speak to or go near the sick brought infection and a common death to the living; and moreover, to touch the clothes or anything else the sick had touched or worn gave the disease to the person touching them."

Varying Reactions to Disaster

"...Such fear and fanciful notions took possession of the living that almost all of them adopted the same cruel policy, which was entirely to avoid the sick and everything belonging to them. By so doing, each one thought he would secure his own safety.

Some thought that moderate living and the avoidance of all superfluity would preserve them from the epidemic. They formed small communities, living entirely separate from everybody else. They shut themselves up in houses where there were no sick, eating the finest food and drinking the best wine very temperately, avoiding all excess, allowing no news or discussion of death and sickness, and passing the time in music and other such pleasures. Others thought just the opposite. They thought the sure cure for the plague was to drink and be merry, to go about singing and amusing themselves, satisfying every appetite they could, laughing and jesting at what happened. They put their words into practice, spent day and night going from tavern to tavern, drinking immoderately, or went into other people's houses, doing only those things which pleased them. This they could easily do because everyone felt doomed and had abandoned his property, so that most houses became common property and any stranger who went in made use of them as if he had owned them. And with all this bestial behaviour, they avoided the sick as much as possible.

In this suffering and misery of our city, the authority of human and divine laws almost disappeared, for, like other men, the ministers and the executors of the laws were all dead or

sick or shut up with their families, so that no duties were carried out. Every man was therefore able to do as he pleased.

Many others adopted a course of life midway between the two just described. They did not restrict their victuals so much as the former, nor allow themselves to be drunken and dissolute like the latter, but satisfied their appetites moderately. They did not shut themselves up, but went about, carrying flowers or scented herbs or perfumes in their hands, in the belief that it was an excellent thing to comfort the brain with such odours; for the whole air was infected with the smell of dead bodies, of sick persons and medicines.

Others again held a still more cruel opinion, which they thought would keep them safe. They said that the only medicine against the plague-stricken was to go right away from them. Men and women, convinced of this and caring about nothing but themselves, abandoned their own city, their own houses, their dwellings, their relatives, their property, and went abroad or at least to the country round Florence, as if God's wrath in punishing men's wickedness with this plague would not follow them but strike only those who remained within the walls of the city, or as if they thought nobody in the city would remain alive and that its last hour had come."

The Breakdown of Social Order — Brother Abandoned Brother

"One citizen avoided another; hardly any neighbour troubled about others, relatives never or hardly ever visited each other. Moreover, such terror was struck into the hearts of men and women by this calamity, that brother abandoned brother, and the uncle his nephew, and the sister her brother, and very often the wife her husband. What is even worse and nearly incredible is that fathers and mothers refused to see and tend their children, as if they had not been theirs.

Thus, a multitude of sick men and women were left without any care, except from the charity of friends (but these were few), or the greed, of servants, though not many of these could be had even for high wages. Moreover, most of them were coarse-minded men and women, who did little more than bring the sick what they asked for or watch over them when they were dying. And very often these servants lost their lives and their earnings. Since the sick were thus abandoned by neighbours, relatives and friends, and while servants were scarce, a habit sprang up which had never been heard of before. Beautiful and noble women, when they fell sick, did not scruple to take a young or old man-servant, whoever he might be, and with no sort of shame, expose every part of their bodies to these men as if they had been women, for they were compelled by the necessity of their sickness to do so. This, perhaps, was a cause of looser morals in those women who survived."

Mass Burials

"The plight of the lower and most of the middle classes was even more pitiful to behold. Most of them remained in their houses, either through poverty or in hopes of safety, and fell sick by the thousands. Since they received no care and attention, almost all of them died.

Many ended their lives in the streets both at night and during the day; and many others who died in their houses were only known to be dead because the neighbours smelled their decaying bodies. Dead bodies filled every corner. Most of them were treated in the same manner by the survivors, who were more concerned about getting rid of their rotting bodies than moved by charity towards the dead. With the aid of porters, if they could get them, they carried the bodies out of the houses and laid them at the door; where every morning quantities of the dead might be seen. They then were laid on biers or, as these were often lacking, on tables.

Such was the multitude of corpses brought to the churches every day and almost every hour that there was not enough consecrated ground to give them burial, especially since they wanted to bury each person in the family grave, according to the old custom. Although the cemeteries were full they were forced to dig huge trenches, where they buried the bodies by hundreds. Here they stowed them away like bales in the hold of a ship and covered them with a little earth, until the whole trench was full [4]".

The Great Plague of London, 1665

During the Great Plague of London (April–October 1665), many markets were cancelled and street stalls banned. Forty thousand dogs and 80,000 cats were slaughtered—a desperate measure for a desperate situation even though this last move actually made things worse, as the plague-carrying rats were then free of predators. By the end of July, more than 1,000 Londoners were dying each week [5].

Napoleon's Troops and the Black Death, 1799

Early in 1799, the Ottoman Empire declared war on France. Napoleon Bonaparte expected a Turkish attack on Egypt. He decided to enter Syria (now Israel and Syria) to disrupt any Turkish action against Egypt. Bonaparte personally led 13,000 French soldiers into Syria, quickly taking the coastal towns of El Arish, Gaza, Jaffa, and Haifa from Mameluke, Arab, and Turkish defenders. By August 1799 when he returned to France to meet his fate, he had lost most of his soldiers to plague. During Napoleon's Syrian campaign, the mortality rate from plague was 92% [1].

Immunity from Plague

We know from the historian Thucydides in the fifth century B.C. that people knew then that because survivors of plague were 'never attacked twice - never at least fatally', such people were involved in caring for those sick or dying from the disease [6].

Plague confers natural immunity after an attack but unfortunately, there are still no effective vaccines against the disease.

Conclusion

Plague illustrates vividly again man's response to a fatal and highly infectious disease like plague. Though man has known for centuries that survivors of plague are conferred with lifelong immunity against another attack, man is yet to develop effective vaccines against the disease.

References

[1] http://entomology.montana.edu/historybug/napoleon/plague_syria.htm

[2] http://www.medicinenet.com /plague/article.htm

[3] Boccaccio, Giovanni, The Decameron vol. I (translated by Richard Aldington illustrated by Jean de Bosschere) (1930); Gottfried, Robert, The Black Death (1983).

[4] "The Black Death, 1348," Eyewitness to History, www.eyewitnesstohistory.com (2001).

[5] http://www.channel4.com/history/microsites/H/history/plague/story.html

[6] Richard Crawley's translation, bk. 2, chap. 7 of Thucydides' *The History of the Peloponnesian War.*

Chapter IV

Variolation

Abstract

Smallpox, a highly infectious disease with high mortality and morbidity rates has been known to humanity for a very long time. It is responsible for the deaths of millions. Attempts were made to protect people from the scourge by a process called variolation, the intentional introduction of a mild form of the disease to protect people from the scourge itself; this came from the observation that survivors of the disease never get a second attack. Of course there were dangers associated with variolation; sometimes it results in smallpox with some fatalities, and it tended to start epidemics of the disease, also. Nevertheless, the practice spread from Asia to Europe and, later, to the New World. The desperate measure of variolation was a desperate measure to combat the more dangerous smallpox itself. Eventually, it was outlawed when a better protective remedy was developed by Edward Jenner in the twilight years of the 18th Century.

Introduction

Smallpox (Variola or the speckled death) is a highly infectious disease that causes severe morbidity (blindness, hearing loss, unsightly and permanent pock scars on the skin especially of the face, etc.) with about 30% mortality rate. Like the plague, it had been known since antiquity that survivors of smallpox do not get a second attack.

Smallpox was a leading cause of death in the 18th century, respecting no social class. Many of the patients who recovered from it were disfigured.

The only means of combating the disease was the so-called inoculation—intentionally infecting a healthy person with the "matter" taken from a patient sick with a mild attack of smallpox. This practice, which originated in the East, had been introduced into England early in the eighteenth century. A person in good health was inoculated with matter from smallpox pustules and was thus given what was usually a mild case of the disease in order to confer immunity against further smallpox infection. The practice was dangerous, however, since smallpox thus induced could be severe or fatal, and it tended to spread smallpox among the population.

Smallpox was a killer disease; infants and young children formed the majority of its victims. The name smallpox is very misleading. Except for the skin lesions, there is nothing small about smallpox. The name was introduced to differentiate it from the big pox or the great pox, syphilis.

In the seventeenth century, it killed more than 60 million people in Europe alone, and in the twentieth century, before it was eradicated, it killed more than 300 million—three times the number of deaths from all the century's wars and battles combined. Smallpox was a major reason that the European population grew only slowly in the centuries before 1800.

Smallpox has been one of mankind's greatest scourges since time immemorial. It is believed to have appeared at the time of the first agricultural settlements in northeastern Africa, around 10,000 B.C. It probably spread from Africa to India by means of Egyptian merchants in the last millennium B.C.

The earliest evidence of skin lesions resembling those of smallpox is found on the faces of mummies from the time of the 18th and 20th Egyptian Dynasties (1570 to 1085 B.C.). The mummified head of Pharaoh Ramses V who died around 1156 B.C. bears evidence of the disease. The first recorded smallpox epidemic occurred in 1350 B.C. during the Egyptian-Hittite war.

Ancient Sanskrit texts of India referred to the disease, pointing to its existence in Hindustan at least 1000 B.C.

During the epidemic in Athens in 430 BC, Thucydides noted that those who survived the disease were later immune to it. These observations were reiterated by Rhazes (Abu Bakr Muhammad Ibn Zakariya al-Razi), to whom we owe the first medical description of smallpox, *De variolis et morbillis commentarius*, which was written in about A.D. 910.

Rhazes also noted that the illness was transmitted from person to person. His explanation of why survivors of smallpox do not develop the disease a second time is the first theory of acquired immunity.

Smallpox for Biological Warfare?

Smallpox greatly and adversely affected the development of western civilization. The first stages of the decline of the Roman Empire, around A.D. 180, coincided with a large-scale epidemic, the plague of Antonine, which killed between 3.5 and 7 million persons. The Arab expansion, the Crusades, and the discovery of the West Indies all contributed to the spread of the illness.

Unknown in the New World, smallpox was introduced by Spanish and Portuguese explorers. It decimated the local population and was instrumental in the fall of the empires of the Aztecs and the Incas.

When the Spanish arrived in 1518, Mexico had about 25 million inhabitants; by 1620, this number had diminished to 1.6 million. This devastating effect of smallpox gave rise to one of the first examples of biological warfare.

In a letter written to Colonel Henry Bouquet in 1763, Sir Jeffrey Amherst, commander-in-chief of British forces in North America, suggested grinding the scabs of smallpox pustules into blankets that were to be distributed among disaffected tribes of Indians.

The History of Variolation

In Asia, practitioners developed the technique of variolation—the deliberate infection with smallpox. Dried smallpox scabs were blown into the nose of an individual who then contracted a mild form of the disease. Upon recovery, the individual was immune to smallpox. One to two percent of those variolated died as compared to 30 percent who died when they contracted the disease naturally.

By 1700, variolation had spread to Africa, India and the Ottoman Empire.

In contrast to Asians and Africans who inoculated by blowing dried smallpox scabs up the nose, Europeans and their American cousins tended to inoculate through a puncture in the skin [1].

In China

Smallpox was described in China as early as in 1122 B.C. Attempts to combat the scourge started in China with variolation, or inoculation that originated in the southern province of Szechuan. From China this procedure spread to Europe and became the foundation for modern scientific immunology.

The Chinese were familiar with the fact that inoculation has certain advantages and dangers that separate it from the later technique of vaccination. When the virus has been introduced into the body, it causes life-long immunity—if you are lucky. But the process can also cause a direct contagion, producing smallpox.

Inoculation against smallpox at first glance may look like madness. Were not people infected all the time? The answer is no, and here we meet the subtlety of the Chinese inoculators. They used several methods to attenuate the deadly virus, so that the danger of catching the disease was minimized and the chance of acquiring immunity was maximized.

In China, 100 years before Edward Jenner, healthy persons took pills made from the fleas of cows to prevent smallpox; this is the first recorded example of oral vaccination.

The Chinese preferably did not use smallpox matter from smallpox patients, but from persons who had been inoculated and developed a few scabs. The Chinese also knew the difference between the two types of smallpox, Variola major and Variola minor, and chose matter from the latter, which was a less virulent form.

It is believed that 80 percent of the smallpox virus used by the Chinese for inoculation were dead and could not infect anybody with smallpox. Instead they aimed for, like in vaccination, to stimulate the body intro producing antibodies against smallpox, as well as the substance interferon which strengthens the immune system in general.

Despite all this knowledge, according to the author Yü T'ien Ch'ih, inoculation against smallpox was not generally known and practiced on a large scale before the period 1567-1572, the Ming dynasty.

In India

In India, variolation took several forms, the most common of which was the application of scabs or pus from a person with smallpox to the intact or scarified skin of a healthy person.

In Europe

Caravaners spread the technique of variolation from China and India to Europe.

Variolation was known and practiced frequently in the Ottoman Empire, where it had been introduced by Circassian traders around 1670. From there, the practice came to Europe at the beginning of the 18th century with the arrival of travellers returning from Istanbul.

The person responsible for the introduction of variolation into England was the English aristocrat Lady Mary Wortley Montagu (1689–1762). In 1717, Lady Mary Wortley Montagu, the wife of the British ambassador, learned about variolation in Constantinople. In 1721, at the urging of Montagu and the Princess of Wales, several prisoners and abandoned children were inoculated by having smallpox inserted under the skin. Several months later, the children and prisoners were deliberately exposed to smallpox. When none contracted the disease, the procedure was deemed safe and members of the royal family were inoculated. The procedure then became fashionable in Europe [1].

The primary side effect of the procedure was the appearance of smallpox itself; however, in 1722, in one of the first applications of statistics to a medical and social problem, James Jurin (1684–1750) observed that the smallpox-associated case-fatality rate was 1:14 in non-inoculated children and 1:91 in inoculated children.

With new improvements that reduced the likelihood of serious infection, the technique became widespread in England and reached towns and rural communities by the 1740s. In 1745, the London Smallpox and Inoculation Hospital was founded; this centre was dedicated exclusively to the treatment and prevention of smallpox.

Variolation was also practiced in Greece, Russia, and Sweden.

Over to the New World

African slaves introduced variolation into America. In Massachusetts, Cotton Mather learned about the practice from his slave, Onesimus. Mather publicized the technique and the procedure was first tried during a smallpox epidemic in Boston in 1721 [1].

James Kilpatrick, an early American physician, was the author of an essay on inoculation, occasioned by smallpox being brought into South Carolina in the year 1738.

Variolation was never risk-free. Not only could the patient die from the procedure but the mild form of the disease which the patient contracted could spread, causing an epidemic. Victims of variolation could be found at all levels of society; King George III lost a son to the procedure as did many others.

In Edward Jenner's Days

Jenner himself was variolated at the age of 8. When he began medical practice at Berkeley, he was frequently asked to inoculate persons against smallpox. His invention later of vaccination against smallpox was the medical breakthrough which saved most lives before the era of antibiotics.

The Demise of Variolation

In variolation, a healthy person was inoculated with matter from smallpox pustules and was thus given what was usually a mild case of the disease in order to confer immunity against further smallpox infection. The practice was dangerous, however, since smallpox thus induced could be severe or fatal, and it tended to spread smallpox among the population. Variolation was eventually outlawed in America and England because some of those variolated died of smallpox [2, 3].

Conclusion

Variolation, though effective if the recipient survived, is not safe enough to be used for trying to prevent smallpox. The safety of any disease remedy, vaccines inclusive, is of prime importance.

References

[1] http://www.nlm.nih.gov/exhibition/smallpox/sp_variolation.html

[2] Barquet N, Domingo P (1997). Smallpox: The Triumph over the Most Terrible of the Ministers Death. *Annals of Int Med*, 127:635-642

[3] http://www.whonamedit.com/doctor.cfm/1818.html

Chapter V

Edward Jenner and His Vaccine

Abstract

Once upon a time, about 200 years ago, there lived in the English Countryside County of Gloucestershire a man called Edward Jenner. His work on the smallpox scourge then contains many useful lessons for us in the struggle against the HIV/AIDS scourge now facing us. His first considerations were human life and health, and nothing else. That was the motivating force that enabled him to tame the smallpox monster, even though he was not at risk from the disease because he had been violated at the age of eight. Virtually all the steps he took on his smallpox adventure were desperate ones taken for the desperate situation created by smallpox epidemics. He had no idea what caused the disease smallpox; he did not know why and how his approach worked. All that mattered was that it worked, and he went ahead to continue to give his remedy to those who were interested even though his colleagues, as they still do today, sat in London in criticism of Jenner. They refused to publish his work. Jenner got it published at his own expense. It took several years before the British Parliament decided to recognize Jenner's work. Read on and determine for yourself whether history is repeating itself with this dreadful and dreaded HIV/AIDS in our days and before our own eyes or not.

Introduction

Many including the author consider the English Surgeon Edward Jenner the pioneer of Immunology, Public Health and Vaccinology. The author is an unrepentant believer in history because he believes great treasures of knowledge lie therein; knowledge that would assist us immensely if we are confronted with similar problems that our forebears faced. Accordingly, the author has randomly selected just five accounts on Edward Jenner for this book in the hope that when they are read together, they would give us a reasonable panoramic recollection of the events before and after his death.

The First of Five Accounts of Edward Jenner [1]

How Listening to a Milkmaid's Story Can Change the World

Edward Jenner has a place among the immortals in preventive medicine. His invention of vaccination against smallpox was the medical breakthrough which saved most lives before the era of antibiotics. Before him, smallpox was a killer disease, the majority of its victims infants and young children. And, except for the skin lesions, there is nothing small about smallpox. In the twentieth century alone it killed more than 300 million, three times the number of deaths from all the century's wars and battles combined. The last reported case of smallpox occurred in Somalia. There, on October 26, 1977, a youth named Ali Maow Maalin recovered from a rash caused by the disease. He was pronounced the last case of natural smallpox in the world. In 1980, as a result of Jenner's discovery, the World Health Assembly officially declared "the world and its peoples" free from endemic smallpox. *(Earlier, on December 9, 1979, the chief scientists of the WHO had declared that smallpox as a naturally occurring disease had been eradicated from this planet [2]).*

A Country Boy

Edward Jenner (1749–1823) was born and brought up in Berkeley in the English farming county of Gloucestershire, about 240 kilometres northwest of London. He was the sixth and youngest child of the Reverend Stephen Jenner (1702–1754), Master of Arts from Oxford, rector of Rockhampton and vicar of Berkeley, a small market town in the Severn Valley in Gloucestershire. His mother was a daughter of the Reverend Henry Head, a former vicar of Berkeley. In addition to his church offices, Jenner's father owned a considerable amount of land in the vicinity of Berkeley. In 1754, when Edward was five years old, both parents died within a few weeks of each other and he came under the guardianship of his elder brother, the Reverend Stephen Jenner, who had succeeded their father as rector of Rockhampton.

Jenner's first schooling was received from the Reverend Mr. Clissold at the nearby village of Wotton-under-Edge. Later he was sent to the grammar school of Dr. Wasbourn in Cirencester. He was then placed in the care of a clergyman in Wooden-under Edge who gave him an introduction to classical knowledge.

Growing up in the depths of the countryside, surrounded by nature and men of the country, Jenner developed a love for nature which he preserved during his life. As a boy he could recognize the cry of every bird and name every plant that grew alongside the Castle brooks and streams. One of his favourite boyhood activities was searching for fossils among the oolite rocks of the countryside.

A Surgeon's Apprentice

Despite his initial interest in classical studies, Jenner early decided to study medicine, and in 1761, at 13 years of age, he was apprenticed to Abraham Ludlow, a surgeon of

Sodbury, near Bristol. In the ensuing years Jenner received a thorough introduction to medical and surgical practice. It was during this time he heard a dairymaid say, "I shall never have smallpox for I have had cowpox. I shall never have an ugly pockmarked face." This belief was part of common lore.

In those days, studies at the medical faculty of a University were both expensive and rather theoretical, and thus the best opportunity for further education was at one of the London Hospitals. London then had no University.

At 21 years of age, in 1770, after completing his apprenticeship, Jenner went to London to study anatomy and surgery under John Hunter as surgical dresser at St. George's Hospital. Hunter had just taken over the large house of his brother William on Jermyn Street, and Jenner was one of Hunter's first boarding pupils. With Hunter, Jenner learned surgical techniques and, more importantly, the use of the scientific method, which his instructor summarized as follows "Why think; why not try the experiment?"

Jenner also served as Hunter's anatomical assistant and, while with Hunter, arranged the zoological specimens brought back by Joseph Banks from the first voyage of the H.M.S. Endeavour under Captain James Cook (1728–1779) in 1772. The close friendship between the two lasted until Hunter died of angina pectoris in 1793. Before this, Jenner had made observations on angina pectoris, but because of his concern for John Hunter whom he knew suffered from the disease, he did not publish them.

Jenner declined Cook's offer to take part in the second voyage and, after two years in London, in 1773, he returned to Berkeley where he lived with his elder brother and built a very successful practice as a village surgeon. He was capable, skilful and popular.

Jenner's medical practice at Berkeley left him enough leisure time for activity in local medical societies. He was a member of the Gloucestershire Medical Society, which assembled three times a year in Rodborough near Stroud; and of the Convivio-Medical Society that met in Alveston every Wednesday. Of these the first was the more important. There, he met old friends, former classmates and student mates like Caleb Hillier Parry (1755–1822), to whom Jenner was later to dedicate his work on cow pox, and Daniel Ludlow, the son of Jenner's old master.

He played the violin in a music society, and as a natural scientist he made numerous observations, particularly on the nesting habits of the cuckoo and migrations of birds. He also wrote verse, a poetry which sometimes has a simple beauty, his best poems being 'Address to a Robin' and 'The Signs of Rain', both showing his love of the countryside.

The Naturalist

Hunter continually encouraged Jenner's studies in natural history, for instance, by asking him to obtain particular specimens and to investigate temperatures of hibernating animals. Hunter incorporated many of Jenner's observations in his own papers, published in the Philosophical Transactions of the Royal Society and in his book Observations on certain Parts of the animal Economy (London, 1786).

Many of Hunter's letters to Jenner have been preserved, but Jenner's letters to Hunter have unfortunately been lost.

In 1786 Jenner wrote a paper on the breeding habits of the cuckoo and Hunter submitted it to the Royal Society. Jenner had shown that when a cuckoo's egg, laid in the nest of another bird such as the hedge sparrow, was hatched, the eggs or nestlings of the foster parent were thrown out of the nest, apparently by their own parents. Jenner had no explanation for this seemingly unnatural behaviour. The paper was read before the society on March 29, 1787 and was accepted for publication in the Philosophical Transactions. Then, on June 18, 1787, Jenner discovered that it was the newly hatched cuckoo which ejected from the nest of its own "foster parent" the hedge sparrow's own unhatched eggs and nestling. Accordingly, Jenner withdrew his original paper before publication and revised it. On December 27, 1787 he sent the revised report to Hunter, and it was read before the Royal Society on March 13, 1788.

Jenner and Variolation

When Jenner began medical practice at Berkeley, he was frequently asked to inoculate persons against smallpox. Inoculation was evidently not a common practice in the English countryside until about 1768, when it was improved by Robert Sutton of Debenham, Suffolk. Sutton required the patient to rest and maintain a strict diet for two weeks before inoculation. He inoculated by taking, on the point of a lancet, a very small quantity of fluid from a developing (unripe) smallpox pustule and introducing it between the outer and inner layers of the skin of the upper arm without drawing blood. He used no bandage to cover the incision.

Jenner began to inoculate against smallpox using Sutton's method, but he soon found some patients to be completely resistant to the disease. On inquiry he found that these patients had previously had cowpox. Jenner, however, familiar with this folklore, concluded that cowpox not only protected against smallpox, but could be transferred from one human being to another as a deliberate mechanism of protection.

As early as 1780 Jenner learned that the eruptions of the teats of infected cows differed. All were called cowpox and all could be communicated to the hands of those that milked the cows, but only one kind created a resistance to smallpox. He called this type "tru cowpox". Jenner subsequently found that even true cowpox conferred immunity against smallpox only when matter was taken from the cowpox pustules before they were too old (as had been the case with Sutton's smallpox fluid). At that period of time, smallpox was at low ebb in the Vale of Berkeley and it was some time before he could put his theory to the test.

In 1791 one Mary Barge, who had had cowpox many years previously, was inoculated with smallpox. A pale red inflammation appeared at the inoculation site and spread extensively, but it disappeared within a few days. Jenner noted how remarkable it was that the smallpox virus should produce such inflammation more rapidly than it could produce smallpox itself. He also observed that although cowpox gave immunity to smallpox, it did not confer similar immunity to the cowpox itself.

Breakthrough

The story of the great breakthrough is well known. In May 1796 a farm in Jenner's district was struck with cowpox, and Jenner met a young maid, Sarah Nelmes, who had fresh scars of cowpox on her finger. Sarah was described as a Berkeley milk maid but in fact was from an old highly respected local family, and certainly no peasant.

On May 14, 1796 Jenner obtained consent for a risky experiment from the parents of James Phipps, an eight-year-old boy with no known history of either cowpox or smallpox. Removing pus from Sarah, Jenner deposited it over scratches he had made on the boy's arms. The boy developed cowpox symptoms a week later, and then recovered shortly afterward.

On July 1, 1796, Jenner performed a more daring experiment. He inoculated Phipps, this time with pus from a smallpox patient. James did not develop smallpox, even after repeated inoculations. The protection was complete.

Some of Jenner's medical colleagues awaited the results with excitement while others condemned him for the risk he was taking. James Phipps, however, lived to a ripe old age.

Sir Walter Farquhar said to Jenner that if he chose to keep this a secret he might make one hundred thousand pounds by it, but Jenner was determined to give it to the world, and he was as good as his word.

As early as 1881, Louis Pasteur honoured Jenner by christening the process "vaccination", for the vaccinia virus of cowpox.

"Lest it should injure his established credit."

After conducting the experiment successfully on thirteen more patients, Jenner at the end of 1796 submitted a report describing this to the Royal Society. However, Sir Joseph Banks, the President of the Royal Society, and Sir Everard Home rejected the manuscript for publication in Philosophical Transactions of this august body. The Council of the Royal Society repulsed Jenner because he was "in variance with established knowledge" and "incredible." Jenner was further warned: "He had better not promulgate such a wild idea "lest it should injure his established credit." The title words of his manuscript were: "An Inquiry into the Natural History of a Disease Known in Glostershire by the Name of the Cow-pox."

One of the first persons he inoculated was his own one-year-old son. Jenner was the family physician of the Berkeley's at Berkeley Castle, and their own son was among the first people to be vaccinated.

Jenner was not able to resume his experiments until the spring of 1798 because no new cases of cowpox were recorded in the vicinity. In June 1798, he published at his own expense a small 75-page book based on twenty-three cases in which cowpox had conferred lasting immunity to smallpox, *"An Inquiry into the Causes and Effects of the Variolae Vaccinae, a Disease Discovered in Some of the Western Counties of England, Particularly Gloucestershire, and Known by the Name of the Cow Pox"*. In it, Jenner described 10 cases of vaccination and 13 persons who had had cowpox in whom variolation was unsuccessful.

To describe the matter producing cowpox, Jenner introduced the term "virus", contending that the cowpox virus had to be acquired from the cow and that it gave permanent

protection from smallpox. Case IV in Jenner's book also described a kind of reaction now known as anaphylaxis, an allergic hypersensitivity reaction of the body to a foreign protein or drug.

But, Mr. Pearson . .

Jenner's publication was not immediately well received, and his work was subjected to fierce criticism. Some physicians were sceptical; others had a financial interest in variolation. He went to London to find volunteers for vaccination, but after three months he had found none.

In London, vaccination was made popular by others, in particular the surgeon Henry Cline (1750–1827), whom Jenner had given some of his inoculation matter, and the physicians George Pearson (1751–1828) from St. George's Hospital, and William Woodville (1752–1805), head of the London Smallpox and Inoculation Hospital. Some difficulties arose, of which some were very unpleasant. Pearson, who began vaccinating in 1799 and proved Jenner's findings, attempted to steal the honour from Jenner.

In 1799, Jenner was seriously attacked by William Woodville, who vaccinated about 600 persons in the first 6 months of 1799. Woodville had contaminated the cowpox material he was using for vaccination with smallpox stuff, and thus inadvertently inoculated his patients with smallpox when he attempted to vaccinate them, a misfortune which produced serious cases of smallpox and at least one death.

During this early stage of the development of the vaccine, it is probable that mistakes were made. On many occasions, smallpox rashes were confused with cowpox rashes, presumably leading to the use of smallpox material for vaccination. Another possible source of error was the contamination of the cowpox pustule fluid with the smallpox virus. This was always a danger because the same lancets were used for variolation and for vaccination.

Vaccinations Conquer the World

Jenner's procedure had proved its value, and Jenner became extremely active in promoting vaccination. The method was taken up not only by medical practitioners but also by country gentlemen, clergymen, and schoolmasters. Jenner found that lymph taken from smallpox pustules might be dried in a glass tube or quill and kept for as long as three months without losing its effectiveness. The dried vaccine could thus be sent long distances. Jean de Carro, a Swiss physician living in Vienna, introduced vaccination on the continent of Europe and was instrumental in sending vaccine virus into Italy, Germany, Poland, and Turkey.

In 1801, Lord Elgin, British ambassador at Constantinople (known for having removed the frieses—now called the Elgin Marbles—from Acropolis, and brought them to the British Museum in London), sent vaccine received from de Carro overland to Bussora (Basra) on the Persian Gulf, and thence to Bombay. The marquis of Wellesley, governor general of India, actively promoted the distribution of the vaccine and many thousands of people were vaccinated in India during the next few years.

In Massachusetts, Benjamin Waterhouse (1754-1846), professor of the theory and practice of Physics at Harvard Medical School, was among the first to be convinced of the value of Jenner's work, and introduced vaccination to America with vaccine received from Jenner. On July 8, 1800, he vaccinated his five-year-old son, Daniel Oliver Waterhouse, who thus became the first person to be vaccinated in America. After he successfully vaccinated his son and two slaves, they were inoculated with smallpox, with negative results. Jenner also sent vaccine to President Thomas Jefferson, who had 18 members of his family and some of their neighbours at Monticello vaccinated. On this occasion, the last Mohican was also vaccinated. He was later immortalized by James Fenimore Cooper's book *The Last of the Mohicans* (1826) which has been filmed.

The US President's Letter to Jenner in 1806

Letter from Thomas Jefferson, 3rd President of the United States (1801–1809) read:

"SIR, - - I have received a copy of the evidence at large respecting the discovery of the vaccine inoculation which you have been pleased to send me, and for which I return you my thanks. Having been among the early converts, in this part of the globe, to its efficiency, I took an early part in recommending it to my countrymen. I avail myself of this occasion of rendering you a portion of the tribute of gratitude due to you from the whole human family. Medicine has never before produced any single improvement of such utility. Harvey's discovery of the circulation of the blood was a beautiful addition to our knowledge of the animal economy, but on a review of the practice of medicine before and since that epoch, I do not see any great amelioration which has been derived from that discovery. You have erased from the calendar of human afflictions one of its greatest. Yours is the comfortable reflection that mankind can never forget that you have lived. Future nations will know by history only that the loathsome small-pox has existed and by you has been extirpated.

Accept my fervent wishes for your health and happiness and assurances of the greatest respect and consideration.

Monticello, May 14, 1806."

The British Parliament

In 1802 the British Parliament voted Jenner a grant of £10,000 in recognition of his discovery and in 1806 an additional grant of £20,000. In 1803 the Royal Jennerian Society was founded at London to promote vaccination of the poor and Jenner took a large part in its affairs; it was superseded in 1808 by a national vaccination program, National Vaccine Establishment.

Although Great Britain and France were at war, in 1804 Napoleon had a medal struck in honour of Jenner's discovery and in 1805 he made vaccination compulsory in the French army. During the Napoleonic wars Jenner wrote to Napoleon requesting the release of a relative of his, captain Milman. Napoleon said: "*Ah, c'est Jenner, je ne peut rien refuser à Jenner*".

Despite some errors and occasional chicanery, the process of vaccination spread rapidly and the death rate from smallpox plunged. Complications however, were many. Vaccination seemed simple, but the vast number of persons who practiced it did not necessarily follow the procedure that Jenner had recommended, and deliberate and unconscious innovations often impaired the effectiveness. Pure cowpox vaccine was not always easy to obtain, nor was it

easy to preserve or transmit. Furthermore, the biological factors that produce immunity were not yet understood.

Surgeon Turned Doctor

In 1785 Jenner acquired The Chantry, a comfortable Georgian country house at Berkeley, where he resided, except for intervals at London and Cheltenham, where he bought an estate in 1810, for the rest of his life. Following an unhappy love affair in 1778, Jenner in 1788, aged 39 years, married Katherine Kongscote.

In 1792 Jenner obtained the medical doctorate—by way of correspondence—from the University of St. Andrews in Fife, Scotland. He then abandoned the less reputed and poorer paid profession of surgery for that of a physician. Until 1815 he practiced as a balneologist at the spa Cheltenham.

In 1813 the University of Oxford awarded Jenner an honorary M.D. degree.

Later Years

Jenner, although he received worldwide recognition and many honours, made no attempt to enrich himself through his discovery and actually devoted so much time to the cause of vaccination that his private practice and his personal affairs suffered. Jenner not only received honours but also aroused opposition and found himself subjected to attacks and calumnies, despite which he continued his activities on behalf of vaccination. When his wife, who bore him four children, fell ill with tuberculosis, and died in 1815, Jenner retired from public life. One of his sons was mentally retarded and died in 1810.

He resumed his study of natural history and finished an article on bird migrations, in which he showed that birds appeared to migrate into England in summer for the purpose of reproduction, and that the ovaries of the female and testes of the male were enlarged at that time. The article was first published after his death. Jenner also served as Justice of the Peace at Berkeley.

A kind and gentle man, Jenner built a cottage for his first vaccination patient, James Phipps, and personally planted the rose garden.

The day before his death he walked to a neighbouring village, where he ordered that fuel be provided for certain poor families. In 1820 he had suffered a mild stroke, and on January 25, 1823, he was found unconscious on the floor of his library. His right side was completely paralyzed. He died early the next morning.

Edward Jenner was buried near the altar in Berkeley church. The principal monument to commemorate his great contribution is in Kensington Gardens. He sits there reflectively, chin in hand, but only the name "Jenner" was inscribed on his pedestal. The statue is virtually forgotten. It was sculptured by William Calder Marshall, RA.

Edward Jenner must be considered the founder of immunology. In vaccination he was the first to use attenuated virus for immunization. For his coining the term virus, his efforts to describe the natural history of the cowpox virus, and his description of anaphylaxis, he must

be considered the first pioneer in the new science of virology, and made possible the extermination of smallpox.

Edward Jenner was a free mason—Worshipful Master Royal Berkeley Lodge of Faith and Friendship Berkeley, Gloucestershire 1812. In 1825 his lodge brothers raised a monument to him in Gloucester Cathedral.

Here are some written excerpts by Edward Jenner:

> Shall I, who even in the morning of my days sought the lowly and sequestered paths of life, the valley and not the mountains; shall I now my evening is fast approaching, hold myself up as an object for fortune and fame? Admitting it as a certainty that I obtain both, what stock should I add to my little fund of happiness? My fortune, with what flows in from my profession, is sufficient to gratify my wishes; indeed, so limited is my ambition ... that were I precluded from further practice, I should be enabled to obtain all that I want. And as for fame, what is it? A gilded butt forever pierced with the arrows of malignancy.
>
> Letter to John Hunter

> The scepticism that appeared, even among the most enlightened of medical men when my sentiments on the important subject of cow-pox were first promulgated, was highly laudable. To have admitted the truth of a doctrine, at once so novel and so unlike any thing that ever had appeared in the annals of medicine, without the test of the most rigid scrutiny, would have bordered upon temerity.
>
> A Continuation of Facts and Observations Relative to the Variolae Vaccinae, or Cow-Pox

> The joy I felt at the prospect before me of being the instrument destined to take away from the world one of its greatest calamities . . . was so excessive that . . . I have sometimes found myself in a kind of reverie.
>
> Quoted by John Baron in Life of Edward Jenner, volume I, chapter 4

> The deviation of man from the state in which he was originally placed by nature seems to have proved to him a prolific source of diseases.
>
> An Inquiry into the Causes and Effects of the Variolae Vaccine...

> I shall endeavour still further to prosecute this inquiry, an inquiry I trust not merely speculative, but of sufficient moment to inspire the pleasing hope of its becoming essentially beneficial to mankind.

> I hope that some day the practice of producing cowpox in human beings will spread over the world—when that day comes, there will be no more smallpox.

The word vaccination comes from vaccinae, which is derived from the Latin 'vacca', meaning cow. Cowpox was also called vaccinia.

The disease has also been called Variola, from the Latin word 'varius', meaning "stained," or from 'varus', meaning "mark on the skin. The word was used for the first time by Bishop Marius of Avenches (near Lausanne, Switzerland) in AD 570.

To describe the matter producing cowpox Jenner introduced the term "virus" that does not carry the same meaning as in our days.

It was Louis Pasteur who, as early as 1881, honoured Edward Jenner by christening the process "vaccination", for the vaccinia virus of cowpox [1].

The Second of Five Accounts of Edward Jenner [3]

Edward Jenner, *FRS, (May 17, 1749 – January 26, 1823*) was an English scientist who studied his natural surroundings in *Berkeley, Gloucestershire, England.* He is famous as the first doctor to introduce and study the *smallpox vaccine*, although *Benjamin Jesty*, a farmer, earlier had vaccinated with *cowpox* to induce immunity to *smallpox*. It is believed that Jenner discovered it independently.

His Early Life

Jenner trained in *Chipping Sodbury,* Gloucestershire as an apprentice to Dr. Ludlow, a surgeon, for eight years from the age of 14. In 1770 Jenner went up to London to study surgery and anatomy under the *surgeon John Hunter* and others at *St George's, University of London*. Hunter was a noted experimentalist, and later a fellow of the *Royal Society.*

William Osler records that Jenner was a student to whom Hunter repeated *William Harvey*'s advice, very famous in medical circles (and characteristically Enlightenment), "Don't think; try." Jenner therefore was early noticed by men famous for advancing the practice and institutions of medicine. Hunter remained in correspondence with him over natural history and proposed him for the Royal Society. Returning to his native countryside, by 1773 he became a successful *general practitioner* and surgeon, practicing in purpose-built premises at Berkeley.

Jenner and others formed a medical society in Rodborough, Gloucestershire, meeting to read papers on medical subjects and dine together. Jenner contributed papers on *angina pectoris*, *ophthalmia* and valvular disease of the heart and commented on *cowpox*. He also belonged to a similar society which met in Alveston, near Bristol.[1]

He was elected Fellow of the *Royal Society* in 1788, following a careful study combining observation, experiment and dissection into a description of the previously misunderstood life of the *cuckoo* in the nest.

Jenner's description of the newly-hatched cuckoo pushing its host's eggs and fledglings from the nest was confirmed in the 20th century when photography became feasible. Having observed the behaviour, he demonstrated an anatomical adaptation for it—the baby cuckoo has a depression in its back which is not present after 12 days of life, in which it cups eggs and other chicks to push them out of the nest. It had been assumed that the adult bird did this, but the adult (Figure 5-1) does not remain in the area for sufficiently long. His findings were published in the Philosophical Transactions of the Royal Society in 1787.

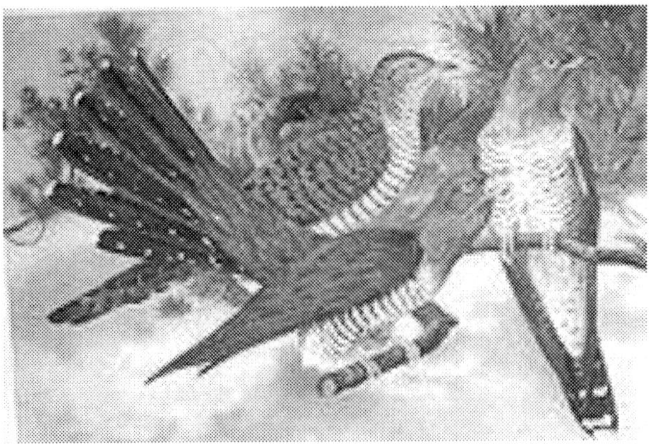

Figure 5-1. The common cuckoo [1].

He married Catherine Kingscote (died 1815 from *tuberculosis*) in March 1788 having met her when *balloons* were hot science, and he and other Fellows were experimenting with them. His trial balloon descended into Kingscote Park, owned by Anthony Kingscote, Catherine being one of his three daughters.

In 1792, he obtained his M.D. from the *University of St Andrews.*

Smallpox

Around this time *smallpox* was greatly feared, as one in three of those who contracted the disease died, and those who survived were commonly badly disfigured. *Voltaire,* a few years later, recorded that 60% of people caught smallpox, with 20% of the population dying of it. In the years following 1770 there were at least six people in England and Germany (Sevel, Jensen, Jesty 1774; Rendall, Plett 1791) who had successfully tested the possibility of using the cowpox vaccine as an immunization for smallpox in humans. For example, *Dorset* farmer, *Benjamin Jesty*, had successfully *induced immunity* in his wife and two children with cowpox during a smallpox epidemic in 1774, but it was not until Jenner's work some twenty years later that the procedure became widely understood. Indeed it is generally believed that Jenner was unaware of Jesty's success and arrived at his conclusions independently.

Jenner's Initial Theory

In fact he thought the initial source of infection was a disease of horses, called "the grease", and that this was transferred to cows by farm workers, transformed, and then manifested as cowpox. From that point on he was correct, the complication probably arose from coincidence.

Noting the common observation that milkmaids did not generally get smallpox, Jenner theorized that the pus in the blisters which milkmaids received from *cowpox* (a disease similar to smallpox, but much less virulent) protected the milkmaids from smallpox. He may

have had the advantage of hearing stories of *Benjamin Jesty* and perhaps others deliberately arranging cowpox infection of their families and of a reduced risk in those families.

On *May 14, 1796*, Jenner tested his theory by inoculating *James Phipps,* a young boy of 8 years old, with material from the cowpox blisters of the hand of Sarah Nelmes, a milkmaid who had caught cowpox from a cow called Blossom[3]. Phipps was the 17th case described in Jenner's first paper on vaccination.

Jenner inoculated Phipps with cowpox pus in both arms on one day, by scraping the pus from Nelmes' blisters onto a piece of wood then transferring this to Phipps' arms. This produced a fever and some uneasiness but no great illness. Later, he injected Phipps with *variolous material,* which would have been the routine attempt to produce immunity at that time. No disease followed. Jenner reported that later the boy was again challenged with variolous material and again showed no sign of infection.

Known: that smallpox was more dangerous than variolation and cowpox less dangerous than variolation.

The hypothesis tested: That infection with cowpox would give immunity to smallpox.

The test: If variolation failed to produce an infection, Phipps was shown to be immune to smallpox.

The consequence: Immunity to smallpox could be induced much more safely.

He continued his research and reported it to the Royal Society, which did not publish the initial report. After improvement and further work, he published a report of twenty-three cases. Some of his conclusions were correct, and some erroneous—modern microbiological and microscopic methods would make this easier to repeat. The medical establishment, as cautious then as now, considered his findings for some time before accepting them. Eventually vaccination was accepted, and in 1840 the British government banned variolation and provided vaccination free of charge.

Jenner's continuing work on vaccination prevented his continuing his ordinary medical practice. He was supported by his colleagues and the King in petitioning Parliament and was granted £10,000 for his work on vaccination. In 1806 he was granted another £20,000 for his continuing work.

In 1803 in London he became involved with the Jennerian Institution, a society concerned with promoting vaccination to eradicate *smallpox*. In 1808, with government aid, this society became the National Vaccine Establishment. Jenner became a member of the Medical and Chirurgical Society on its foundation in 1805, and subsequently presented to them a number of papers. This is now the *Royal Society of Medicine.*

Returning to London in 1811 he observed a significant number of cases of smallpox after vaccination occurring. He found that in these cases the severity of the illness was notably diminished by the previous vaccination. In 1821 he was appointed Physician Extraordinary to *King George IV,* a considerable national honour, and was made Mayor of Berkeley and Justice of the Peace. He continued his interests in natural history. In 1823, the last year of his life, he presented his Observations on the Migration of Birds to the Royal Society.

He was found in a state of *apoplexy* on *25 January 1823*, with his right side paralysed. He never rallied, and died of what was apparently a stroke (he had suffered a previous stroke) on *26 January 1823,* aged 73. He was survived by one son and one daughter, his elder son having died of tuberculosis at the age of 21.

His Legacy

In 1980, the *World Health Organization* declared smallpox an eradicated disease. This was the result of coordinated public health efforts by many people, but vaccination was an essential component. Although it was declared eradicated, some samples still remain in laboratories in *Centres for Disease Control and Prevention* (CDC) in *Atlanta, Georgia* in the United States, and *State Research Centre of Virology and Biotechnology VECTOR* in *Koltsovo, Novosibirsk Oblast*, Russia [3].

The Third of Five Accounts of Edward Jenner [4]

"Edward Jenner was an English country doctor who pioneered vaccination. Jenner's discovery in 1796 that inoculation with cowpox gave immunity to smallpox was an immense medical breakthrough and has saved countless lives.

Edward Jenner was born on May 17, 1749 in the small village of Berkeley in Gloucestershire. From an early age Jenner was a keen observer of nature and after nine years as a surgeon's apprentice he went to St George's Hospital, London to study anatomy and surgery under the prominent surgeon John Hunter. After completing his studies, he returned to Berkeley to set up a medical practice where he stayed until his death in 1823.

How Did Edward Jenner Discover Vaccination?

Jenner worked in a rural community and most of his patients were farmers or worked on farms with cattle. In the 18th century *smallpox* was a very common disease and was a major cause of death. The main treatment was by a method which had brought success to a Dutch physiologist Jan Ingenhaus and was brought to England in 1721 from Turkey by Lady Mary Wortly Montague. This method involved inoculating healthy people with substances from the pustules of those who had a mild case of the disease, but this often had fatal results.

In 1788 an epidemic of smallpox hit Gloucestershire and during this outbreak Jenner observed that those of his patients who worked with cattle and had come in contact with the much milder disease called *cowpox* never came down with smallpox. Jenner needed a way of showing that his theory actually worked.

Jenner was given the opportunity on the 14 May 1796, when a young milkmaid called Sarah Nelmes came to see him with sores on her hands like blisters. Jenner identified that she had caught cowpox from the cows she handled each day. Jenner now had the opportunity to

obtain the material and try out his theories. He carefully extracted some liquid from her sores and then took some liquid from the sores of a patient with mild smallpox.

Jenner believed that if he could inject someone with cowpox, the germs from the cowpox would make the body able to defend itself against the dangerous smallpox germs which he would inject later.

Jenner approached a local farmer called Phipps and asked him if he could inoculate his son James against smallpox. He explained to the farmer that if his theory was correct, James would never contract smallpox. Surprisingly, the farmer agreed.

Jenner made two small cuts on James's left arm. He then poured the liquid from Sarah's cowpox sores into the open wounds which he bandaged.

James went down with cowpox but was not very ill. Six weeks later when James had recovered, Jenner vaccinated him again, this time with the smallpox virus.

This was an extremely dangerous experiment. If James lived Jenner would have found a way of preventing smallpox. If James developed smallpox and died he would be a murderer.

To Jenner's relief James did not catch smallpox. His experiment had worked.

In 1798 after carrying out further successful tests, he published his findings: *An Inquiry into the Causes and Effects of the Variola Vaccinae, a Disease Known by the Name of Cow Pox*. Jenner called his idea “vaccination" from the word *vaccinia* which is Latin for cowpox.

Jenner also introduced the term *virus*.

Jenner found a great deal of scepticism to his ideas and was subject to much ridicule. A cartoon was drawn, showing cows coming out of various parts of people's bodies after they had been vaccinated with cowpox.

However, Jenner persevered and eventually, doctors found that vaccination did work and by 1800 most were using it. Jenner was awarded £30 000 by Parliament to enable him to continue carrying out his tests.

Deaths from smallpox plummeted and vaccination spread through Europe and North America.

Jenner died in Berkeley on January 26, 1823 aged 74 [4].

The Fourth of Five Accounts of Edward Jenner [5]

Edward Jenner is alongside the likes of *Joseph Lister, Robert Koch* and *Louis Pasteur* in *medical history*. Edward Jenner was born in 1749 and died in 1823. Edward Jenner's great gift to the world was his vaccination for smallpox. This disease was greatly feared at the time as it killed one in three of those who caught it and badly disfigured those who were lucky enough to survive catching it.

Edward Jenner was a country doctor who had studied nature and his natural surroundings since childhood. He had always been fascinated by the rural old wives' tale that milkmaids could not get smallpox. He believed that there was a connection between the fact that milkmaids only got a weak version of smallpox—the non-life threatening cowpox—but did not get smallpox itself.

A milkmaid who caught cowpox got blisters on her hands and Jenner concluded that it must be the pus in the blisters that somehow protected the milkmaids.

Jenner decided to try out a theory he had developed. A young boy called James Phipps would be his guinea pig. He took some pus from cowpox blisters found on the hand of a milkmaid called Sarah. She had milked a cow called Blossom and had developed the tell-tale blisters. Jenner 'injected' some of the pus into James. This process he repeated over a number of days gradually increasing the amount of pus he put into the boy. He then deliberately injected Phipps with smallpox. James became ill but after a few days made a full recovery with no side effects. It seemed that Jenner had made a brilliant discovery.

He then encountered the prejudices and conservatism of the medical world that dominated London. They could not accept that a country doctor had made such an important discovery and Jenner was publicly humiliated when he brought his findings to London. However, what he had discovered could not be denied and eventually his discovery had to be accepted – a discovery that was to change the world.

So successful was Jenner's discovery, that in 1840 the government of the day banned any other treatment for smallpox other than Jenner's.

Jenner did not patent his discovery as it would have made the vaccination more expensive and out of the reach of many. It was his gift to the world. A small museum now exists in his home town. It was felt that this was appropriate for a man who shunned the limelight and London. In the museum are the horns of Blossom the cow. The word vaccination comes from the Latin 'vacca' which means cow – in honour of the part played by Blossom and Sarah in Jenner's research. A more formal statue of Jenner is tucked away in one of the more quiet areas of Hyde Park in London.

As a young man, Jenner also wrote about what he had seen cuckoos doing. His were the first written records to describe a baby cuckoo pushing the eggs and the young of its host out of the nest so that the baby cuckoo was the only one to receive food from its foster parents. This was only confirmed many years later but it stands as a testament to the importance of the countryside for Jenner. If he had gone to a city to further his career, would he have been in the right environment to make his famous discovery? In 1980, the World Health Organisation declared that smallpox was extinct throughout the world.

However, as medical treatment was far too expensive for the poor (and it would be the poor who lived in the least hygienic areas) it would be many more years before smallpox was finally eradicated from Britain.

The irony is that Jenner gave his cure to the world for free rather than patent it for himself, though doctors could charge their patients for services rendered [5].

The Fifth of Five Accounts of Edward Jenner [6]

Smallpox (Figure 5-2) is an *infectious disease* unique to humans, caused by either of two *virus* variants named *Variola major* and *Variola minor*.

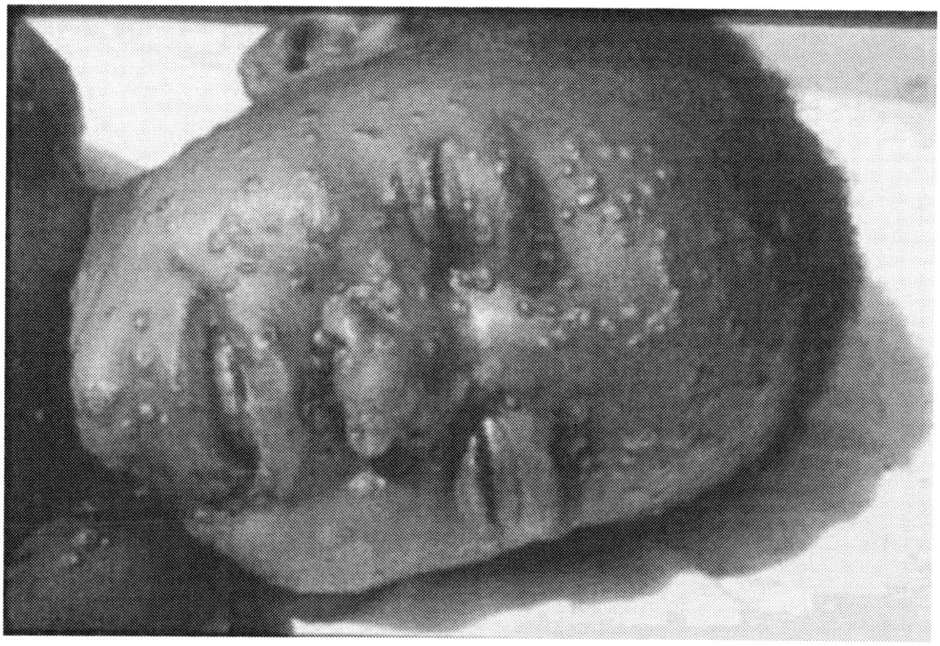

Figure 5-2. A child infected with smallpox [6].

The disease is also known by the *Latin* names *Variola* or *Variola vera*, which is a derivative of the Latin *varius*, meaning spotted, or *varus*, meaning "pimple". The term "smallpox" was first used in Europe in the 15th century to distinguish variola from the great pox (*syphilis*). Smallpox localizes in small *blood vessels* of the skin and in the mouth and throat. In the skin, this results in a characteristic *maculopapular* rash, and later, raised fluid-filled *blisters*. *V. major* produces a more serious disease and has an overall mortality rate of 30–35%. *V. minor* causes a milder form of disease (also known as alastrim, cottonpox, milkpox, whitepox, and Cuban itch) which kills ~1% of its victims.

Long-term complications of *V. major* infection include characteristic scars, commonly on the face, which occurred in 65–85% of survivors. *Blindness* resulting from *corneal ulceration* and scarring, and limb deformities due to arthritis and *osteomyelitis* are less common complications, seen in about 2–5% of cases.

Smallpox is believed to have emerged in human populations about 10,000 B.C. The disease killed an estimated 400,000 Europeans each year during the 18th century (including five reigning *monarchs*), and was responsible for a third of all blindness. Between 20 and 60% of all those infected—and over 80% of infected children—died from the disease.

During the 20th century, it is estimated that smallpox was responsible for 300–500 million deaths. As recently as 1967, the *World Health Organization* (*WHO*) estimated that 15 million people contracted the disease and that two million died in that year. After successful *vaccination* campaigns throughout the 19th and 20th centuries, the WHO certified the eradication of smallpox in 1979. To this day, smallpox is the only human infectious disease to have been completely eradicated from nature.

Cause

Smallpox is caused by infection with variola virus, which belongs to the genus *Orthopoxvirus,* the family *Poxviridae*, and subfamily chordopoxvirinae. It affects mostly babies and young children. Variola virus is a large brick-shaped virus measuring approximately 302 to 350 *nanometers* by 244 to 270 nm, with a single linear *double stranded DNA genome* consisting of 186 *kilobase pairs* (kbp) and containing a *hairpin loop* at each end (Figure 5-3).

The two classic varieties of smallpox are variola major and variola minor. The closest viral relative is *molluscum contagiosum*, which like smallpox, infects only humans.

However, unlike variola species, molluscum infection is benign. The lifecycle of poxviruses is complicated by having multiple infectious forms, with differing mechanisms of cell entry. Poxviruses are unique among DNA viruses in that they replicate in the *cytoplasm* of the cell rather than in the *nucleus*. In order to replicate poxviruses produce a variety of specialized proteins not produced by other *DNA viruses*, the most important of which is a viral-associated *DNA-dependent RNA polymerase*. Both *enveloped* and nonenveloped virions are infectious. The viral envelop is made of modified *Golgi* membranes containing viral-specific polypeptides, including *hemagglutinin*. Infection with either variola major or variola minor confers immunity against the other.

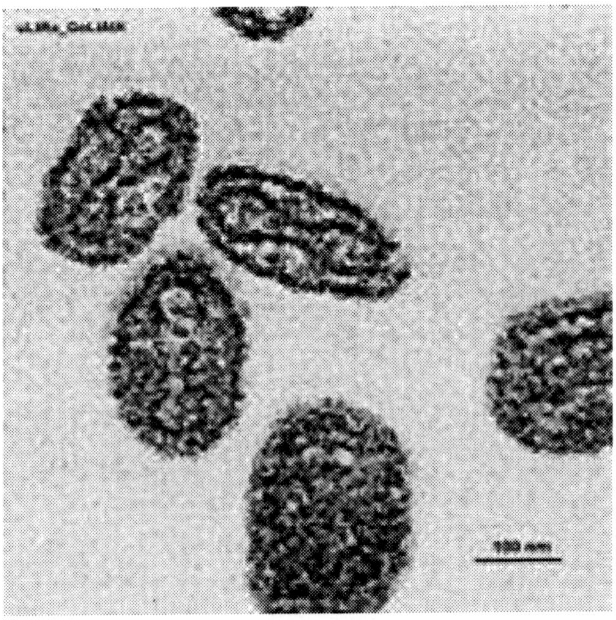

Figure 5-3. Electron micrograph of smallpox virus [6].

Four orthopoxviruses cause infection in humans: variola, *vaccinia, cowpox,* and *monkeypox*. Variola virus infects only humans in nature, although primates and other animals have been infected in a laboratory setting. Vaccinia, cowpox, and monkeypox viruses can infect both humans and other animals in nature.

Documented smallpox epidemics in the New World [6]

Year	*Location*	*Description*
1520–1527	Mexico, Central America, South America	Smallpox kills millions of native inhabitants of Mexico. Unintentionally introduced at Veracruz with the arrival of Panfilo de Narvaez on *April 23, 1520* and was credited with the victory of Cortes over the Aztec empire at Tenochtitlan (present-day Mexico City) in 1521. Kills the Inca ruler, *Huayna Capac*, and 200,000 others and destroys the Incan Empire.
1617–1619	North America northern east coast	Killed 90% of the Massachusetts Bay Indians
1674	Cherokee Tribe	Death count unknown. Population in 1674 about 50,000. After 1729, 1738, and 1753 smallpox epidemics their population was only 25,000 when they were forced to Oklahoma on the Trail of Tears.
1692	Boston, MA	
1702–1703	St. Lawrence Valley, NY	
1721	Boston, MA	
1736	Pennsylvania	
1738	South Carolina	
1770s	West Coast of North America	Kills out 30% of the West Coast Native Americans
1781–1783	Great Lakes	
1830s	Alaska	Reduced *Dena'ina Athabaskan* population in *Cook Inlet* region of south-central *Alaska* by half. Smallpox also devastated *Yup'ik Eskimo* populations in western *Alaska*.
1860–1861	Pennsylvania	
1865–1873	Philadelphia, PA, New York, Boston, MA and New Orleans, LA	Same period of time, in Washington D.C., Baltimore, MD, Memphis, TN, Cholera and a series of recurring epidemics of Typhus, Scarlet Fever and Yellow Fever
1877	Los Angeles, CA	

Famous Sufferers and Survivors

Famous historical figures who contracted smallpox include *Ramesses V*, the *Kangxi Emperor*, *Shunzhi Emperor* and *Tongzhi Emperor* of China (official history), *Date Masamune* of Japan (who lost an eye to the disease), and the Incan emperor *Huayna Capac* in 1527. More recent public figures also include: *Guru Har Krishan* 8th Guru of the Sikhs in 1664, *Peter III of Russia* in 1744.and *Maximilian III Joseph, Elector of Bavaria*.

Prominent families prominent throughout the world often had several people infected by and/or perish from the disease. For example, several relatives of *Henry VIII* survived the disease but were scarred by it. These include his sister *Margaret, Queen of Scotland*, his fourth wife, *Anne of Cleves*, and his daughter, *Elizabeth I of England* in 1562 (as an adult she would often try to disguise the pockmarks with heavy makeup). A more distant relative, *Mary Queen of Scots*, contracted the disease as a child but had no visible scarring.

In Europe, deaths from smallpox often impacted dynastic succession. *Louis XV of France* succeeded his great-grandfather *Louis XIV* through a series of deaths of smallpox or measles among those earlier in the succession line. He himself died of the disease in 1774. The only surviving son of Henry VIII, *Edward VI,* likely died from complications shortly after apparently recovering from the disease, thereby rendering his sire's infamous efforts to provide England with a male heir moot. (His immediate successors were all females.) *William III* lost his mother to the disease when he was only ten years old in 1660, and named his uncle Charles as legal guardian: her death from smallpox would indirectly spark a chain of events that would eventually lead to the permanent ousting of the Stuart line from the British throne.

Both *George Washington* and *Abraham Lincoln*, Presidents of the United States, contracted and recovered from the disease. *Joseph Stalin*, who was badly scarred by the disease early in life, often had photographs retouched to make his pockmarks less apparent. Crime figure *Lucky Luciano* contracted the disease in 1907 at the age of ten, upon coming to New York from Sicily.

Indian actress Geeta Bali died of smallpox in 1965 [6].

Conclusion

The author strongly believes there are interesting and important lessons for us from the history of Jenner and his smallpox vaccines. In his view, such lessons should include, but not be limited to the following:

Human lives and health should always be our first consideration. Jenner's first consideration was how to deal with the smallpox scourge and save humanity from its morbidity and mortality. He himself was not at risk of the scourge since he had already been variolated.

He took desperate measures for the desperate situation on hand in his days. With the consent of Phipp's dad, he proceeded to use the boy as guinea pig in order to try and save humanity from the dreadful claws of smallpox. The author is one of the many who believe

Jenner would have used himself instead of his nephew for his experimentation if he had neither been variolated nor suffered smallpox.

Jenner had no idea about how and why his vaccine worked. All that mattered was that it worked. Faced with such a calamity for mankind, one should not be wasting time and energy and resources on how and why any candidate treatment works, or whether any candidate remedy has satisfied any other conditions, animal experimentation, immunogenicity tests, guidelines or protocols. The primary aim should be to get a safe and effective remedy; the how and why the remedy works should, at best, take the secondary status.

Jenner's grace is that the world continues to hail him for his brilliant work that has led not only to the control of, but also to the eradication of smallpox. However, had Jenner lived today and done what he did, he would not only have lost his medical license but would have been tried and likely jailed for life, if not executed, for unethical medical practice and crimes against humanity. Unimpressed by Jenner's efforts, his peers refused to publish his work. In addition, the public ridiculed him and his smallpox vaccine. He had to arrange to get it published at his expense. Jenner's case was indeed one of moving from grass to grace. Are most of the experts and researchers of our day not behaving like their peers in Jenner's days?

References

[1] http://www.whonamedit.com/doctor.cfm/1818.html
[2] Bazin H (2000). The Eradication of Smallpox. Academic Press, San Diego.
[3] http://en.wikipedia.org/wiki/Edward_Jenner
[4] http://www.zephyrus.co.uk/edwardjenner.html
[5] http://www.historylearningsite.co.uk/edward_jenner.htm
[6] http://en.wikipedia.org/wiki/Smallpox

Chapter VI

Louis Pasteur and His Vaccines

Abstract

Louis Pasteur was not a medical doctor but a renowned Chemist and Bacteriologist (the existence of viruses as we now know them was unknown in his days). Like Jenner who lived about 100 years before him, Pasteur had many diseases ravaging cattle, poultry and man in his days. He made tremendous breakthroughs in the prevention and treatment of these epidemics. Under the threat of his life and legal action, he applied his remedy for rabies on a chap that had been mauled by a rabid dog because Pasteur knew, as his critics also did, that the boy would definitely die if left untreated. With Pasteur's remedy, the boy had a chance. Pasteur opted to give the boy that chance, and the boy made it. His remedy involved giving the boy preparations he had made in his lab from the spinal cord of rabid rabbits! If Pasteur had lived and done that today in the US, Britain or his own country France, the author leaves the reader to imagine what his lot would be especially when, to begin with, he was not licensed to practice medicine. Desperate situations call indeed for desperate actions, and that was exactly what Pasteur did. Has humanity been facing a desperate situation about HIV/AIDS since 1984? Who has really taken any desperate actions anywhere in order to prevent or cure HIV/AIDS? The author put his life on the line in a desperate plunge to deal with the HIV/AIDS calamity and succeeded, but he has been the subject of criticism, blackmail, backstabbing, orchestrated falsehood, condemnation and humiliation by those who have still not contemplated taking any such actions in a bid to try and deal with the HIV/AIDS monster! Is history not again repeating itself before our very eyes? Read on.

Introduction

Louis Pasteur *(December 27, 1822 – September 28, 1895*) was a *French chemist* and *microbiologist* best known for his remarkable breakthroughs in the causes and prevention of disease. His experiments supported the *germ theory of disease*, also reducing mortality from *puerperal fever* (childbed), and he created the first *vaccine* for *rabies.* He was best known to the general public for inventing a method to stop milk and wine from causing sickness—a process that came to be called *pasteurization.* He is regarded as one of the three main

founders of *microbiology,* together with *Ferdinand Cohn* and *Robert Koch.* He is also credited with dispelling the theory of spontaneous generation with his experiment employing chicken broth and a goose neck flask. He also made many discoveries in the field of chemistry, most notably the *asymmetry of crystals*. He is buried beneath the Institut Pasteur, an incredibly rare honour in France, where being buried in a cemetery, is mandatory save for the fewer than 300 "Great Men" who are entombed in the *Pantheon.*

Early Life and Biography

Louis Jean Pasteur was born on *December 27, 1822* in *Dole* in the *Jura* region of *France* and grew up in the town of *Arbois*. There he later had his house and laboratory, which is a Pasteur museum today. His father, Jean Pasteur (1791-1864), was a poorly educated *tanner* and a decorated *Sergeant-Major* of the *Grande Armee*. Louis's aptitude was recognized by his college headmaster, who recommended that the young man apply for the *École Normale Supérieure*, which accepted him. After serving briefly as *professor of physics* at Dijon Lycée in 1848, he became professor of *chemistry at Strasbourg University*, where he met and courted Marie Laurent, daughter of the university's *rector* in 1849. They were married on May 29, 1849 and together they had five *children*, only two of whom survived to *adulthood.* Throughout his life, Louis Pasteur remained an ardent *Catholic*. A well-known *quotation* illustrating this is attributed to him: "The more I know, the more nearly is my *faith* that of the Breton peasant. Could I but know all I would have the faith of a Breton peasant's wife."

Work on Chirality and the Polarization of Light

Pasteur separated the left and right *crystal* shapes from each other to form two piles of crystals: in solution one form rotated light to the left, the other to the right, while an equal mixture of the two forms cancelled each other's rotation. Hence, the mixture does not rotate *polarized light.*

In Pasteur's early works as a *chemist*, he resolved a problem concerning the nature of *tartaric acid* (1849). A solution of this compound derived from living things (specifically, *wine lees*) rotated the plane of *polarization* of light passing through it. The mystery was that *tartaric acid* derived by *chemical synthesis* had no such effect, even though its chemical reactions were identical and its elemental composition was the same.

Upon examination of the minuscule *crystals* of Sodium ammonium tartrate, Pasteur (Figure 6-1) noticed that the crystals came in two asymmetric forms that were mirror images of one another. Tediously sorting the crystals by hand gave two forms of the compound: solutions of one form rotated polarized light clockwise, while the other form rotated light counter clockwise. An equal mix of the two had no polarizing effect on the light. Pasteur correctly deduced the molecule in question was asymmetric and could exist in two different forms that resemble one another as would left- and right-hand gloves, and that the biological source of the compound provided purely the one type. This was the first time anyone had demonstrated *chiral* molecules.

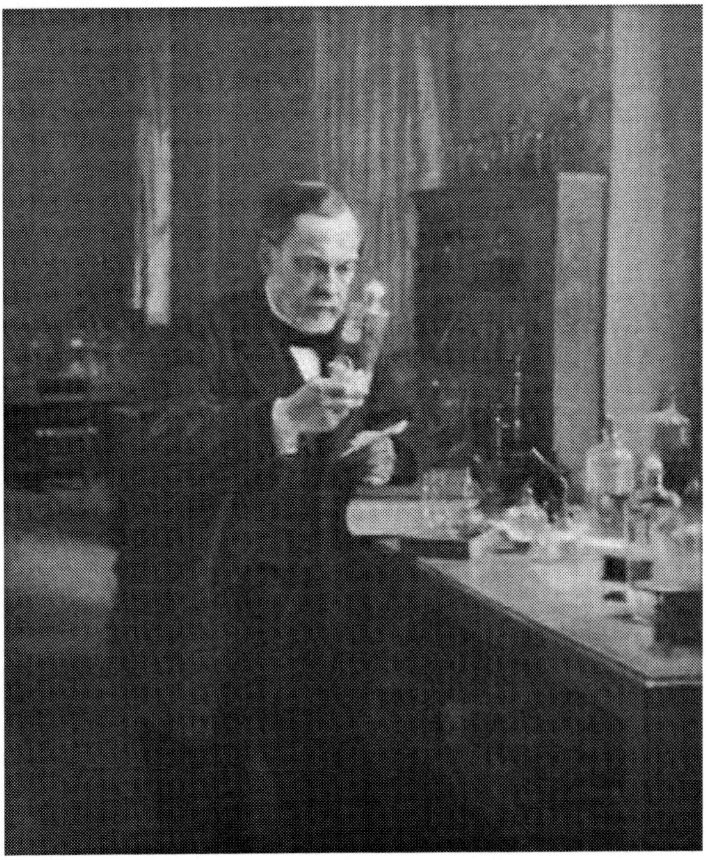

Figure 6-1. Louis Pasteur in his laboratory, painting by A. Edelfeldt in 1885 [1].

Pasteur's doctoral thesis on *crystallography* attracted the attention of M. Puillet and he helped Pasteur garner a position of professor of chemistry at the *Faculté* (College) of *Strasbourg*.

In 1854, he was named Dean of the new Faculty of Sciences in Lille. In 1856, he was made administrator and director of scientific studies of the *École Normale Supérieure*.

Immunology and Vaccination

Chicken Cholera

Pasteur's later work on diseases included work on chicken *cholera.* During this work, a culture of the responsible *bacteria* had spoiled and failed to induce the disease in some *chickens* he was infecting with the disease. Upon reusing these healthy chickens, Pasteur discovered that he could not infect them, even with fresh bacteria; the weakened bacteria had caused the chickens to become *immune* to the disease, even though they had only caused mild symptoms.

His assistant *Charles Chamberland* had been instructed to inoculate the chickens after Pasteur went on holiday. Chamberland failed to do this, but instead went on holiday himself.

On his return, the month-old cultures made the chickens unwell, but instead of the infection being fatal, as it usually was, the chickens recovered completely. Chamberland assumed an error had been made, and wanted to discard the apparently faulty culture when Pasteur stopped him. Pasteur guessed the recovered animals now might be immune to the disease, as were the animals at *Eure-et-Loir* that had recovered from anthrax.

Anthrax

In the 1870s, he applied this immunization method to *anthrax,* which affected *cattle,* and aroused interest in combating other diseases.

Pasteur publicly claimed he had made the anthrax vaccine by exposing the bacillus to oxygen. His laboratory notebooks, now in the *Bibliotheque Nationale* in Paris, in fact show Pasteur used the method of rival *Jean-Joseph-Henri Toussaint*, a *Toulouse veterinary surgeon*, to create the anthrax vaccine. This method used the oxidizing agent *potassium dichromate*. Pasteur's oxygen method did eventually produce a vaccine but only after he had been awarded a *patent* on the production of an anthrax vaccine.

The notion of a weak form of a disease causing immunity to the virulent version was not new; this had been known for a long time for *smallpox*. Inoculation with smallpox was known to result in far less scarring, and greatly reduced mortality, in comparison to the naturally acquired disease. *Edward Jenner* had also discovered *vaccination*, using *cowpox* to give cross-immunity to smallpox (in 1796), and by Pasteur's time this had generally replaced the use of actual smallpox material in inoculation. The difference between smallpox vaccination and *cholera* and *anthrax* vaccination was that the weakened form of the latter two disease organisms had been *generated artificially*, and so a naturally weak form of the disease organism did not need to be found.

This discovery revolutionized work in infectious diseases, and Pasteur gave these artificially weakened diseases the generic name of *vaccines*, to honour Jenner's discovery.

Rabies

Pasteur produced the first vaccine for *rabies* by growing the virus in rabbits, and then weakening it by drying the affected nerve tissue.

The rabies vaccine was initially created by *Emile Roux,* a French doctor and a colleague of Pasteur who had been working with a killed vaccine produced by desiccating the spinal cords of infected rabbits. The vaccine had only been tested on eleven dogs before its first human trial.

This vaccine was first used on 9-year old *Joseph Meister*, on *July 6, 1885*, after the boy was badly mauled by a rabid dog. This was done at some personal risk for Pasteur, since he was not a licensed physician and could have faced prosecution for treating the boy. However, left without treatment, the boy faced almost certain death from rabies. After consulting with colleagues, Pasteur decided to go ahead with the treatment. The treatment proved to be a spectacular success, with Meister avoiding the disease; thus, Pasteur was hailed as a hero and

the legal matter was not pursued. The treatment's success laid the foundations for the manufacture of many other vaccines. The first of the *Pasteur Institutes* was also built on the basis of this achievement.

Allegations of Deception

In 1995, the centennial of the death of Louis Pasteur, the *New York Times* ran an article titled "Pasteur's Deceptions". After having thoroughly read Pasteur's lab notes the science historian *Gerald L. Geison* declared that Pasteur had given a misleading account of the experiment on anthrax vaccine at Pouilly-le-Fort.

Honours and Final Days

Pasteur won the *Leeuwenhoek medal, microbiology*'s highest honour, in 1895. He was a *Grand Croix of the Legion of Honor* - one of only 75 in all of France. He died in 1895, near Paris, from complications of a series of strokes that had started in 1868. He died while listening to the story of *St Vincent de Paul,* whom he admired and sought to emulate.

He was buried in the *Cathedral of Notre Dame*, but his remains were reinterred in a crypt in the *Institut Pasteur,* Paris, where he is remembered for his life-saving work. Both Institut Pasteur and *Université Louis Pasteur* were named after him. Pasteur was ranked #12 in the 1978 edition of *Michael H. Hart*'s controversial book, *The 100:* A Ranking of The Most Influential Persons in History. However, Pasteur was promoted to no. 11, replacing *Karl Marx* in the 1992 revised edition of the book [1].

Conclusion

Unlike Jenner, Louis Pasteur was not a medical doctor; he was a great chemist and a renowned bacteriologist.

The existence of viruses, as we now know them, was still unknown to humanity even during Pasteur's days. It was about 5 years after Pasteur's death that a scientist postulated the existence of viruses.

The momentous discoveries of Louis Pasteur in the second half of the nineteenth century completely revolutionized agriculture, chemistry, medicine (human and veterinary), hygiene, and surgery. Though Pasteur's discoveries were accepted and applied very quickly by their users (industrialists for pasteurization, farmers for veterinary vaccines against fowl cholera and anthrax, people bitten by rabid animals for his rabies vaccine), they were accepted much later by the scientists (human and veterinary doctors) because they could not explain the mode of action of the vaccines.

Surgeons who had been practising for many years without any rules of hygiene would not accept Pasteur's new rules of hygiene even though they had been infecting most of their patients. Only the English Surgeon Joseph Lister (1827-1912) was greatly influenced by

Pasteur's researches, and was the first to introduce antiseptic measures in his surgical practice with very rewarding results.

Pasteur was the first person to produce a vaccine (a weakened form of fowl cholera bacilli) in the laboratory even though he knew little about the mechanism by which the bacilli killed fowls. Later, Pasteur produced in his laboratory effective human rabies vaccines using weakened and killed rabies virus obtained in slices of the spinal cord of rabid rabbits. It had been known even before Pasteur's days that rabies was, for all practical purposes, a uniformly fatal disease. With the onset of the symptoms of rabies, the sufferer invariably died agonizingly within the next 10 days.

Europe was under siege by rabies at the time of Pasteur. He used the spinal cord of rabid rabbits to prevent people bitten by rabid animals, and were therefore infected with the lethal rabies virus, from developing rabies. The first demonstration of the efficacy of his vaccine was on the 9-year old lad, *Joseph Meister* brought to him for his remedy after severe rabid dog bites.

The doctors of his days rose in severe opposition, threatening that if the boy died after Pasteur's treatment, they would kill Pasteur (as if the boy had any chance of survival without Pasteur's treatment!). Pasteur ignored both the ranting of the doctors and the threat of legal action against him, and treated the boy. The boy never developed rabies. Later, patients bitten by rabid dogs were brought to Pasteur in Paris even from as far away as Russia, a journey of several days then. With Pasteur's therapy, most of them survived [2].

Let us recall again that viruses were not known to man in Pasteur's days; yet, he single-handedly developed a safe and effective therapeutic vaccine against rabies, a viral infection that is still regarded as uniformly fatal in any person who develops clinical signs of the disease. Like Jenner, Pasteur who was not the person that isolated the causative agent of rabies developed a safe and effective vaccine against the disease. The rabies vaccines in use up till today are just modifications of Pasteur's rabies vaccine.

Again the lesson is clear—one need not know how or why a vaccine works provided it works. The opposition from doctors against Pasteur's vaccines was unjustified. Pasteur rightly ignored them and proceeded, prompted only by his interest in preventing the victim from dying of rabies. Any new discovery receives severe criticism because man is always opposed to change. One should ignore such opposition against new medical remedies that are safe and effective. Ethical considerations, protocols and the how or why a remedy works should not take the front seat whenever there is a new but safe and effective remedy against any human epidemic; the only two important and crucial things are safety and efficacy.

References

[1] http://en.wikipedia.org/wiki/ Louis_Pasteur

[2] Plotkin S.A, Orenstein W.A., Editors (2003). *Vaccines* (4th Edition), Elsevier Books, Oxford.

Chapter VII

Jonas Salk and His Vaccine

Abstract

Polio, like smallpox, plague and rabies, has been man's visitor for millenniums. The causative agent was only isolated about 100 years ago. Polio visited the New World many times especially in the last century. Again, the response of the citizenry to the unwelcome polio visits was dramatic and desperate. President Roosevelt, a polio victim, played a key role in the fight against the evil unwelcome visitor. Researchers everywhere went all out to tame the polio visitor, dead or alive. Jonas Salk was the first to achieve it. Who was the man? How did he achieve the feat? What were his dividends? How did his colleagues treat him? Are there any lessons for us from all this? This chapter attempts to address these and other questions.

Introduction

Poliomyelitis or Infantile Paralysis (which does not only afflict infants) is a disease that has been known to man for several millenniums. In the last century, it caused several epidemics in the US that really brought out from the citizenry desperate responses that are beyond imagination. President Roosevelt was himself paralysed at the age of 39 by polio. He used the tremendous influence of his office to bring polio to the front seat of the nation's consciousness. Funds poured in for a vaccine to prevent the disease. Jonas Salk, one of the marathoners for the polio vaccine, was the first to cross the finish line. Read the following accounts of the great Salk, and reach your own conclusions.

The First of Four Accounts of Jonas Salk [1]

In America in the 1950s, summertime was a time of fear and anxiety for many parents; this was the season when children by the thousands became infected with the crippling disease poliomyelitis, or polio. This burden of fear was lifted forever when it was announced

that Dr. Jonas Salk had developed a vaccine against the disease. Salk became world-famous overnight, but his discovery was the result of many years of painstaking research.

Jonas Salk was born in New York City. His parents were Russian-Jewish immigrants who, although they themselves lacked formal education, were determined to see their children succeed, and encouraged them to study hard. Jonas Salk was the first member of his family to go to college. He entered the City College of New York intending to study law, but soon became intrigued by medical science.

While attending medical school at New York University, Salk was invited to spend a year researching influenza. The virus that causes flu had only recently been discovered and the young Salk was eager to learn if the virus could be deprived of its ability to infect, while still giving immunity to the illness. Salk succeeded in this attempt, which became the basis of his later work on polio.

After completing medical school and his internship, Salk returned to the study of influenza, the flu virus. World War II had begun, and public health experts feared a replay of the flu epidemic that had killed millions in the wake of the First World War. The development of vaccines controlled the spread of flu after the war, and the epidemic of 1919 did not recur.

In 1947, Salk accepted an appointment to the University of Pittsburgh Medical School. While working there, with the National Foundation for Infantile Paralysis, Salk saw an opportunity to develop a vaccine against polio, and devoted himself to this work for the next eight years.

In 1955 Salk's years of research paid off. Human trials of the polio vaccine effectively protected the subject from the polio virus. When news of the discovery was made public on April 12, 1955, Salk was hailed as a miracle worker. He further endeared himself to the public by refusing to patent the vaccine. He had no desire to profit personally from the discovery, but merely wished to see the vaccine disseminated as widely as possible.

Salk's vaccine was composed of "killed" polio virus, which retained the ability to immunize without running the risk of infecting the patient. A few years later, a vaccine made from live polio virus was developed, which could be administered orally, while Salk's vaccine required injection. Further, there was some evidence that the "killed" vaccine failed to completely immunize the patient. In the U.S., public health authorities elected to distribute the "live" oral vaccine instead of Salk's. Tragically, the preparation of live virus infected some patients with the disease, rather than immunizing them. Since the introduction of the original vaccine, the few new cases of polio reported in the United States were probably caused by the "live" vaccine which was intended to prevent them.

In countries where Salk's vaccine has remained in use, the disease has been virtually eradicated.

In 1963, Salk founded the Jonas Salk Institute for Biological Studies, an innovative centre for medical and scientific research. Jonas Salk continued to conduct research and publish books, some written in collaboration with one or more of his sons, who are also medical scientists.

Salk's published books include *Man Unfolding* (1972), *The Survival of the Wisest* (1973), *World Population and Human Values: A New Reality* (1981), and *Anatomy of Reality* (1983).

Dr. Salk's last years were spent searching for a vaccine against AIDS. Jonas Salk died on June 23, 1995. He was 80 years old [1].

The Second of Four Accounts of Jonas Salk [2]

Jonas Edward Salk *(October 28, 1914 – June 23, 1995*) was an *American biologist* and *physician* best known for the research and development of a killed-virus *polio vaccine,* the *eponymous Salk vaccine.*

During his life, Salk worked in *New York, Michigan, Pittsburgh* and *California.* In his later career, he devoted much energy toward the development of an *AIDS vaccine.*

While being interviewed by *Edward R. Murrow* on *See It Now* in 1955, Salk was asked: "Who owns the patent on this vaccine?" Surprised by the question's assumption of the requirement of a profit motive for his creation, he responded: "There is no patent. Could you patent the sun?"

Biography

Jonas Salk was born in *New York City* to *Russian-Jewish* immigrant parents, Dora and Daniel B. Salk. He had two brothers, Lee and Herman Salk. Herman became a *veterinarian,* and Lee became a *clinical psychologist.* Jonas graduated from *Townsend Harris High School* and then went to the *City College of New York,* where he earned a *B.Sc.* He received a *medical degree* from the *School of Medicine* at *New York University* in June 1939.

While in college he met his future wife, Donna Lindsay, whom he married on *June 9, 1939.* They had three children: Peter, Darrell, and Jonathan. In *1968,* they divorced, and in *1970* Salk married *Françoise Gilot,* the former mistress of *Pablo Picasso.*

As a child, Salk did not show any interest in medicine or science in general. He says in an interview with the *Academy of Achievement:*

> "As a child I was not interested in human anatomy. I was merely interested in things human, the human side of nature, if you like, and I continue to be interested in that. That's what motivates me. And in a way, it's the human dimension that has intrigued me."

His first desire was to become a lawyer and only due to his mother's persuasion (which included her telling him he wouldn't be good at it), he changed from a pre-law student to a pre-med student. During his first year in medical school, he was offered the chance to do research and teach biochemistry. He recalls this experience in the previously mentioned interview:

> "At one point at the end of my first year of medical school, I received an opportunity to spend a year in research and teaching in biochemistry, which I did. And at the end of that year, I was told I could, if I wished, switch and get a Ph.D. in biochemistry but my preference was to stay with medicine. And I believe that this is all linked to my original ambition, or desire, which was to be of some help to humankind, so to speak, in a larger sense than just on a one-to-one basis."

While attending the NYU School of Medicine, he heard two lectures that would change his life forever. Salk reflected on the lectures in 1990:

> "In the first lecture, we were told that it was possible to immunize against diphtheria and tetanus by the use of a chemically treated toxin [to kill it]... In the very next lecture, we were told that in order to immunize against a virus disease it was necessary to go through the experience of infection. It was not possible to kill the virus... The light went on at that point. I said that those two statements can't possibly both be true. One has to be false."

In 1938, while still in college, Salk began working with Dr. Thomas Francis, Jr., on an influenza vaccine. In 1941, Francis was appointed the head of the epidemiology department at the newly formed School of Public Health at the University of Michigan, and Salk, who in 1942 won a research fellowship, followed him. Together they worked to develop an influenza vaccine at the behest of the United States Army. Salk advanced to the position of assistant professor of epidemiology and continued his work on virology.

After medical school, Salk first worked as a staff physician at the Mount Sinai School of Medicine in New York City. Later, he worked for Dr. Francis's virus lab at the University of Michigan in Ann Arbour. In 1947, he moved to Pittsburgh, where he led the Virus Research lab at the University of Pittsburgh.

During the 1950s, Salk developed, tested and refined the first successful killed-virus polio vaccine, using inactive (dead) poliovirus cells that were injected into the body. In 1955 he began immunizations at Pittsburgh's Arsenal Elementary School in the Lawrenceville neighbourhood. (Hilary Koprowski had already in 1950 initiated the use of an oral attenuated-live-virus polio vaccine, which would prove to be the future of polio immunization.)

In 1965, Salk struck out on his own, leaving the University of Pittsburgh and establishing the Salk Institute for Biological Studies in La Jolla, California, where the major focus of study was molecular biology and genetics. The first faculty included many distinguished members such as Jacob Bronowski and Francis Crick. Salk directed the institute until his retirement in 1985.

During Salk's last years, he co-founded The Immune Response Corporation with Kevin Kimberlin to search for a vaccine against AIDS, and patented a p24- vaccine as "Remune".

Salk died on June 23, 1995 in La Jolla, CA, at the age of 80 due to heart failure.

Polio Vaccine

In 1947, Salk received a position at the *University of Pittsburgh,* as the head of the Virus Research lab. Though he continued his research on improving the influenza vaccine, he set his sights on the *poliomyelitis* virus. Although about 99% of cases of polio are asymptomatic, the *polio virus* can attack the *nervous system* and within a few hours of infection, *paralysis* can occur. The *death rate* for paralytic cases is about 5–10%. Death usually occurs when the breathing muscles become paralyzed. Polio was sometimes hard to diagnose because of its *flu*-like symptoms, which include stiff neck, fever, and headache.

At that time, it was believed that immunity can come only after the body has survived at least a mild infection by live virus. In contrast, Salk observed that it is possible to acquire

immunity through contact with inactivated (killed) virus. Using formaldehyde, Salk killed the polio virus, but kept it intact enough to trigger the necessary immune response. Salk's research caught the attention of Basil O'Connor, president of the National Foundation for Infantile Paralysis (now known as the March of Dimes Foundation). The organization decided to fund Salk's efforts to develop a killed virus vaccine.

The vaccine was first tested in monkeys, and then in patients at the D.T. Watson Home for Crippled Children. After successful tests, in 1952, Salk tested his vaccine on volunteering parties, including himself, the laboratory staff, his wife, and his children. In 1954, national testing began on two million children, ages six to nine, who became known as the *Polio Pioneers*. This was one of the first double-blind placebo-controlled tests, which has since become standard: half of the treated received the vaccine, and half received a placebo, where neither the individuals nor the researchers know who belongs to the control group and the experimental group. One-third of the children, who lived in areas where vaccine was not available, were observed in order to evaluate the background level of polio in this age group. On April 12, 1955, the results were announced: the vaccine was safe and effective. The patient would develop immunity to the live disease due to the body's earlier reaction to the killed virus.

Salk's vaccine was instrumental in beginning the eradication of polio, a once widely-feared disease. Polio epidemics in 1916 left about 6000 dead and 27,000 paralyzed in the United States. In 1952, 57,628 cases were recorded in the U.S. After the vaccine became available, polio cases in the U.S. dropped by 85–90 percent in only two years. Unfortunately, some drug companies manufactured contaminated polio vaccine containing live virus, and this error cost dozens of lives.

However, the live-virus oral vaccine developed by Albert Sabin became the preferred alternative after a sometimes intense clash between the two scientists and their adherents. The Salk vaccine, which is injected, proved to be effective in sharply reducing the number of polio cases in the United States. A disadvantage to Salk's vaccine was that booster shots had to be taken periodically. The Sabin vaccine had the advantage of easier delivery and became accepted in the United States after the testing abroad. It was licensed in 1961 and eventually became the vaccine of choice in most parts of the world. The last indigenous case of polio in the U.S. was reported in 1991. Partly because of that fact, only inactivated, Sabin-type polio vaccines have been recommended for use in the United States since 2000.

The Salk vaccine was based upon plasmid DNA. Esther M. Zimmer Lederberg and Jonas Salk were colleagues and friends. However, Lederberg had expressed reservations concerning polio and the Salk vaccine. Esther Lederberg was quite well aware that from an epidemiological viewpoint it was possible that Salk's vaccine was not as effective as he thought. Specifically, the incidence of polio was noted to occur in waves. Thus, Lederberg wondered whether the marked reduction in polio cases was due to Salk's vaccine or the end of a wave of infection (and Salk's vaccine having little effect). Lederberg felt that Salk could have done more to elucidate this possible ambiguity had he kept better records.

Honors

In 1956, he was awarded the Lasker Award; in 1958, The Bruce Memorial Award; in 1975, The Jawaharlal Nehru Award and the Congressional Gold Medal.

In 1977, he was awarded the Presidential Medal of Freedom from President Jimmy Carter, with the following statement accompanying the medal:

> "Because of Doctor Jonas E. Salk, our country is free from the cruel epidemics of poliomyelitis that once struck almost yearly. Because of his tireless work, untold hundreds of thousands who might have been crippled are sound in body today. These are Doctor Salk's true honours, and there is no way to add to them. This Medal of Freedom can only express our gratitude, and our deepest thanks."

In the late 1950s Salk was elected to the Polio Hall of Fame, which was dedicated in Warm Springs, Georgia, on January 2, 1958.

On December 5, 2007, California Governor Arnold Schwarzenegger and First Lady Maria Shriver inducted Salk into the California Hall of Fame, located at the California museum for History, Women and the Arts.

There are schools in Bolingbrook, Illinois; Levittown, New York; Old Bridge, New Jersey; and Sacramento, California, named for him.

Special Quotes:

> "Always be the best you can be." [2]

The Third of Four Accounts of Jonas Salk [3]

> *I feel that the greatest reward for success is the opportunity to do more.*
> Jonas Salk (Figure 7-1)

When Dr. Jonas Salk envisioned the idea of the Salk Institute for Biological Studies, it was with the idea of creating a vibrant, intellectual community, dedicated to pursuing the kinds of scientific achievements that had made him an international figure only five years before.

Salk came to La Jolla following a career in clinical medicine and virology research. After obtaining his M.D. degree at the New York University School of Medicine in 1939, he was a staff physician at Mount Sinai Hospital in New York City.

He then joined his mentor, Dr. Thomas Francis, as a research fellow at the University of Michigan. There, he worked to develop an influenza vaccine at the behest of the U.S. Army. In 1947, he was appointed director of the Virus Research Laboratory at the University of Pittsburgh School of Medicine.

It was in Pittsburgh that Salk began to put together the techniques that would lead to his polio vaccine.

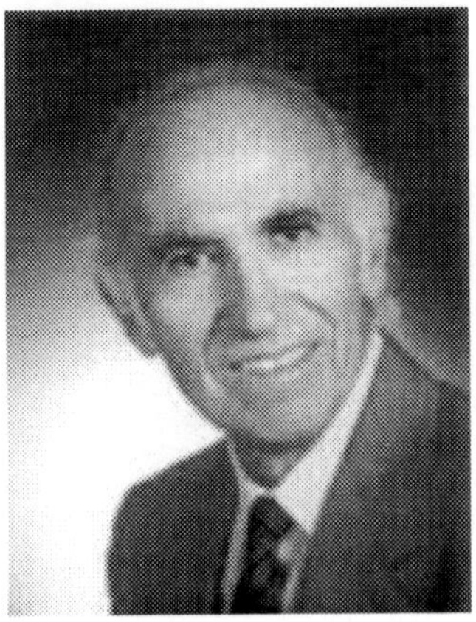

Figure 7-1. Jonas Salk [3].

He was already struck by the principle of vaccination: that if the body is artificially exposed to a harmless form of a disease virus, the body will produce antibodies that resist or kill the dangerous form of the virus if later exposed. In contrast to the Pasteurian dogma of the times, Salk believed that protective immunity could be induced without infection by a living virus such as those used in the vaccines against smallpox and rabies. In developing the influenza vaccine, he had observed that protection could be established using non-infectious, inactivated (killed) viruses.

Salk's research caught the attention of Basil O'Connor, president of the National Foundation for Infantile Paralysis (now known as the March of Dimes Birth Defects Foundation). The organization decided to fund Salk's efforts to develop a killed virus vaccine against the most frightening scourge of the time: paralytic poliomyelitis.

Using formaldehyde, Salk killed the poliovirus, but kept it intact enough to trigger the necessary immune response. His work was enabled by a key achievement made by Harvard researcher John Enders. Enders and his team had figured out how to grow poliovirus in test tubes. This step was necessary to obtain the quantities of pure virus needed to develop and manufacture a vaccine.

The resulting injectable vaccine was tested first in monkeys and then in patients at the D.T. Watson Home for Crippled Children (now The Watson Institute), who already had polio.

Next, vaccine was given to volunteers who had not had polio, including Salk, his laboratory staff, his wife and their children. The volunteers developed anti-polio antibodies and none had bad reactions to the vaccine. Finally, in 1954, national testing began on one million children, ages six to nine, who became known as *the Polio Pioneers*: half received the vaccine, and half received a placebo. One-third of the children, who lived in areas where vaccine was not available, were observed to evaluate the background level of polio in this age group. On April 12, 1955, the results were announced: the vaccine was safe and effective. In the two years before vaccine was widely available, the average number of polio cases in the U.S. was more than 45,000. By 1962, that number had dropped to 910. Salk never patented the vaccine, nor did he earn any money from his discovery, preferring to see it distributed as widely as possible.

Given the fear and anxiety that polio caused during the first half of the century, the vaccine's success in 1955 made Salk an international hero, and he spent the late 1950s refining the vaccine and establishing the scientific principles behind it. By 1960, however, Salk was ready to move on. Salk's dream was to create an independent research centre where a community of scholars interested in different aspects of biology—the study of life—could come together to follow their curiosity.

For more than a year, Salk toured the country in search of the right location for his research centre. Finally, wooed by San Diego Mayor Charles Dail, who had had polio, he was drawn to 27 acres on a mesa in La Jolla, just west of the proposed site for the new University of California campus then planned for San Diego. With a gift of the land from the citizens of San Diego and with initial financial support from the National Foundation/March of Dimes, Salk was able to proceed. To bring his concept of free-flowing labs and quiet studies to life, Salk recruited architect Louis Kahn. The resulting collaboration is a series of elegant concrete structures that overlook the Pacific Ocean.

Under Salk's direction, the Institute began research activities in 1963 and gradually expanded its faculty and the areas of their research interests. Salk's personal research activities included multiple sclerosis and autoimmune diseases, cancer immunology, improved manufacture and standardization of killed poliovirus vaccine, and the development of an AIDS vaccine. He published several philosophical books and advocated cooperative rather than confrontational approaches to addressing human needs.

Completed in 1967, the original Institute buildings were declared an historic landmark in 1991. During Salk's tenure as Founding Director, a major building addition consistent with his and Louis Kahn's original architectural vision was designed and constructed. The Institute now has 57 faculty members and a scientific staff of more than 850, with labs that house research on everything from cancer, diabetes and birth defects to Alzheimer's disease, Parkinson's disease, AIDS and plant biology.

The Salk Institute truly reflects the broad, humanistic interests of its namesake.

Salk died at age 80 on June 23, 1995. A memorial at the Institute with a statement from Salk captures his vision: "Hope lies in dreams, in imagination and in the courage of those who dare to make dreams into reality." [3]

The Fourth of Four Accounts of Jonas Salk [4]

Many scientists were racing to make a polio vaccine in the '50s — but he got there first
By Wilfred Sheed

How many cases make an epidemic? Survivors of the great polio plagues of the 1940s and '50s will never believe that in the U.S. the average toll in those years was "only" 1 victim out of every 5,000 people. Was that really all it took to scare the nation out of its wits, sending families scurrying in all directions—to the mountains, to the desert, to Europe—in vain hope of sanctuary.

Perhaps polio's other name, infantile paralysis, had something to do with it. Images of babies in wheelchairs and tots on crutches tend to skew one's perception. And just in case

anyone wasn't scared enough, the National Foundation for Infantile Paralysis hammered the nightmare home with photos that seemed to show up everywhere of sad-looking children in leg braces. "Please give to the March of Dimes." Oh yes, indeed, five times at the same movie —or so it sometimes felt.

It was inevitable that whoever was first to allay such fears would become a national hero. "The Man Who Saved the Children" should be good for a statue in every town in the world. And since the odds of a microbiologist becoming even a little bit famous are a lot worse than 5,000 to 1, it was perhaps inevitable that this hero's achievements would immediately be disputed. In a scientific field so heavily manned, findings routinely crisscross and even minor discoveries can leave a trail of claims and counterclaims, not to mention envy and acrimony that are truly incurable.

Thus a monument to the conquest of polio faithful to the facts would consist of not one man in a white lab coat but two of them glaring at each other. Both Drs. Jonas Salk and Albert Sabin could and did make convincing cases for themselves and pretty good ones against each other, too. But since the public usually prefers one hero to two and since Salk did get there first, he got the monument.

Between occasional shouts of "Eureka!" even the heroes of science tend to have quiet careers. But Salk's career stands out in at least two respects: the sheer speed with which he outraced all the other tortoises in the field and the honours he did not receive for doing so. How could the Man Who Saved the Children be denied a Nobel Prize? Or summarily be turned down for membership in the National Academy of Sciences? What was it about Salk that so annoyed his fellow scientists?

That he was fast, there was no doubt. And hungry, too. After taking brilliant advantage of the amazing public education available to New Yorkers in the first half of this century, this son of Orthodox Polish-Jewish immigrants whizzed through his medical training to fetch up at the University of Michigan an enviable fellowship to study virology under the distinguished Dr. Thomas Francis—who, incidentally, would remain in Salk's corner for life, politics or no politics.

Salk's major patron at Michigan, however, proved to be no one man but the whole U.S. Army, which needed a flu vaccine at once to help win World War II and was happy to complete Salk's education in speed under pressure. After that, it was a snap for him to set up his own peacetime lab at the University of Pittsburgh and equip it to the gills for the Great Crusade—the one that every immunologist in the world then had his eye on—against the Great White Whale itself, poliomyelitis.

Fortunately, Salk had somehow found time to do basic research on the virus and write a few theoretical papers, and it was these that caught the eye of Basil O'Connor, the zealous head of the Infantile Paralysis Foundation, who decided to play a hunch and shove some dimes in Salk's direction with instructions to get going.

With that, the seeds of resentment, deep and abiding, were sown. By then, dozens of worthy researchers had been toiling far longer than Salk in the fields of polio and would have given their microscopes for such funding and freedom. Who was this hired gun who appeared from nowhere with a bankroll the size of a special prosecutor's, plus free use of all the backbreaking work that had gone before?

In fact, the key piece of research, available to all, was completed a few years earlier by the one undisputed hero of this story, Harvard's John Enders. It was his team that figured out how to grow polio in test tubes—suddenly giving vaccine hunters everywhere enough virus to work with.

Now the goal was truly in sight, and who got there first was largely a matter of speed—Salk's forte—and luck. "Salk was strictly a kitchen chemist," Sabin used to gripe. "He never had an original idea in his life." But imaginative people perennially underrate efficient ones, and at the time, the kitchen chemist—who prepared his vaccine by marinating the virus in formalin—was just what the doctor ordered.

Salk and Sabin came from the two competing schools of vaccine research. Sabin, like Louis Pasteur, believed the way to produce immunity was to create a mild infection with a "live" but crippled virus, and he concocted his competing vaccine accordingly. Salk, from his flu-fighting days, knew the immune system could be triggered without infection, using deactivated, or "killed," viruses. And, as it turned out, his quick-and-dirty killed viruses were better suited to a crash program than Sabin's carefully attenuated live ones. By 1954, Salk and Francis were ready to launch the largest medical experiment yet carried out in the U.S., vaccinating more than 1 million kids ages six to nine, some with the vaccine, some with a placebo. The children weren't told which they were getting.

The vaccine worked. But the world of science has a protocol for releasing such findings: first publish them in a medical journal, and then spread the credit as widely as possible. Salk took part in a press conference and went on radio but gave credit to nobody, including himself—of course, he was going to get the credit anyway. And that was the mistake that would haunt him.

Radio was right; vanity was wrong. This was not some breakthrough in carbuncle research but hot news that couldn't wait one more minute. Within the brotherhood of researchers, however, Salk had sinned unforgivably by not saluting either Enders or, more seriously, his colleagues at the Pittsburgh lab. Everything he did after that was taken as showboating—when he opened the Salk Institute, a super lab in La Jolla, Calif., for the world's scientists to retreat to and bask in, and even when not long before his death in 1995, he started a search for an AIDS vaccine, to a flourish of trumpets and welcome new funding.

Just as some politicians are at their best when running for office, so Salk came into his own as a spokesman for vaccination. Although it is generally accepted in the field that the real man on the monument should be Enders (who in 1954 shared the only Nobel Prize given for polio research), it seems unlikely that either he or the pugnacious Sabin would have performed half so patiently as Salk the ceremonial chores expected of monuments or would have sat so politely through so many interviews and spread the gospel of disease prevention quite so far and wide and indefatigably.

And one last thing. Like the millions of American veterans who have never ceased thanking Harry Truman for dropping the Bomb and ending World War II, the folks who got their polio shot between the first Salk vaccine and the Sabin model have never had any quarrel with Salk's high place in history. (The two vaccines are now given in alternating booster shots.) [5].

(Author's remarks: Since 1998 however, only the inactivated polio vaccine IPV, otherwise popularly called Salk vaccine is recommended to prevent polio in the United States.)

There are times when even genius has to give way to the old Yankee virtues of know-how and can do. And if in this instance these happened to be embodied in the son of a couple of Polish-Jewish immigrants... well, a lot of that kind of thing happens in America. [4]

The Visits to the USA of the Ancient Disease Polio

Poliomyelitis, one of man's ancient diseases, was known as far back as 1580—1350 B.C, as recorded in an Egyptian stele during the 18th Dynasty [6]. The author hopes that the following account of the unwelcome, nay dreaded visits of poliomyelitis (infantile paralysis) to the USA would provide an illuminating background to the work of Jonas Salk on polio. The cases quoted are new cases reported in the US [7].

1894 - Polio killed 18 children in Rutland County, Vermont, and paralyzed 114 others, the largest outbreak in the US at that date.

1899 - Scientists in Vienna showed that polio was spread by an infectious agent.

1908 - Landsteiner isolated the polio virus, an enterovirus, but did not develop any safe and effective polio vaccine..

1911 - After 18 months work on polio virus, Flexner, an American, predicted that within 6 months a remedy would be announced. His prediction was not correct.

1916 - Over 27,000 cases and 7,179 deaths. There was panic in New York where over 2,000 died. (People fled Manhattan, only to meet armed robbers in the suburbs. Some hospitals refused to admit cases for fear of infecting others. Cities impounded cats and dogs because authorities mistakenly thought they could transmit the virus to humans. Parents sealed windows and doors and refused to let their children outside to play. Miracle cures like ox and frog blood, cedar shavings, and radium water abounded.)

1921 - Franklin Delano Roosevelt (1882–1945), the 32nd President (1933–1945) of the US was, at 39, crippled by polio in 1921.

1934 - This year marked the beginning of the personal involvement of President Roosevelt in raising funds for polio victims. He established the President's Birthday Ball Commission for Infantile Paralysis (polio) that was renamed The Commission for Infantile Paralysis the following year. In 1937, he replaced it with the National Foundation for Infantile Paralysis.

1935 - Maurice Brondie of New York University reported he had protected monkeys with a killed poliovirus vaccine. Using funds he received from the Commission for Infantile Paralysis, he distributed his vaccines to hospitals and health departments. More than 9,000 children received the vaccine. John Kolmer of Temple University claimed about the same time that he had developed attenuated poliovirus vaccine with which, private physicians assisting, he vaccinated about 11,000 kids. It was alleged that some of the vaccinees had developed polio with paralysis, and that some died of the disease. It was concluded that both

were ineffective and dangerous. Some suspect that Brodie's death in 1939 was suicidal even though the official cause of death was coronary infarction.

1938 - 1,705 cases. Working under Thomas Francis Jr. at New York University until 1940, Jonas Edward Salk (1914-1995) acquired experience in isolating influenza virus from mice and inactivating it with ultraviolet light.

1942- Salk began research on prophylactic viral immunization using the $2,100 fellowship he had obtained from the National Foundation for Infantile Paralysis.

1948- 27,726 cases. Salk moved to Polio vaccine research. Isabel Morgan of Johns Hopkins University in Baltimore successfully protected monkeys against one type of poliovirus with a killed-virus vaccine.

1949 - 42,033 cases. John Enders, Children's Hospital, Boston developed the technique of growing polio virus in monkey testicles or kidneys instead of the nervous tissue cultures in use before then.

1950- 33,000 cases. Salk had developed his own polio virus tissue-culturing system. Hilary Koprowski successfully developed live attenuated polio vaccine by growing the virus in the brains of cotton rats. The vaccine boosted anti-polio virus antibody production. Koprowski and his boss took their vaccines without ill effect. Later, Koprowski vaccinated 20 institutionalized children with his polio vaccine, with their parents' consent. The children developed antibodies to the virus without illness. Scientists, however, still claimed Koprowski had been brash and reckless.

1951 - 28,386 cases

1952 - With funding from the National Foundation. Salk developed in his laboratory killed (Formalin inactivated) polio vaccine against the 3 strains of the virus, and successfully tested it in monkeys. He was ready for human trials (no ethicists in his University and no FDA in those days). All he needed were willing participants. Salk's public relations officer had stated publicly that Salk never tested his polio vaccine on himself. However, Salk was reported to have later admitted to a friend that he had actually tested the vaccine on himself. Salk secretly tested the vaccine on a few dozen polio sufferers with their parents' consent to see if the vaccine boosted antibody production. The vaccine indeed boosted effective antibody production that neutralized the virus in tissue culture.

1953 - 35,592 cases. The National Foundation and the National Institute of Health (NIH) spent $2 million and $72,000 respectively on polio research. Salk announced his achievement on the polio vaccine at a February press conference during which he said scientific publication would follow later. Salk drew the ire of his colleagues for going public before scientific publication.

1954 - 38,476 cases. The National Foundation organized field trials in 44 States when 1,830,000 school children received the (unregistered) Salk vaccine. 20,000 doctors and public health officials, 40,000 registered nurses, 14,000 school principals, 50,000 teachers and 200,000 lay volunteers participated in the field trials.

1955- 28,985 cases. At a crowded press conference in April, Thomas Francis Jr. announced that from 144 million separate pieces of data collected and analyzed, the Salk vaccine had at least 60% efficacy, and had not caused any significant harm to a single child. The Department of Health, Education and Welfare licensed the vaccine just 2 hours later. The US and the world 'exploded with joy, dancing and singing and hugging, and blasting,

ringing, and clinking anything that would make noise. ... During the next few weeks, letters, telegrams, phone calls, and in-the-flesh well-wishers descended on Salk. ... There was no end to the awards, honorary degrees, and donations. It was a train of elation, with ever more cars hooking on'. Just 13 days after the Salk vaccine was publicly declared safe and effective, the bubble burst. Unfortunately, Cutter Laboratories of Berkeley, California, had accidentally produced the vaccine that contained live virus, causing at least 149 cases of polio out of which 10 died. The Cutter incident, as it was called, frightened many parents away from giving their children Salk vaccine.

1956 - 15,140 cases.

1957 - 5,485 cases. The US Government stopped financing mass immunizations. The USSR started mass vaccination with Sabin vaccine, the oral attenuated polio vaccine.

1958 - 5,787 cases.

1959 - 8,425 cases.

1960 - 3,190 cases.

1961 - 1,312 cases. Licensing one strain at a time, the US Government registered the 1st strain of Sabin vaccine in August.

1962 - In March, the US Government licensed the 3rd strain of Sabin vaccine.

1998 - Only the inactivated polio vaccine IPV, otherwise popularly called Salk vaccine is recommended to prevent polio in the United States [5].

In the US now, polio is no longer an important disease. The country has less than 30 cases annually.

The following Table summarizes the major milestones of polio vaccine development in the US.

Table summarizing cases of US cases of polio and the milestones of polio vaccine development

Year	No. of U.S. Polio Cases	Remarks
1911		Flexner, after 18 months work with the poliovirus, said a polio vaccine would be ready in 6 months
1916	27,000	Panic in New York
1938	1,705	
1948	27,726	Morgan protected monkeys using a killed polio vaccine
1949	42,033	Enders developed monkey testes or kidney tissue culture for poliovirus
1950	33,000	Koprowski vaccinated 20 children with attenuated polio vaccine
1951	28,386	
1952		Salk's success in monkeys, himself and few dozen children with 3 strains of killed poliovirus
1953	35,592	Salk announced his polio vaccine success at a press conference
1954	38,476	1,830,000 children immunized with Salk vaccine in 44 States
1955	28,985	Salk vaccine declared safe and was licensed immediately. Cutter incident.

Table (Continued)

Year	No. of U.S. Polio Cases	Remarks
1956	15,140	
1957	5,485	US Govt stopped financing mass vaccinations. USSR started mass vaccination with Sabin vaccine.
1958	5,787	
1959	8,425	
1960	3,190	
1961	1,312	US Govt licensed the 1st strain of Sabin vaccine
1962		US Govt completed licensing Sabin vaccine by licensing the 3rd strain, but only the Salk vaccine is recommended for polio prevention in the US since 1998.
Total	302,242	

Conclusion

Let us note that:

- Then US President Roosevelt, himself a polio victim, was instrumental in raising funds for polio, and he started doing so the year after he became President.
- Almost 2 million children were immunized in the US in 1954 with an unregistered Salk vaccine.
- The vaccine was only registered the following year after the massive field trial of the previous year showed it was safe and had at least 60 percent efficacy. The Cutler incident occurred 13 days after this.
- When the Sabin vaccine was introduced in the US, many US experts were vociferous in condemning the Salk vaccine; they actually advocated that the US use only the Sabin vaccine. However, after about 40 years of using both the Salk and Sabin polio vaccines, only the Salk vaccine is recommended in the US for polio prevention since 1998. There are always those who are experts at criticism of new discoveries even though some of them hardly attempt to work to solve the problem at hand.
- Undoubtedly, it was the Salk vaccine, not the Sabin oral vaccine that was responsible for the control of polio in the US. We should also remember that the polio virus was not isolated by either Salk or Sabin.
- In New York in 1916 when over 2,000 died from polio, some hospitals refused to admit cases for fear of infecting others; cities impounded cats and dogs because authorities mistakenly thought they could transmit the virus to humans; parents sealed windows and doors and refused to let their children outside to play; and miracle cures like ox and frog blood, cedar shavings, and radium water abounded. Again, desperate measures for a desperate situation.

With millions of new cases and millions of deaths annually from HIV/AIDS, would it not be reasonable to embrace any safe and effective HIV vaccine that will reduce this global burden, even if it is only 10 percent efficacious?

References

[1] http://www.achievement.org/autodoc/page/sal0bio_1
[2] http://en.wikipedia.org/wiki/Jonas_Salk
[3] http://www.salk.edu/jonas/jonas_about.php?sid=jonas
[4] www.time.com/time/time100/scientist/profile/salk.html
[5] http://www.chop.edu/consumer/jsp/division/generic.jsp?id=75724
[6] Schaechter M, Medoff G, Eisenstein BI (1993). *Mechanisms of Microbial Disease*. 2nd Edition. Baltimore: Williams and Wilkins 31:408.
[7] Cohen J (2001). Chapter 2 'The Next Breakthrough' in *Shots in the dark: the wayward search for an AIDS vaccine*. W.W. Norton and Company, New York. The quotations are from the author's copy that he kindly emailed to the author in September 2004 after *Vaccine* published our report.

People enrolled in these studies are usually healthy adults with a low risk for the infection. This study usually includes less than 100 participants.

Phase II

If a vaccine passes the Phase I studies, larger Phase II studies are designed. They are based on information gained from the Phase I study. Phase II studies are usually done in the type of people who will ultimately use the vaccine. Typically, these studies enrol a few hundred participants. If the vaccine is determined to be unsafe or doesn't consistently induce an immune response, it will not be further developed. Again, the assumption is that researchers know beforehand the sort of induced immune response required and how to evaluate it.

Phase III

Phase III studies determine whether vaccines work and include thousands to tens of thousands of people studied for many years. In many cases, more than one Phase III trial will be performed. Often, these trials are done across a large geographic area to ensure that the vaccine is working in people with different backgrounds and lifestyles. Phase III studies typically include more than 5,000 people.

In the US for instance, if a vaccine appears to be safe and to work, all of the data will be submitted to scientists and regulatory personnel at the U.S. Food and Drug Administration (FDA). They will check the data to be sure the studies were done correctly and the results were consistent.

While much of the early research is done in academic research laboratories using grants obtained from foundations or the government (e.g., the National Institutes of Health), Phase I, II and III studies are performed by pharmaceutical companies. These studies typically cost hundreds of millions of dollars.

Once a vaccine has been reviewed by the FDA and considered to be safe, it is still not ready to be given to people. All of the information generated about how the vaccine works in people is then provided to members of a recommending group of scientists and doctors that advise the Centres for Disease Control and Prevention (CDC). This group, called the Advisory Committee on Immunization Practices or ACIP, then recommends how the vaccine should be used and by whom. The CDC, as well as the American Academy of Paediatrics (AAP) and the American Academy of Family Physicians (AAFP), then make a final recommendation that doctors and healthcare professionals can follow in deciding who should receive the new vaccine.

Phase IV (After Licensure)

Once the vaccine begins to be distributed, additional studies occur. These studies are called Phase IV studies. Because some rare side effects may not have been detected in the phase III trials, vaccine safety is continually monitored by the CDC. These studies take at least four forms. First, the CDC will have certain health departments (usually in areas where there is a high occurrence of disease and hence, high vaccine distribution) monitor every person who receives the vaccine and report to it regularly. Second, the CDC monitors disease that is reported to every health department in the country, so they will see if there are any abnormal occurrences of disease after the vaccine is introduced and consider whether the two events may be related. Third, there is a Vaccine Adverse Events Reporting System (or VAERS). If a doctor, nurse or consumer believes that a person who received a vaccine had a significant negative side effect, he or she can file a report in this system, which is continuously monitored for trends in the data. Fourth, the Vaccine Safety Data link (VSD) includes about 6 million people in six large HMOs on the West Coast to look at who did and did not receive the vaccine and answer safety questions. The VSD is one of the most effective post-licensure measures that we have. These systems proved their utility in 1999 when a newly licensed rotavirus vaccine was found to be a rare cause of intussusception, a folding of the intestine into itself that may require emergency surgery and can result in death if untreated. Once the relationship was confirmed, the rotavirus vaccine was discontinued." [3]

NEWSWEEK, The International Newsmagazine, June 11, 2001 carried a special report on pages 38 - 48 on "*AIDS AT 20*". That special report describes eight methods of producing vaccines, thus:

"Eight Routes to a Vaccine"

Because no one recovers from HIV infection, scientists aren't sure what it will take to make people immune. Here are some of the approaches now under investigation.

1) *Live attenuated HIV:* Weakened version of the virus triggers a robust immune response, but the vaccine itself could cause AIDS. Human tests unlikely.
2) *Whole killed HIV*: Safer than live virus but less effective because virus doesn't generate proteins. Vaccines based on pieces of HIV are easier to prepare.
3) *Recombinant HIV proteins*: Molecules mimicking HIV's outer surface trigger the production of antibodies, but the antibodies may not block infection.
4) *Peptide epitopes:* Tiny fragments of HIV proteins are easy to make and safe to use, but may not elicit a broad-enough response to handcuff the virus.
5) *Live bacterial vectors*: Genetically altered bacteria generate HIV proteins, which the immune system learns to recognize and destroy. Safe, simple.
6) *Live viral vectors*: Harmless viruses are engineered to generate HIV proteins, which elicit an immune response. More stable than bacterial vectors.
7) *Naked DNA*: HIV genes are introduced into the recipient's cells, which then produce the viral proteins needed to activate the immune system.

8) *Combinations*: Researchers hope that cocktails incorporating more than one element will elicit the broad immune response needed to ward off infection."

Of course, these methods are not exclusive. Other methods may be developed with the passage of time and more research. The author's HIV vaccines are not produced in any of the ways listed here.

Procedure Before Bringing a New Vaccine to the Market in an Emergency

The author cannot find any document on the procedure to be followed for vaccine development in the face of an epidemic of an infectious disease for which a vaccine does not exist. However, there are many documented cases of what humanity did in such circumstances. Using polio as an example, let us see how the disease and its vaccine when it was eventually developed were handled in and by the USA.

"(Jonas) Salk may well have been overly enthusiastic about the prospects of an old-fashioned killed-virus vaccine thwarting HIV. *But his grander point was right on target: Past successes offer powerful lessons that could speed modern vaccine development. And all too often, these lessons are given lip service and then blithely ignored.*

Among Greek, Etruscan, and Roman Art in Copenhagen's Ny Carlsberg Glyptotek museum resides an Egyptian stele of the Eighteenth Dynasty that depicts a young priest and a woman, offerings in hand. The stone carving appears typical of its era, 1580–1350 B.C., except for one detail: the priest's right leg is gnarled and shortened, telltale deformities of poliomyelitis.

Though this is the first recorded evidence of polio, no epidemics were charted until the mid-1800s. Hard-hit cities like Stockholm, Oslo, and Lyon were befuddled when the disease began its assault, much in the same way AIDS took San Francisco, New York, and Kinshasa by surprise. Many Americans probably first learned of polio in 1894, the year the disease killed 18 children in Rutland County, Vermont, and paralyzed 114 others, the largest outbreak to that date.

Nearly 15 years passed before scientists in Vienna showed that polio was spread by an infectious agent. In the signal experiment, the researchers caused monkeys to develop polio by inoculating their brains with spinal cord tissue taken from a human who had died of the disease. Just as the isolation of HIV spawned the AIDS vaccine search, so did the isolation of poliovirus. By 1910, investigators had fashioned experimental polio vaccines.

The pioneers of polio vaccinology knew little about poliovirus—or, for that matter, any virus. Shaped like a minuscule soccer ball, poliovirus contains a single strand of ribonucleic acid (RNA), which holds the virus's genetic code. Poliovirus enters the body through the mouth and nose from droplets, such as saliva, or from microscopic pieces of faeces. The virus then slides into the gut and reproduces. Normally the immune system can limit this infection before it causes serious disease, but on rare occasions, the virus travels through the blood and into the central nervous system, causing meningitis. Paralysis occurs only if the virus then enters nerve cells. Scientists now estimate that in an unvaccinated population, wild poliovirus paralyzes only 1% to 2% of the people it infects.

The first prototype polio vaccines worked, to a degree, in experiments with animals, though the results ultimately were inconclusive. Still, the fact that these scientists, for the most part working in the dark, had any success is instructive. Vaccinology at the turn of the 20th century was largely an empirical art. If the vaccine worked, it worked. How or why a vaccine protected a person from disease was relevant but not all-important. Vaccinologists aimed to stop human suffering and the loss of farm animals. If these investigators had an understanding of how a potion performed its magic, so much the better.

The drive to develop a polio vaccine paradoxically owes much to the success that late 19th century populations had at eliminating poliovirus from their environments. For centuries, polio kept a low profile because human behaviour successfully exploited the immune system. The umbilical cord supplies foetuses with blood from their mothers. In addition to passing blood-borne germs—such as HIV—from mother to baby, this natural bridge helps newborns, too, by providing them with maternal antibodies that can ward off many diseases. Breast milk also can supply a baby with a mother's antibodies. But these "passively" acquired antibodies disappear within a few months, meaning the protection they offer is temporary. Still, if poliovirus infected an infant while a mother's antibodies were there, the baby not only would clear the infection unscathed; its immune system would "actively"—and safely—learn how to make antibodies against the bug. Owing to a phenomenon called immunologic memory, the child's immune system would never forget this active lesson. In essence, then, babies used to routinely receive what amounts to a natural polio vaccine.

But then came sanitation, which catapulted polio from obscurity to plague status. Indoor plumbing, the germ theory, and other advances of the industrial age reduced the exposure of infants to poliovirus, creating more and more people susceptible to infection and disease. Most often, the disease struck these "susceptibles" early in life, earning polio the moniker infantile paralysis.

By 1916 the pool of susceptibles in the United States had so deepened that the disease afflicted more than 27,000 Americans, killing 7,179. *Panic hit especially hard in New York City, where more than 2,000 died. People fled Manhattan, only to meet unwelcoming committees of gun totters in the suburbs. Some hospitals refused to admit cases for fear of infecting others. Cities impounded cats and dogs, which authorities mistakenly thought could transmit the virus to humans. Parents sealed windows and doors and refused to let their children outside to play. Miracle cures like ox and frog blood, cedar shavings, and radium water abounded.*

Poliovirus crippled the 39-year-old Franklin Delano Roosevelt in 1921. Just as the news in 1985 that Rock Hudson had AIDS would later stoke public concern about that disease, Roosevelt's condition changed the public's perception of polio and became a catalyst for increased scientific research.

Beginning in 1934, President Roosevelt staged charity balls on his birthday (January 30) "to dance so others may walk" - and, more to the point, to pay off the debts accrued at the Warm Springs Foundation, a polio centre that he had established eight years before in the pine-studded hills of Warm Springs, Georgia. Under the direction of Basil O'Connor,

Chapter VIII

Other Vaccines

Abstract

Yellow fever epidemics caused much panic and fear in the US in the past, but now that the cause is known and an effective preventive vaccine developed against it, there is no more fear or dread from this disease in the US. The same thing has befallen many other diseases as we saw in the chapter dealing with vaccines.

Introduction

In this short chapter, we will just take a glance at yellow fever and other vaccines. They all have nothing very different from the other vaccines that we have looked at in some detail. The author feels that he must mention them for completeness.

Yellow Fever

Yellow fever was also exotic. Epidemics prior to 1793 all seemed to be exceptions. Philadelphia, for example, had epidemics in 1699, 1741 and 1762.

From 1793 to 1822 yellow fever was one of the most dreaded diseases in the port cities of the United States. Statistically, one can dismiss it as inconsequential in comparison to tuberculosis and smallpox. Yellow fever did not kill that many people, but during that period, it struck with such ferocity in principal cities that it spread gloom and fear throughout the country. Doctors were uncertain of the cause of yellow fever and the factors that led it to reach epidemic proportions. That uncertainty was not unique. The causes of other diseases were also unknown. But doctors and patients then had an acute understanding of fever.

Today, fever is a symptom that can usually be controlled with over-the-counter medicines. Then, fever was tantamount to disease itself. Fever was far more than a question of body temperature and discomfort. It was a state in which a person's whole being was reordered. Two hundred years ago it was conceived in much the same way that we conceive of cancers. Just as today, when one discusses cancer, death is assumed to be a likely consequence, then when one discussed fever, death was assumed to be a likely consequence.

It was this view of morbidity that made yellow fever so feared simply because in the experience of these people who were so sensitive to fevers, yellow fever was most powerful and horrible.

Indeed during the 1793 epidemic it became clear to many that an epidemic in New York City in 1791 was yellow fever. The city establishment had suppressed almost all discussion about the epidemic. However, in 1793 New York as well as most other cities in the nation instituted strong quarantines against people fleeing from Philadelphia, turning them away at gunpoint in some places. Baltimore had one of the strictest quarantines. And not without gratification to some in Philadelphia, in 1794 Baltimore was struck with an epidemic.

We know today that yellow fever is caused by a Flavivirus spread by the Aedes aegypti mosquito. This mosquito has peculiar habits which we are continuing to learn about. Its most distinguishing feature from other mosquitoes is its preference for urban habitat. It breeds best in relatively clean standing water and cisterns were a prominent feature among many city houses in that day before indoor plumbing. It also feeds during the day, and so must have quite enjoyed the bustling scenes common at the quays of the major port cities of the 18th century. Finally, it has no trouble adapting to life inside a house. Thus in a day when window screens were unknown, it had ready access to relatively protected environments [1].

Fortunately for us today, a safe and effective yellow fever vaccine, developed using live attenuated virus, is available for those at risk. Attenuation is achieved by repeated culture in chick embryos. A single shot of the vaccine provides protection for approximately 10 years.

Other Vaccines

We have several other safe and effective vaccines in use today. They include MMR, DPT, BCG, Hepatitis A and B, Hib, Influenza, typhoid, rotavirus, JEV, anthrax, meningococcus, pneumococcus, Varicella and HPV vaccines. They are made either from inactivated (killed) micro-organisms, or live attenuated viruses, or inactivated toxins (toxoids) or recombinant technology/genetic engineering techniques. As shown in the next chapter, virtually all these vaccines generate high titres of binding and specific antibodies against the causative infectious agent or their toxins.

Conclusion

Understandably, fear, too, was associated with yellow fever epidemics in years past, especially when no one had any idea of the cause of the disease. Eventually, the cause of the disease was isolated and an effective attenuated vaccine developed against it. Similarly, effective preventive vaccines were also developed against many other diseases.

Reference

[1] http://www.geocities.com/bobarnebeck/history.html

Chapter IX

Some Key Features of 25 Human Vaccines

Abstract

The author wishes to end this Section by taking a holistic look at most of the vaccines in human medical practice today with the aim of highlighting some of their key features such as how each vaccine is produced, the mode of action of the vaccine, the efficacy of the vaccine, whether the benefits of giving the vaccine outweigh the risks of not giving the vaccine, the causative agent of the diseases, the first person to isolate the causative agent, and the first person to produce the vaccine against the disease. The author hopes that these summaries would provide relevant facts to those who may need to get such information quickly. A quick look at the value worthiness of vaccines precedes the conclusion.

Introduction

The author hopes that readers will find this chapter handy for whoever wants to get the key facts about any of the vaccines currently in use in human medical practice. Readers may also find it interesting to compare the first isolation of the causative agent of the diseases with the first development of safe and effective vaccines against the disease. These are all historical facts that we cannot alter or ignore. The author is presenting them with the hope that they will guide us in our present travails with the HIV/AIDS holocaust.

Table summarizing the production method, mode of action and efficacy of 25 human vaccines [1]

Ser. No.	Type of Vaccine	How it is Produced	Mode of action of the vaccine	Vaccine Efficacy (%)	Do the benefits Outweigh the risks?

Table (Continued)

1	Anthrax	The bacterial culture containing the toxins is treated with formalin and purified	Antibody production	>92	For military personnel, yes
2	Cholera	Killed cholera bacteria	Antibody production	30-50	For those at risk, Yes
3	DPT (Diphtheria, Pertussis, Tetanus)	Toxins inactivated with formaldehyde (toxoids)	Antibody production	>95	Yes
4	Haemophilus Influenza type b (Hib)	The bacterial poly-saccharide (sugar coat) is joined to a harmless protein to make it immunogenic	Antibody production	>80	Yes
5	Hepatitis A	Using the virus killed (inactivated) with Formaldehyde	Antibody production	70-80	Yes
6	Hepatitis B	Isolating and purifying surface protein of the virus (1980s). Now, the surface protein is produced by yeast cells using recombinant Technology	Antibody production	>95	Definitely, yes
7	Papilloma Virus (HPV)	Virus-like particles (VLPs) Assembled from recombinant HPV coat Proteins	Antibody production		
8	Influenza	The virus is grown in chick embryos, purified inactivated with chemicals like formaldehyde. Another type uses an aerosol of weakened virus grown also in chick embryos.	Antibody production	30-60	Yes
9	Japanese Encephalitis Virus (JEV)	By growing the virus in mice brain followed by purification and Formaldehyde Inactivation	Antibody production	>80	For those at risk, Yes
10	Meningococcus	The polysaccharide coating from different strains is conjugated with a harmless protein to make it Immunogenic	Antibody production	>90	Yes
11	MMR (Measles, Mumps, and Rubella)	Using viruses attenu-ated in chick embryos (Measles and Mumps) or in human embryo fibroblast cells (Rubella)	Antibody production	>95	Yes
12	Pneumococcus	Bacterial polysaccharide + harmless proteins	Antibody production	>90	Yes

13	Polio	The virus is cultured in and killed with formalin (inactivated vaccine, the only one recom-mended for use in the US since 1998) OR The virus is attenuated by culture in monkey kidney cells before purification (oral vaccine, not recom-mended for use in the US since 1998)	Antibody production	>95 >95	Definitely, yes Definitely, yes
14	Rabies	The virus cultured in human diploid cells, chick embryo cells or foetal rhesus lung cells is harvested, purified and inactivated with betapropriolactone.	Antibody production	>90	Yes
15	Rotavirus	Rotavirus isolated, first from a monkey but later from a calf + human Rotavirus proteins to evoke protective antibodies	Antibody production	>90	Yes
16	Shingles	Just a more concentrated version of Varicella vaccine (for those over 60)	Antibody production	>80	Yes
17	Smallpox	From cowpox (Vaccinia)	Antibody production	>90	yes, if there is a risk (the last reported case of the disease was in 1977 from Somalia)
18	Tuberculosis	From a weakened form of bovine tuberculous organisms from a cow	mainly CMI	60-80	Yes
19	Typhoid	From weakened form of the causative bacilli or from polysaccharide of the causative bacilli	Antibody production	50-80	for those at risk, yes

Table summarizing the production method, mode of action and efficacy of 25 human vaccines (Continued)

Ser. No.	Type of Vaccine	How it is Produced	Mode of action of the vaccine	Vaccine Efficacy (%)	Do the benefits Outweigh the risks?
20	Varicella (Chickenpox)	From virus attenuated by culture in human embryo fibroblast cells)	Antibody production	>80	Yes
21	Yellow fever	From the virus weakened by repeated culture in chick embryos	Antibody production	>95	Definitely, yes

Table comparing the first isolation of 25 human infectious agents with the first development of the preventive vaccine for the disease [2]

Ser. No.	Disease	Causative Agent	causative agent		preventive vaccine for the disease	
			was first isolated by	in the year	was first developed by	in the year
1	Anthrax	Bacillus anthracis	Robert Koch (German)	1877	Louis Pasteur and William S. Greenfield	1881
2	Cholera	Vibrio cholera	Filippo Pacini (Italian)	1854	Clua	1885
3	Diphtheria	Corynebacterium Diphtheria	Edwin Klebbs and Friedrich Loffler (Germans)	1884	Behring	1913
4	Haemophilus influenzae type B (Hib)	Haemophilus Influenza	Richard Pfeiffer	1892		1985
5	Hepatitis A	Picornaviridae				1995
6	Hepatitis B	Hepadnaviridae	Baruch Blumberg	1965	Drs. Blumberg and Millman	1969
7	HPV				Merck and Co	2006
8	Influenza	Orthomyxoviridae				1945
9	JEV	Flaviviridae		1935		1930s
10	Measles	Paramyxoviridae	John Enders	1954	Merck and Co	1963
11	Meningococcus	Neisseria meningitides	Weichselbaum	1887		1974
12	Mumps	Rubulaviridae		1945		1948
13	Pertussis	Bordetella pertussis	Bacteriologists Bordet and Gengou	1906	Madsen	1925
14	Plague	Yersinia pestis	Alexandre Emile-Jean Yersin (Swiss bacteriologist) and Shibasaburo Kitasako (Japanese)	1894	No vaccine	
15	Pneumococcus	Streptococcus Pneumonia	George Steinberg (US Army physician) and Louis Pasteur (French chemist)	1881	Robert Austrian	1936 1977 in the US
16	Polio	Enterovirus	Karl Landsteiner	1908	Jonas Salk	1952

Ser. No.	Disease	Causative Agent	causative agent		preventive vaccine for the disease	
			was first isolated by	in the year	was first developed by	in the year
17	Rotavirus	Reoviridae	Ruth Bishop	1973	GlaxoSmithKline	1998
18	Rubella	Togavirus	Parkman and Weller	1962	Parkman and Weller	1969
19	Shingles	Human herpes virus type 3 (HHV-3)	Thomas H. Weller	1954	Merck	2006
20	Smallpox	Poxviridae			Edward Jenner	1796
21	Tetanus	Clostridium tetani	Kitasato Shibasaburo	1889	P. Descombey	1924
22	Tuberculosis	Mycobacterium Tuberculosis	Robert Koch	1882	Albert Calmette (French Bacteriologist) and Camile Guerin (French veterinarian)	1921
23	Typhoid	Salmonella typhi	Karl J. Erberth	1880	Almroth Edward Wright	1897
24	Varicella	Human herpes virus type 3 (HHV-3)	Thomas H. Weller	1954	Michiaki Takahashi	1972
25	Yellow fever	Flaviviridae	Mahaffy and Bauer	1927	Max Theiler	1937

Value Worthiness of Vaccines

Vaccines have indeed changed our lives on this planet. They really work. In the US, for instance, here are the figures to show very clearly the effect of some vaccines on the cases of the disease for which they were developed and used:

- diphtheria vaccine: from 175,855 cases in 1922 to 1 case in 1998
- Hib vaccine: from 20,000 cases in 1982 to 54 cases in 1998
- measles: from 503,282 cases in 1962 to 89 cases in 1998
- mumps: from 152,209 cases in 1968 to 606 cases in 1998
- pertussis: from 147,271 cases in 1925 to 6,279 cases in 1998
- rubella: from 47,745 cases in 1968 to 345 cases in 1998
- smallpox: from 48,164 cases in 1904 to 0 cases in 1998 [3].

Historical Lessons from Vaccines before the Advent of HIV/AIDS

History tells us that the first thing that happens with infectious diseases is the appearance of the disease. It is only after the disease has appeared that man moves to the next stage of either attempting to reduce the morbidity and mortality associated with the disease or thinking of how to prevent the disease, or both. The greater the morbidity and mortality associated with the infectious disease, the more desperate the measures taken by man to handle the disease. If the infectious disease causes an epidemic or epidemics, the more pronounced the desperate measures that society takes against the disease.

In the days of yore when man had no knowledge of the existence of micro-organisms, there was nothing else they could do. Since the advent of microbiology, bacteriology, virology and vaccinology, however, humanity tries to identify the causative agent of the infectious disease, characterize it and do the necessary experiments all in the effort to develop safe and effective remedies, preventive and/or therapeutic.

In this regard, we should note from history that since the advent of microbiology and all its sub-specialties, the first scientist that isolates the causative agent of an infectious disease is unlikely to be the first person to develop an effective vaccine against the disease. From the 25 human vaccines shown in the Tables, the probability that the first scientist to develop an effective vaccine against an infectious agent would be the scientist who first isolated the causative agent of the disease is 2 out of 25, a meagre 8 percent.

History also tells us that when it comes to scientific discoveries including vaccine development, no one has a monopoly of knowledge. The discovery may come from unexpected quarters rather than from the recognized experts of the day. In fact, anything coming out of the established scientific concepts of the day would not be a scientific discovery at all.

As in Jenner's days, approaches that are "in variance with established knowledge" and therefore "incredible" are the fertile grounds for new discoveries. Significant scientific discoveries emanate from minds that swim against the tide of the accepted concepts and dogmas of their day, to wit, Edward Jenner, Louis Pasteur, Robert Koch, the Wright brothers, and many others. It is therefore not surprising that new and significant scientific discoveries are usually received with much criticism by the experts of the day since the discoveries fly in the face of their established knowledge, concepts, dogmas and understanding.

When dealing with infectious diseases, let us remember from history that mere belief and prayers do not help in their control or effective treatment. We are dealing with live infectious agents that neither pray nor are affected by man's prayers and beliefs; we must take appropriate and correct actions to curb the epidemic or infectious agent.

Most infectious diseases that have caused epidemics have had short incubation periods with a short clinical course such that from the time the causative agent enters the host to the time of final resolution of the infection takes a few weeks or months at the longest.

History also tells us that highly specific and binding antibodies against infectious agents have played a pivotal role in man's efforts to prevent or treat these acute infectious diseases. Accordingly and without thinking, we have all become used to thinking of antibodies against infectious agents as our first and main line of protection. If for instance, we are confronted with an infectious viral disease where antibodies are non-protective, we must of necessity completely overhaul our knowledge and understanding of antibodies in that viral infection if we are ever to develop effective vaccines against that virus.

We should also remember from history and basic reasoning that the discovery of any new thing precedes methodology, and not vice versa. Accordingly, it would be absurd and unreasonable, for instance, for anyone to lay down the formula, recipe, guidelines and /or methodology that must be met or complied with before man can conceive the idea and develop or manufacture an unidentified flying object (UFO) if no one had ever succeeded in manufacturing a UFO. Accordingly, it is impossible for us to have an expert or experts in the manufacture of UFOs when no one has ever made a UFO.

Conclusion

When we are discussing safe and effective HIV vaccines therefore, let us always remember that:

1. As long as they are safe and effective, we should not stop or suppress them just because we don't know how and why they work.
2. A mediocre vaccine today would prevent more infections and death than a terrific vaccine introduced five years later.
3. Insistence on understanding the scientific basics and basis for the vaccine is likely to be a scam, an excuse for not finding out whether it works.
4. The measurable end-point for HIV vaccine development should be a vaccine product, not the number of publications in scientific journals or the internationally recognized status of the developer of the vaccine.
5. There will always be those that oppose any scientific advancement, those who want to keep things as they are - to do more research or just wait and see. This is especially inappropriate, if not criminal, at this time with this disease and the vaccine against it. In the US, for instance, three young haemophiliacs were firebombed out of their Florida home when their neighbours learned they were HIV positive in 1987 [4]. For 20 years the United States has been operating a policy that makes it a crime for HIV-positive travellers from other countries to enter the US even for one day [5].
6. The human immune response is far more complex than can be determined by laboratory tests. It may be sheer scientific arrogance for anyone to claim he understands protective immunity.
7. Research is definitely needed but the HIV/AIDS scourge is so devastating that what humanity, especially those afflicted by the disease and those at risk of acquiring the infection, has needed all along are safe and effective vaccines first and foremost. Understanding how such vaccines work comes later.

References

http://www.chop.edu/consumer/jsp/microsite/microsite.jsp?id=75918
This summary is from various sources downloaded from the internet in July 2008.
Downloaded on July 20, 2008 from http://focosi.immunesig.org Vaccines (vaccinology).
Downloaded on July 20, 2008 from http://csm.jmu.edu HIV/AIDS
Downloaded from Yahoo! News on Thursday. July 17, 2008

Section II:
The Era of HIV/AIDS and Its Scourge

Chapter X

AIDS and HIV

Abstract

When the Americans announced at a Press Conference in April 1984 that Gallo's lab in the National Cancer Institutes had isolated the virus that caused AIDS, they were so elated that Gallo went ahead to tell the world his recipe for an AIDS preventive vaccine that would be available for testing within 24 months, and in the market another 12 months later. His recipe was anchored on modern genetic engineering techniques and recombinant technology. Everyone everywhere including the UN fell headlong for Gallo's dummy of an HIV preventive vaccine recipe, implying of course that the developing countries of the world were eliminated since they do not have those modern techniques.

May 2009 marks the 301st calendar month (over 25 years) since the ebullient Americans spontaneously, happily and proudly told the world about their recipe and the 2–3 year time frame for its availability and marketability. Lo and behold, the Americans and their friends in the developed world have been unable to deliver on their promise. The author is not aware they have tendered any apologies to mankind for their false and misleading predictions that have caused humanity not only the loss of millions of lives from the HIV/AIDS pandemic, but also many millions that have been infected with the virus since 1984. Human pride and vanity will not let them apologize.

They have come up with all sorts of gimmicks of explanations for their failure. One of the antics is to develop the costly and toxic antiretrovirals, call them life-saving drugs and force them on humanity every where, telling us it is the best treatment available for now. It would have been more tolerable if they had apologised before forcing the drugs on us, but they did not. They have literally been rubbing salt on the heavy morbidity and mortality wounds that we have been forced to tolerate all these years. Otherwise, how would one justify their looking the other way when they know these vaccines were developed in 1998/99 by a surgeon working single-handedly with only his family's resources in a developing country?

With regards to HIV/AIDS, the developed world has indeed made a great laughing stock of its modern genetic engineering techniques and recombinant technology. Edward Jenner and Louis Pasteur who developed effective vaccines against viral diseases without the facilities that are available even to the poorest countries of the world today may be restless in their graves because of the way we have handled HIV/AIDS and left tens of millions to perish with tens of millions still infected and many more to be infected.

It is gratifying that after more than a quarter of a century had passed since the first publication of the isolation of the causative virus, the HIV that causes AIDS, half of the 2008 Nobel Prize for Medicine was awarded to, and equally shared by two French virologists, Françoise Barré-Sinoussi, 61, and Luc A. Montagnier, 76, for their work that led to the first published report of the isolation of the virus.

In this chapter, the author looks at these developments in more detail.

Introduction

It is man's nature to panic when faced with any serious problem especially fatal diseases including epidemics. To worsen matters, we have been confronted, since the early 1980s with the worst pandemic in history, HIV/AIDS, a pandemic that threatens to unravel societies around the world, just at the time that we have all become interdependent in a "global economy". Accordingly, the search for an effective HIV vaccine is perhaps the most important scientific challenge of our generation, if not the most crucial ever in the history of science [1]. Not surprisingly, therefore, it has indeed been a worldwide pandemonium of panic since the isolation of the HIV as the causative agent of AIDS, a situation that has, sadly, honestly and literally, also paralyzed basic, normal scientific reasoning, approach and open-mindedness.

Alice Park, writing in the *TIME* Magazine's Edition of March 29, 1999 on AIDS, said:

> "For the nearly 35 million people around the world now living with HIV, there may never be a cure. Once cells are infected with HIV, it's excruciatingly difficult—perhaps impossible—to rid them of the virus. The only sure way to stop the epidemic is to prevent infection in the first place and only a vaccine can do that...As scientists learn more about how HIV co-opts the human body to survive, they are realizing that drugs alone may not be enough. To contain the virus effectively, it may take a balance between drug therapy that keeps HIV levels low and a bolstered immune system that can then target and destroy the remaining virus. Until scientists find a vaccine, however, they may control but never cure the century's final scourge."

Unfortunately, neither Alice Park nor any other writer I have come across defines 'cure of HIV infection'.

Later in December 1999, the same *TIME* International Magazine, described the 20th century as

> "...the century that split the atom, probed the psyche, spliced genes and cloned a sheep. It invented plastic, radar and the silicon chip. It built aeroplanes, rockets, satellites, televisions, computers and atom bombs. It overthrew our inherited ideas about logic, language, learning, mathematics, economics and even space and time. And behind each of these great ideas, great discoveries and great inventions is, in most cases, one extraordinary human mind."

Et Tu UNAIDS?

All told, the Joint United Nations Programme on HIV/AIDS (UNAIDS) estimated in June 2000 that sub-Saharan Africa had 15 million deaths from AIDS, 12 million AIDS orphans, and 24.5 million people living with the virus—a whopping 70 percent of the global

AIDS total, even though this region has a mere 10 percent of the world's population. 'Despite millennia of epidemics, war and famine,' stated UNAIDS, 'never before in history have death rates of this magnitude been seen among young adults of both sexes and from all walks of life.' A vaccine, the report concluded, represented 'our best hope' of stemming the epidemic, *(The author agrees so far)* 'but it will take time and a concerted international effort before we have one.' [2]

The author strongly disagrees. How did UNAIDS know it will take time and a concerted international effort? Is it not a clear case of putting the cart before the horse? In the author's view, this is a sheer display of unscientific prejudice, arrogance and pride by UNAIDS. How could UNAIDS say this when it has continued to say loudly, like very many others, that there is still no HIV vaccine anywhere in the world? UNAIDS should not have its cake and eat it, too. If there is no HIV vaccine anywhere in the world, the author beseecheth thee UNAIDS, how do you know that it will take time and a concerted international effort before we have one? Discovery precedes methodology and not vice versa, UNAIDS.

In case somebody somewhere thinks the author is wrong in this matter, the person should note that UNAIDS did not produce any data, control trials or any scientific work, even if haphazard, shoddy or wishy-washy to support its assertion that it 'will take time and a concerted international effort before we have one' HIV vaccine. Since this assertion by UNAIDS has no scintilla of scientific foundation, would one not be justified to discard it as spurious?

On the false claims that no HIV vaccines exist and that no HIV-infected person has been cured anywhere in the world, mankind has (deliberately?) been left at the mercy of HIV/AIDS these past years with the result that the pandemic, described as the worst known to man, has taken the lives of millions, left many orphaned and dislocated numerous societies and their economies; another instance of man's atrocity and inhumanity to man.

The Great Conquests of AIDS and HIV Since Inception

The following account comes from a website [3]:

This year (2000) marks the 19th year since the beginning of the AIDS epidemic. The first reported cases of AIDS appeared in the US in 1981 in 5 young homosexual males diagnosed with *Pneumocystis carinii* pneumonia and other opportunistic infections. Initial conclusions reached were that it was a disease of gay men, particularly those who had many sexual partners. In 1982, cases of AIDS were reported among haemophiliacs and IV drug users. In 1983 the first documented cases of heterosexual transmission were documented. Later that year, AIDS cases were reported in Central Africa with the striking difference that most cases were heterosexually transmitted, rather than homosexually transmitted, as in the U.S.

June 1981 – the CDC reported diseases occurring in gay men that were normally found only in immunosuppressed individuals. The CDC report said that 5 young men in Los Angeles were diagnosed with *Pneumocystis carinii.* They also suggested an association between the disease and the homosexual lifestyle.

July 1981– the CDC reported an uncommon cancer, Kaposi's sarcoma, had been diagnosed in 2 gay men who lived in New York City and California. Because of the connection with gay men, it was initially called GRID (Gay-Related Immune Deficiency)

1981 – Researchers in several laboratories mobilized to try to find the cause of the disease. This included Robert Gallo's lab C at the National Institutes of Health (NIH), and Luc Montagnier's lab at the Pasteur Institute in Paris, France.

1982-83 – AIDS was discovered in drug users, haemophiliacs, heterosexuals, and children. The epidemic was officially recognized [3].

The Centre for Disease Control in the US reacted quite cautiously in 1981 to sound the alarm, for the U.S. citizenry was not quite ready to talk openly about sex, needles, and condoms. Our awareness heightened by the death of well known individuals, such as Rock Hudson in 1985 (Figure 10-1), but ignorance, apathy, and antagonism prevailed. Three young haemophiliacs were firebombed out of their Florida home when their neighbours learned they were HIV positive in 1987.

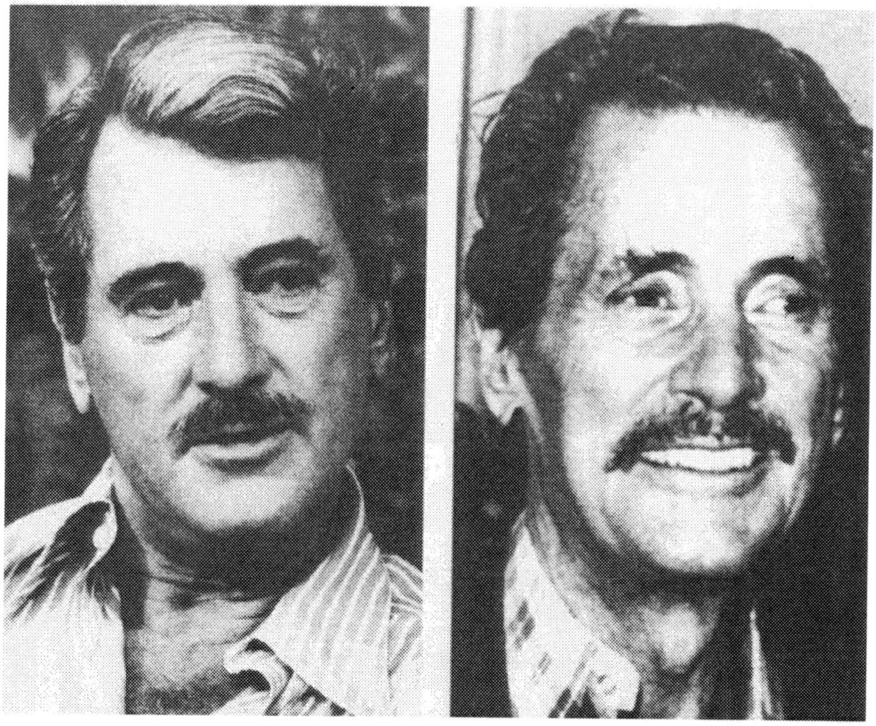

Figure 10-1. Rock Hudson, Movie and Television Star, before and after the developed AIDS. A Hollywood legend and undisclosed homosexual, he was the first major public figure to reveal he had AIDS in 1985. Hudson died in 1985 at the age of 59. (Photograph courtesy of AP/Wide World Photos) [3].

Retrospectively, the earliest confirmed AIDS case in America was that of a 15-year-old male prostitute who demonstrated Kaposi's sarcoma and died in 1969. Frozen tissue sample contained HIV antibodies. In Europe, it was a Danish surgeon who had worked in Zaire before her death in 1976.

The earliest known case is believed to be an African man who died in 1959. Scientists looked for signs of HIV in 1,213 blood samples that were gathered between 1959 and 1982. They found clear signs of the virus in a Bantu man who lived in Leopoldville, Belgian Congo (Kinshasa). Based on this finding, and the known rate of change of HIV, it is estimated that HIV crossed into the human population from an animal reservoir between 1924 and 1946.

In 1985, the epidemic had reached such proportions that scientists, politicians, educators, physicians and concerned individuals started to meet at the International AIDS conference, the most important meeting about AIDS in the world. Though the meetings were quite small at first, over the years they had grown so large that they decided to have it every 2 years. This conference and many other well-publicized AIDS events have served to educate the public regarding AIDS. One such device is the AIDS quilt. It is made up of panels (each one the size of a grave), each one commemorating someone who died of AIDS. In 1987 it was displayed on the mall in D.C. and covered 2 football fields. It had 1,920 panels and took less than 2 hours to read. In 1999, the quilt weighted 55 tons, with 46,000 panels containing 79,000 names. It covers 25 football fields. It is the largest piece of folk art in the world. It was the idea of Cleve Jones of San Francisco. Every day, more panels arrive to be added to the quilt [3].

Isolation of the HIV, the Causative Agent of AIDS [3]

In January 1983, Dr. Luc Montagnier and his colleagues at the Pasteur Institute in France isolated the AIDS virus. In May of that year, they published the first report on a T-cell retrovirus found in a patient with lymphadenopathy (which is one of the early signs of progression to AIDS). He named it LAV, lymphadenopathy-associated virus. Robert Gallo also claimed to have found the virus which, indeed, he had. But it was from a mixture of viruses which had accidentally been contaminated with the virus that Montagnier had sent to his lab. Genetic tests eventually showed that Gallo's virus (HTLV III, human T-cell leukaemia virus type III) was the same virus as Montagnier's. Because of this, the two countries (US and France) negotiated an agreement in which credit was shared between the two men, as well as royalties. Nevertheless, most people outside the US as well as many people in the US give credit to Montagnier (Figure 10-2). Several years after the discovery, there was an investigation into Gallo's lab practices and he was censured. Ultimately, he appealed the censure and it was overturned [3].

Here is the account from another website [4].

In 1984, Gallo and his collaborators published a series of four papers in the research journal *Science* arguing that HIV, a retrovirus that had recently been identified in AIDS patients by Luc Montagnier and his collaborators at the Pasteur Institute in Paris, France, was the cause of AIDS. However, the striking similarity between the first two human immunodeficiency virus type 1 (HIV-1) isolates Lai/LAV (formerly LAV, isolated at the Pasteur Institute) and Lai/IIIB (formerly HTLV-IIIB, reported to be isolated from a pooled culture at the Laboratory of Tumour Cell Biology (LTCB) of the National Cancer Institute), suggested contamination in Gallo's lab and provoked controversy in light of the high level of variability found among subsequent HIV-1 isolates.

Since then, there has been considerable and sometimes acrimonious controversy over the priority for the discovery of HIV, including accusations that Gallo's lab improperly used a sample of HIV produced at the Institut Pasteur. In November 1990, the Office of Scientific Integrity at the National Institutes of Health commissioned a group at Roche to analyze archival samples established at the Pasteur Institute and the Laboratory of Tumour Cell Biology (LTCB) of the National Cancer Institute between 1983 and 1985. Retrospective analyses showed that contamination of a culture derived from patient BRU by one from patient LAI was responsible for the provenance of HIV-1 Lai/LAV; the contaminated culture (M2T-/B) was sent to LTCB in September 1983.

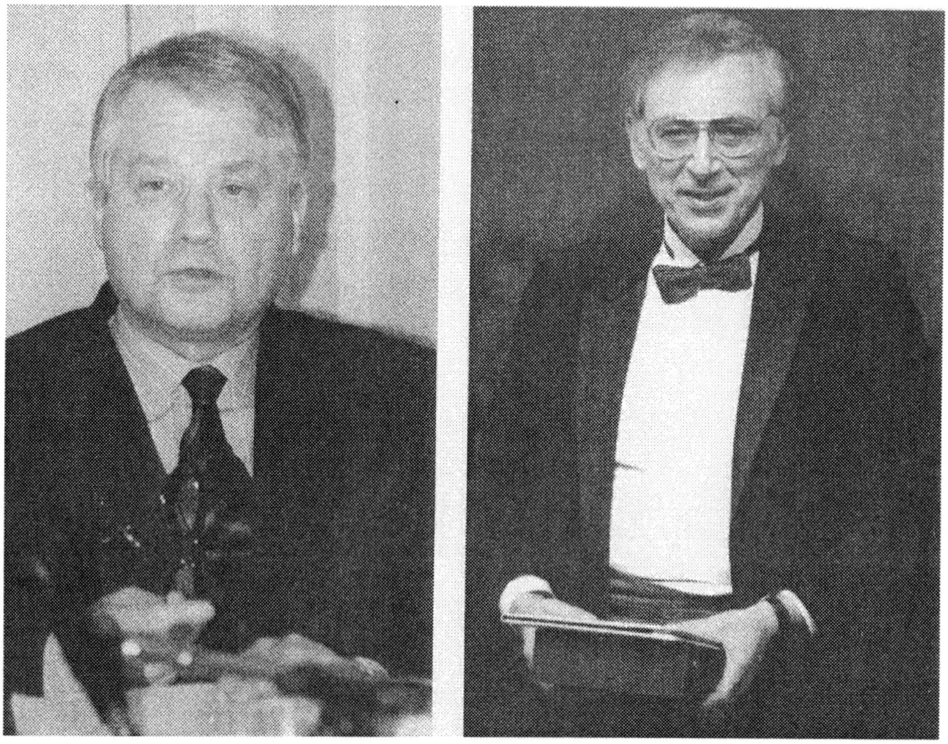

Figure 10-2. Drs. Luc Montagnier of France (left), and Robert Gallo of the US. Were they co-discoverers of the AIDS virus? [3].

Chang et al. (1993) examined archival specimens and reported in *Nature* the detection of six novel HIV-1 sequences in the cultures used to establish the pool: none was closely related to HIV-1 Lai/IIIB. A sample derived from patient LAI contained variants of both HIV-1 Lai/IIIB and HIV-1 Lai/LAV, and a sequence identical to a variant of HIV-1 Lai/IIIB was detected in the contaminated M2T-/B culture. They concluded that the pool, and probably another LTCB culture, MoV, were contaminated between October 1983 and early 1984 by variants of HIV-1 Lai from the M2T-/B culture. Contamination of this kind is common in labs handling viruses, and must be carefully guarded against. In this case, the origin of the HIV-1 Lai/IIIB isolate also was patient LAI.

Today it is generally agreed that Montagnier's group first identified HIV, although Gallo's group is credited with much of the science that made the discovery possible, and to demonstrating that it causes AIDS. Gallo's group also was the first to grow the virus in an immortalized cell line, leading to the development of blood tests for HIV and the ability to screen donated blood for this virus. Also, Gallo insisted the work of Montagnier had relied on a technique previously developed by Gallo for growing T cells in the laboratory by supplementing *interleukin-2*. The two scientists continued to be at the centre of a bitter dispute between the United States and France over royalties from the blood test patent until 1987, when they agreed to share credit for the discovery of HIV. In the November 29, 2002, issue of *Science*, Gallo and Montagnier published a series of articles, one of which was co-written by both scientists, in which they acknowledged the pivotal roles that each had played in the discovery of HIV [4].

Another website [5] says:

Indeed, in January of 1983 Professor Jean-Claude Chermann, internationally renowned retro-virologist and Director of the Retrovirus Laboratory at Institut Pasteur, France, was the first scientist to isolate the AIDS virus, along with his assistant, Françoise Barre-Sinoussi (at that time, Professor Chermann was the director of her thesis). This discovery was done in a laboratory which was attached to the Viral Oncology Unit led by Professor Luc Montagnier.

The honours were initially shared by the three researchers. But, with time, the press and other media only remembered the name of Luc Montagnier, even though the role of Jean-Claude Chermann was essential.

There are not two but three co-discoverers of the AIDS virus. This is corroborated by undeniable facts:

1. The publication of the AIDS virus discovery in the journal *Science*, num 220, dated 20 May 1983:

The first two names are Barre-Sinoussi and Chermann, while Montagnier comes in the twelfth and last position. In a scientific article, this last place is usually for the head of the laboratory. The first two or three places are for the authors who actually did the work described in the article.

2. In every patent, Professor Chermann is cited as co-discoverer:

* In patent # EP0138667 of 24 April 1985 (Method for the Diagnosis of Lymphadenopathy and Acquired Immune Depression Syndrome) the author order is (1) L. Montagnier, (2). J.-C. Chermann, (3) F. Barre-Sinoussi.

* In international patent # AT69650T (Verfahren zur Diagnose von Lymphadenopathie und von Erworbenemimmunddepressionssyndrom)registered by Institut Pasteur on 15 December 1991, Professor Cherman is as well in second position, as inventor.

3. Jean-Claude Chermann was with Luc Montagnier and Francoise Barre-Sinoussi one of the signatories of the Franco-American Agreement of 31 March 1987.

When Prime Minister Jacques Chirac and President Ronald Reagan signed, on 31 March 1987, a compromise giving the discovery of the AIDS virus - and its financial impact - both to France and the United States, the signature of Jean-Claude Chermann was required to valid this treaty.

Against his will, because he did not accept to offer half of the discovery to the U.S., he was forced to affix his signature by the director of the Institut Pasteur. For this reason, he resigned from that institute.

4. Professor Gallo cited Jean-Claude Chermann as the discoverer of the AIDS virus. Speaking of the cytopathic effects of the virus, Dr. Gallo said this to Science magazine: "We just didn't believe that is what this kind of virus could do ... It is certainly true that in that period of time in summer and certainly by early fall (1983), Chermann had recognized the cytopathic effect of that virus and I had not ... As I look back now, I could bang my head against a wall that we were so stubborn in trying to grow those cells long term in IL-2 ... We went through loss of months with that problem" (230, 1985; p. 520) [5].

Diagnosis of HIV/AIDS [3]

Initial diagnosis is by seroconversion. Most people seroconvert within 6–18 weeks. By 6 months, 99 percent of all individuals have seroconverted. Once the initial diagnosis has been made, patients (PWAs) are referred to AIDS specialists (if at all possible) for careful monitoring on an ongoing basis for T-cell count and viral load. A useful indicator developed by David Baltimore is the viral RNA circulating in the bloodstream. This is easily determined via PCR and is directly proportional to viral load, which is much more difficult to assess. Therefore, you often see graphs which have viral RNA as the indicator, rather than virus. The physician carefully monitors these two indicators to determine how to administer the anti-AIDS drugs [3].

Prevalence and Epidemiology of HIV/AIDS [3]

In the US

AIDS is currently the 14th leading cause of death, lagging far behind heart disease and cancer. The major at-risk groups are homosexual/bisexual males and intravenous drug users, though heterosexual contact constitutes a significant and growing percentage.

AIDS is still largely a disease of men. The majority of people who have contracted AIDS have died (60%).

The disease is disproportionately represented in black and Asian ethnic groups. Because of increased awareness about the mode of transmission and changing lifestyles, the rate of infection has decreased, but is still very significant at approximately 50,000 people per year. Only 1% of AIDS-infected individuals reside in the U.S.

In the World

There are approximately 60 million people with AIDS. The vast majority of these are in sub-Saharan Africa. Nearly 40% of babies born in this region are born with HIV. It is rampant, particularly in Africa, but must compete for notoriety with malaria, TB, and measles, all of which are major killers in these populations. AIDS has become a disease of the poor.

The spread of AIDS is much different from the US, with 70% of it being from heterosexual intercourse, 8% from IV drug use, 9% from perinatal causes, and 3 percent from blood transfusion. Women have a much higher chance of becoming infected from unprotected sex. This is because during sex women are exposed to semen carrying lymphocytes (whereas men have limited contact with vaginal fluids), the mucosal surface available for HIV penetration is much larger in women, it is much more likely for the tissue lining the vagina to be torn and abraded than the urethral tissue, and there are many more HIV-infected men than women (in developed countries it's about 6:1) [3].

Transmission of HIV/AIDS [3]

AIDS is transmitted by close contact with bodily fluids and secretions. It can not be transmitted by casual contact or by insect bite. The proof for this is that many people have lived with HIV-positive individuals (family members) and, except for several instances which had explanations (nosebleeds, sharing razors, bloody fight between brothers), not one person has contracted AIDS. In addition, scientists have shown that HIV cannot survive the harsh conditions of the insect gut. AIDS is not transmitted by fomites. There is, however, one documented case of HIV transmission by kissing. This is likely to be because HIV is present in saliva at low concentrations.

The accepted modes of spread are by sexual intercourse, direct injection with HIV-contaminated drugs-needles, etc., and from HIV-infected mother to fetus in utero, during childbirth, from mother to infant, or during breastfeeding. Even if exposed in this way, it is not a foregone conclusion that a person will contract AIDS. This depends on several characteristics of donor, recipient, and portal of entry, but the most important variables appear to be viral load, which subtype and variant of HIV, and the recipient's genetic resistance. By far the largest two modes of transmission are men having sex with men and IV drug use. The efficiency of transmission is greater than 90% for blood transfusion, 20–40% for perinatal transmission and approximately 1% for IV drug use and intercourse. This demonstrates that HIV is not particularly effective at infecting an individual. There are many other indications to this effect. Paul Michael Glaser had normal sexual relations with his wife for 5 years prior to her being diagnosed with AIDS. While their first-born became infected, he did not. Approximately 50% of people who have regular sex with HIV-infected people do not contract the disease. This is not a license for unprotected sex, however. Condoms have been shown to be highly effective at containing the spread of HIV.

Characteristics of HIV [3]

HIV (Figure 10-3) is a retrovirus of the subfamily Lentivirinae. The virus contains an enveloped icosahedral helical capsid, which contains two identical RNA molecules.

These RNA molecules are positive in polarity. The virus possesses a reverse transcriptase, and integrase, as well as other proteins.

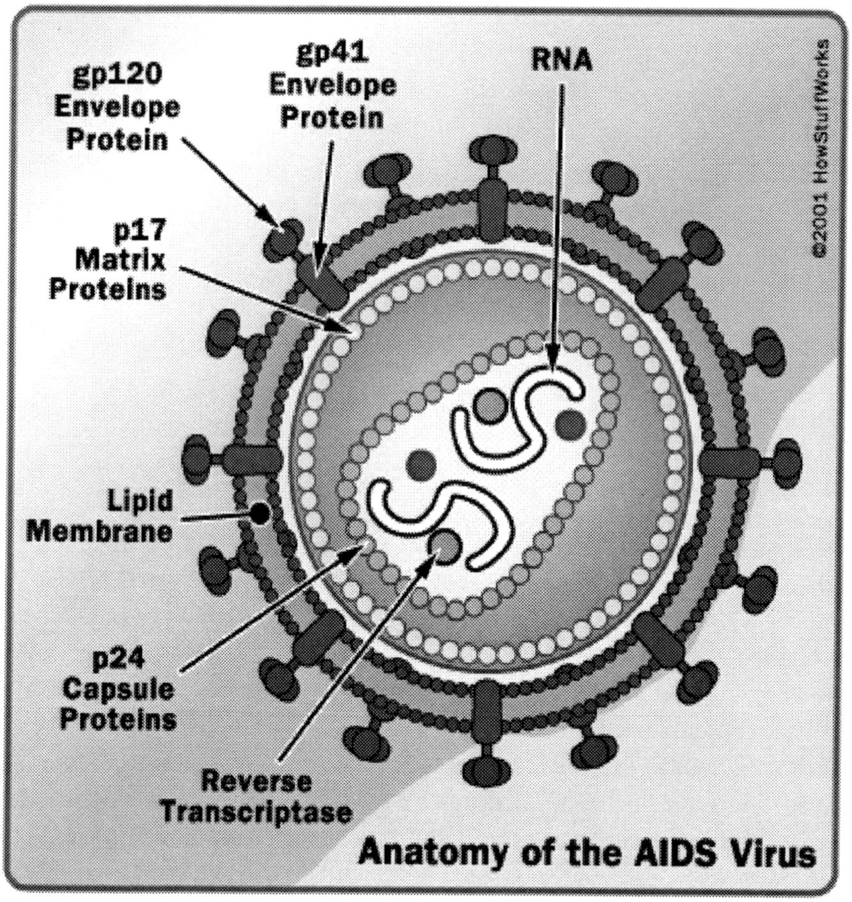

Figure 10-3. Anatomy of the HIV (from a website).

After entering the cell by membrane fusion, the virus RNA is transcribed to a DNA copy. This DNA migrates to the nucleus where it is integrated into the host chromosome via the viral integrase enzyme. There are two distinct phases of transcription. In the early phase, RNA strands or transcripts produced in the cell's nucleus are snipped into multiple copies of shorter sequences by cellular splicing enzymes. When these reach the cytoplasm, they are only about 2,000 nucleotides in length. These early transcripts encode the virus's regulatory proteins. In the second phase of transcription, two new size classes of RNA (long and medium [singly spliced]) are made and go to the cytoplasm. The medium transcripts encode the structural proteins. The long transcripts (full size) become the encapsulated genome. HIV encodes nine genes that are put into three classes, 1) Gag, Pol, and Env – the 3 major structural proteins, 2) Tat, and Rev – two regulatory proteins, and 3) Nef, Vif, Vpu, and Vpr – four accessory proteins.

Genes of the HIV-1 [3]

S/No.	Name(s)	Molecular mass (kDa)	Function
1	GAG (group antigen)	p17 p24 p9, p6	Matrix (protection) Capsid (protection) Nucleocapsid (protection)
2	POL (polymerase)	p10 p31 p50	Protease (enzyme) Endonuclease (enzyme) Reverse transcriptase (enzyme)
3	ENV (envelope)	gp120 gp41	Surface envelope Transmembrane envelope
4	tat (transactivator protein)*	p14	Transactivation of all HIV proteins
5	rev (differential regulator of expression of virus protein)	p13	Increase production of structural HIV protein; transport of spliced/unspliced RNA from nucleus to cytoplasm
6	vif (virus infectivity factor)	p23	Required for infectivity as cell-free virus
7	nef (negative regulator factor)	p27	Retards HIV replication
8	vpr (virus protein R)	?	Triggers cells steroid production to produce HIV
9	vpu (virus protein U)	p16	Required for efficient viral replication and release-budding

*Transactivator gene - the product of their genes influences the function of genes some distance away

Pathophysiology Of HIV/AIDS [3]

HIV primarily infects CD4+ T cells (i.e., T cells that have a CD4+ receptor). To some extent monocytes and macrophages can also be infected (Figures 10-4 and 10-5). HIV binds to the CD4+ receptor and subsequently to the CCKR5 co-receptor (whose normal function is a chemokine receptor). It then enters the cell by fusion with the plasma membrane. It uncoats and the reverse transcriptase makes a DNA copy, which is subsequently used as a template to make a double-stranded DNA (Figures 10-6 and 10-7).

One to three weeks after infection most patients exhibit a brief glandular fever-like illness, which is associated with a high titre of virus in the blood and a decline in CD4+ T cells. A vigorous cellular and humoral immune response commences and within a month or so the viraemia declines to near undetectable levels.

CD8+ cytotoxic T cells, natural killer cells and antibody-dependent cell mediated cytotoxicity may all contribute to this decline by lysing infected cells, while neutralizing antibodies may mop up free virions. After the initial phase, there is a long asymptomatic period of clinical latency, lasting anywhere from 1 to 15 years. During this period, only low titres of virus are demonstrable in blood and only a small number of circulating T cells are infected. However, ten times higher levels are detected in lymph nodes. As time passes there is a steady decline in CD4+ T cells.

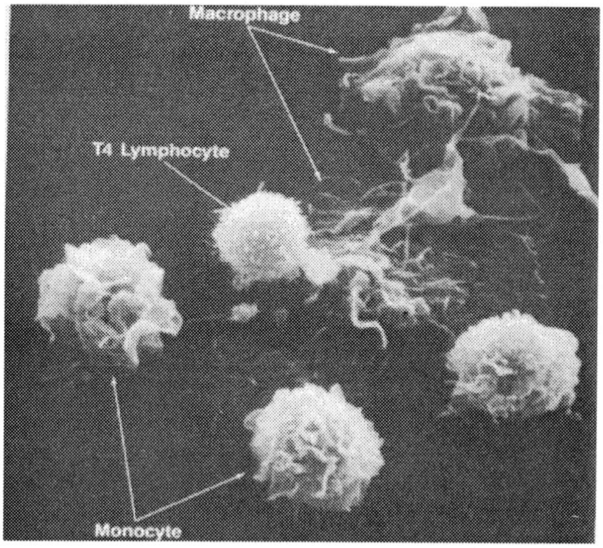

Figure 10-4. Scanning electron micrograph of normal human T4 lymphocytes, monocytes and macrophages magnified x 9,000. T4 white blood cells are the targets of HIV infection. Note that the T4 lymphocyte (round cell at the centre) is adhered to a flattened macrophage. (Photograph courtesy of Dr. M.A. Gonda) [3].

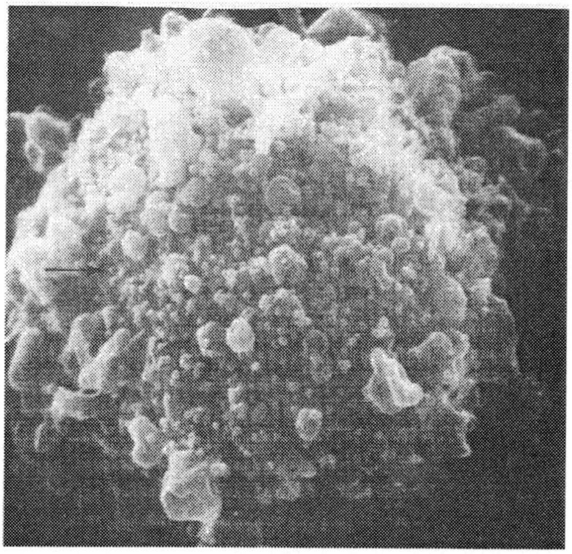

Figure 10-5. Electron micrograph of an HIV-infected T4 lymphocyte. The T cell has produced a large number of HIVs that are located over the entire lymphocyte. Each HIV leaves a hole in the cell membrane. The photograph shows part of the convoluted surface of the lymphocyte magnified 20,000 times. (Courtesy of the National Biological Standards Board, South Mimms, U.K. and David Hockley) [3].

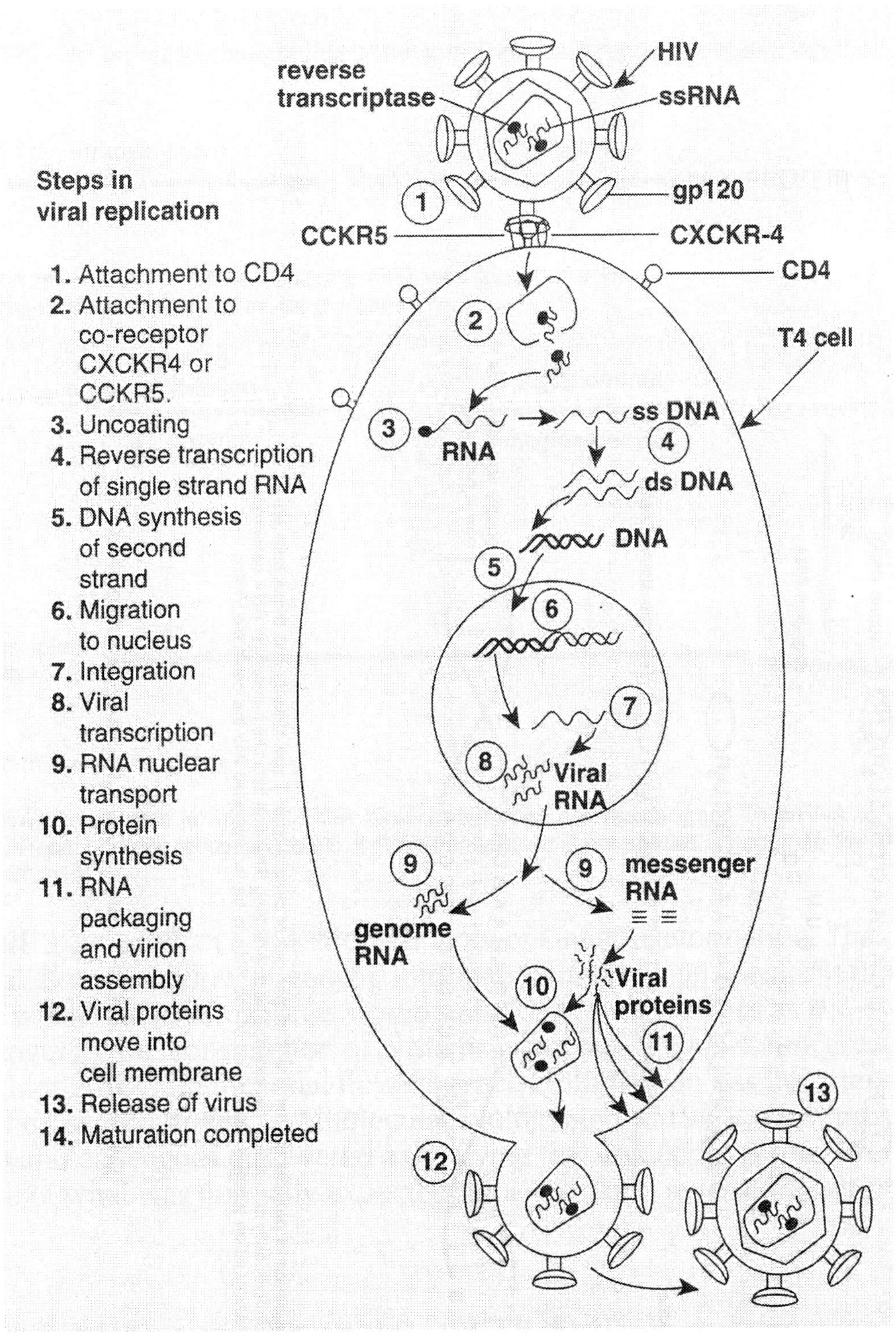

Figure 10-6. The replication cycle of the HIV [3].

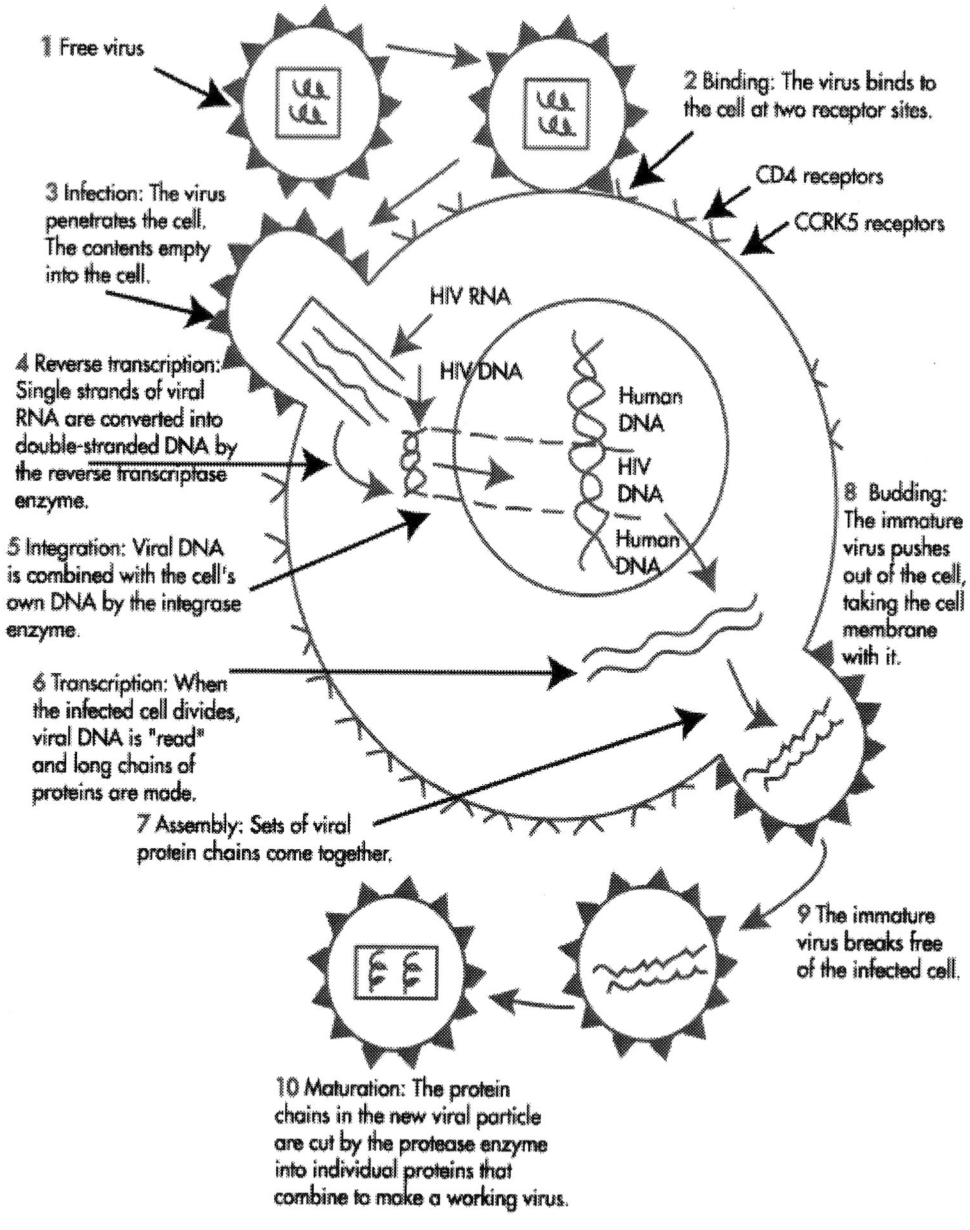

Figure 10-7. The Life Cycle of the HIV (from a website).

When the T cell count falls below 200-400/μL, opportunistic infections with various microorganisms may occur, and eventually the depleted immune system is unable to cope. Activation of CD4+ T cells renders them permissive for HIV replication, and other viruses such as HHV-6, CMV, HTLV, and hepatitis B virus. Death is a result of these and other infections, malignancy, or a cachexia-like state. The average asymptomatic period is 11 years (Figure 10-8).

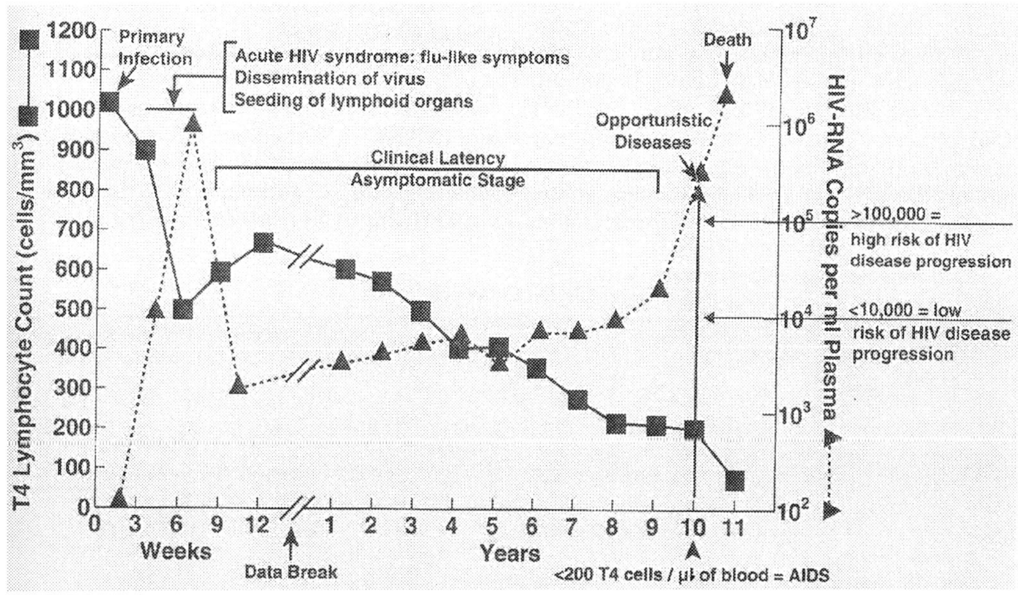

Figure 10-8. Clinical Course of HIV disease as related to T4 cell count and level (number) of HIV RNA copies (viral load) in plasma. During primary infection (the time period between infection and development of HIV antibody), HIV RNA levels spike (triangles) and HIV disseminates (spreads) throughout the body. This is followed by an abrupt drop in measurable HIV RNA in the blood (probably due to the production of HIV antibody), followed by a steady rise in HIV RNA until death. Over these same time periods, there is a continuous loss of T4 cells (squares). Note that the asymptomatic stage can be quite long – on average about 10 to 12 years, at which time T4 cell counts drop and HIV RNA copies increase to levels where there is high risk of opportunistic infections [3].

The Long Chronicity of HIV Infection

One of the more important questions about HIV is 'why does it take so long to cause the disease?' After all, within a few weeks of infection there can be a high viral titre in the blood. The answer, it turns out, is quite complex and not well understood. Many scientists think that the progression to AIDS is a monumental struggle between the HIV and the immune system. In the beginning the immune system is primed and reduces the virus to negligible levels. However, it is not able to totally eradicate the virus because HIV has the advantage of being able to enter the proviral state and exist as nothing more than DNA inside a cell. It does not replicate in resting T cells and prefers to sequester itself in the lymph nodes and not show itself in the bloodstream. Because of this, it can exist for long periods of time. It also has the advantage of being able to move from one cell to another by syncytia formation, thereby evading the immune system. Over a period of time, the virus slowly wins the race and defeats the immune system by destruction of T cells. This is quite noticeable in lymph nodes, which can be nothing but ravaged hulks by the end of the disease.

The mode of destruction of T cells is not exactly known, but there are many theories. They include:

- The virus may leave some of its spike attached to the CD4+ receptor, thereby impairing T-cell function.
- Syncytia formation
- HIV may act as a super antigen, which has the effect of depleting T-cell populations.
- HIV may trigger apoptosis.
- HIV may kill the cell by replication.
- HIV may trick the immune system to kill its own T4 cells (autoimmunity).
- Co-factors (such as HHV-6) may aid in T-cell killing.

One of the more interesting AIDS episodes occurred when two gay men came to the National Institutes of Health, NIH and told the researchers that they had had frequent and unprotected sex, yet they were still HIV-negative. They offered themselves as research models. Scientists determined that these men had a mutation in the CCKR5 co-receptor gene (R-5). Therefore, HIV could not easily enter their T cells [3].

Treatment of HIV/AIDS [3]

Evaluation of drugs is usually done on the basis of an increase in T4 or CD4+ cell number or a reduction in viral load. However, because of day-to-day variability, these are imperfect indicators (but the best we have). In particular, viral load is important because it dictates the aggressiveness of the treatment. In the last 13 years (1987-2000), 15 drugs have received US FDA approval. These fall into 4 general classes, nucleoside reverse transcriptase inhibitors, non-nucleoside reverse transcriptase inhibitors, protease inhibitors, and others.

The side effects of these drugs range from anaemia, nausea, headache and inhibition of mitochondrial DNA replication, peripheral neuropathy (burning pain in hands and feet), pancreatitis, mouth ulcers and hair loss.

For a short time it was thought that antiretroviral drugs (ARVs) could be made more effective by using them in a multidrug cocktail. While this does increase their efficacy slightly, in the end the result is the same.

It is expensive to bring new drugs to market!! Merck estimates that they spent $1,000,000,000 over 10 years to bring Crixivan to market. Recently, it has been found that Crixivan loses its efficacy and has more side effects than a newer competitor... so it is likely that it will not be used within a few years time.

The average cost of protease inhibitors on the market is about $600 per month. Protease inhibitor side effects are different for each drug, but range from rash diarrhoea, stomach discomfort, anorexia, headaches, fatigue, and kidney stones.

Combination Therapy [3]

Though each drug has its failing, if these drugs are used in combination (for instance, a protease inhibitor, a nucleoside analogue, and a non-nucleoside analogue), they can produce significant results, rescuing people from the brink of death. In one instance the viral load went from 98,600 copies per ml of serum to undetectable within 2 weeks.

Combination therapy is based on simple probability. If there is a 1 in 100,000 chance of the virus developing resistance to a single drug, then there is a 100,000 X 100,000 chance (1/10,000,000,000) of a virus developing resistance to two drugs, and a 100,000 X 100,000 X 100,000 chance of a virus developing resistance to three drugs. The cost, however, is significant and substantial. The patients must adhere to a strict regimen of pills (anywhere from 10 to 72 pills per day). If they miss a pill, it can severely hurt their therapy. If they take a pill too early or take too much, it can cause debilitating side effects. The monetary cost is also daunting. For a person that is HIV-positive, but has not yet shown additional symptoms the cost may be approximately $20,000 per year. For a person that has AIDS, the cost may go as high as $150,000 per year. The acronym given for this type of combination therapy is HAART (Highly Active Antiretroviral Therapy).

Anecdotal story: A recovering patient in San Francisco had no measurable HIV in his blood for the 89 weeks he was on the protease inhibitor-AIDS cocktail. He decided to stop the drug therapy; the virus became measurable within 1 week [3].

HIV/AIDS Prevention [3]

Common Sense

HIV Vaccine

No vaccine has yet made it through Phase III trials, and there is only one candidate even in Phase III (AIDSVAX). The primary issues appear to be that cellular immunity is much more important for HIV destruction than previously thought. Most vaccines focus on initiating antibody production. Moreover, HIV mutates very rapidly, overcoming the antibody response. Many of the early vaccines did not stimulate the cellular response strongly enough.

Currently, there are approximately 60 vaccine candidates in various stages of testing [3].

The Continent, not Country of Africa

The author has just remembered that the incumbent Governor of the US State of Alaska Sarah Palin was the Republican vice Presidential candidate in the 2008 Presidential elections. During the election campaign, she referred to Africa as a country! It has just dawned on the author that there may be some others like her who need to be given some basic information about Africa, sub-Saharan Africa and /or Nigeria that are mentioned several times in this Chapter and elsewhere in this book.

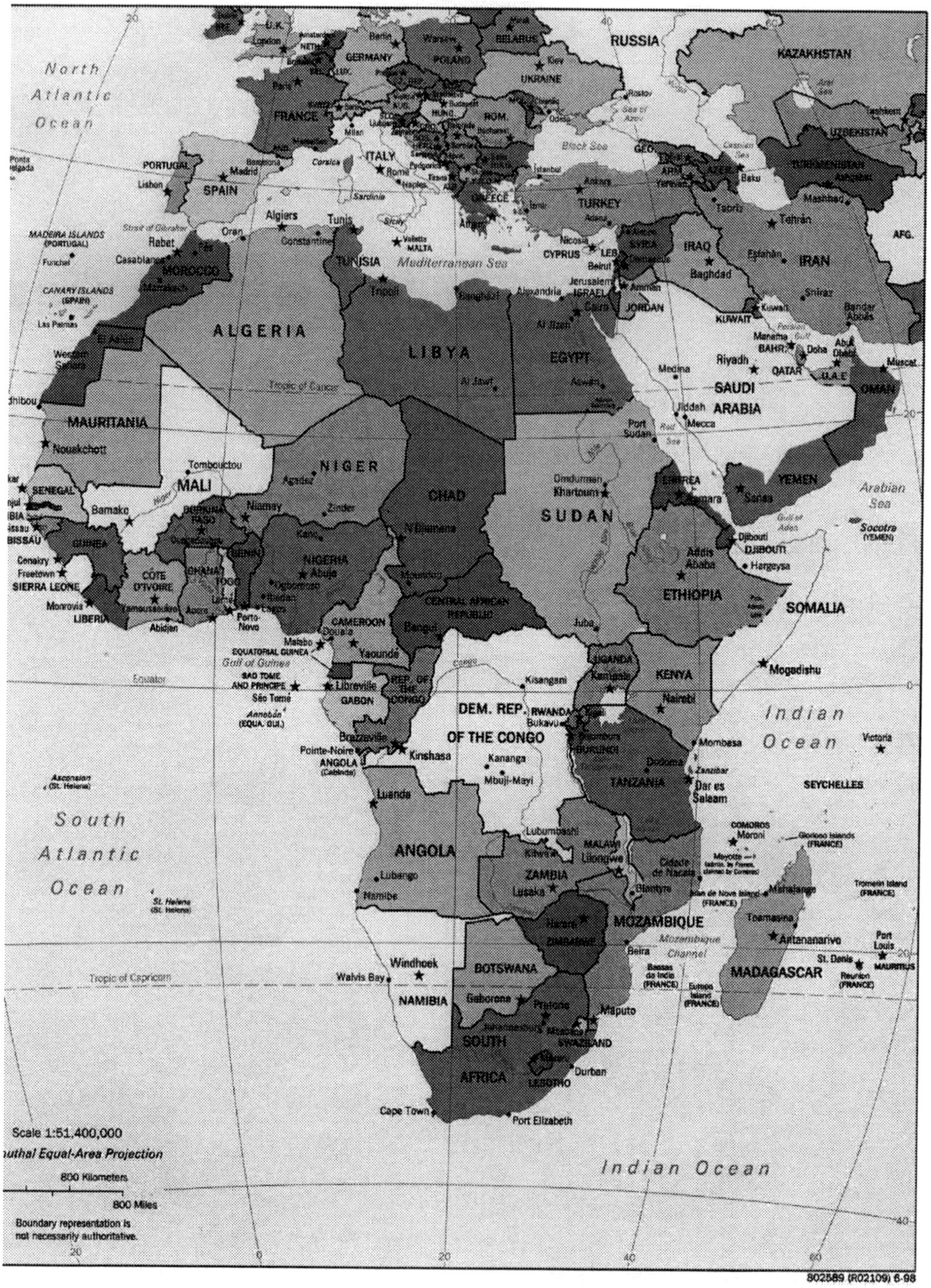

Figure 10-9: A map of Africa showing countries and adjoining countries in Europe and Middle East [5]

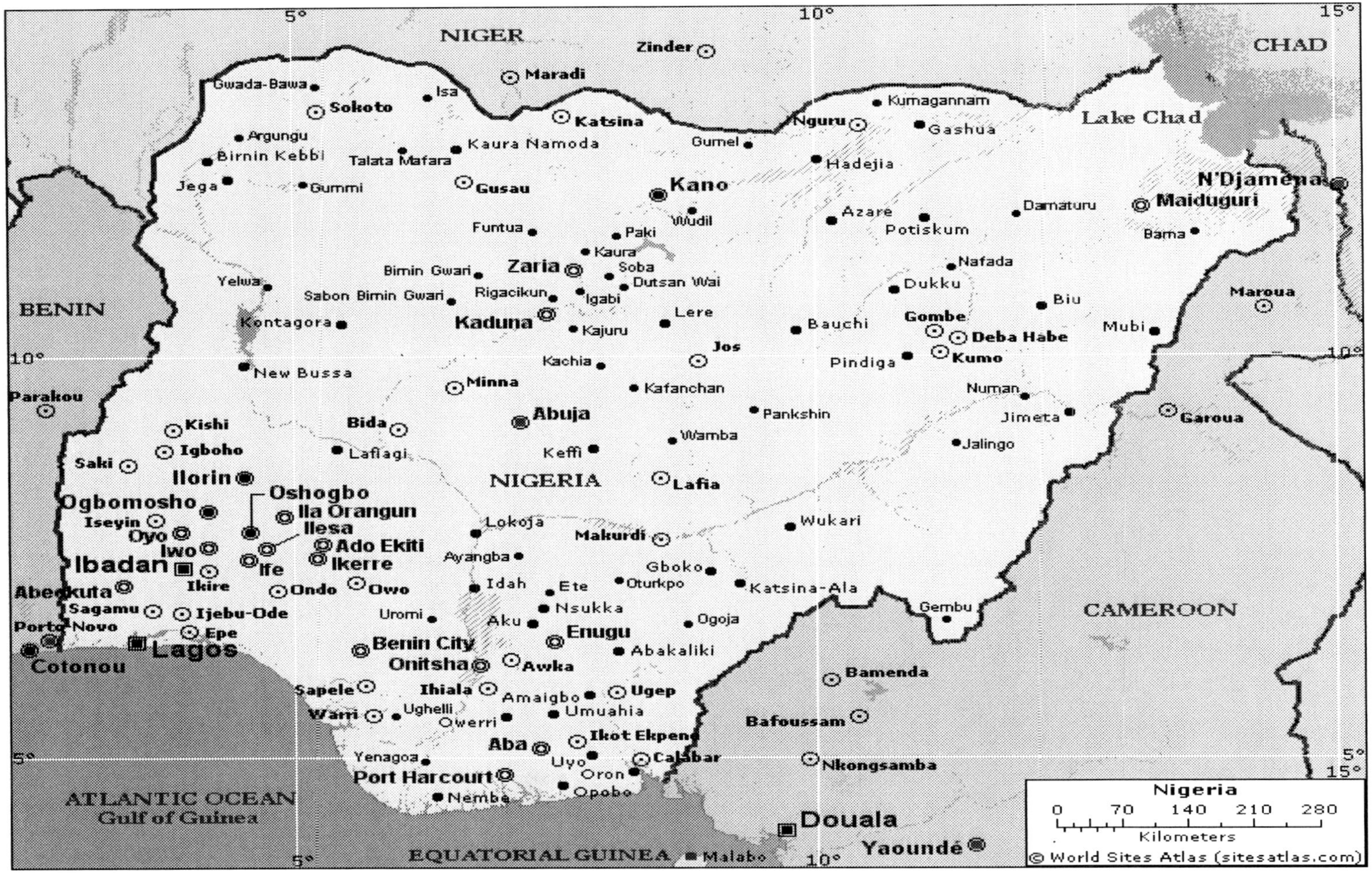

Figure 10-10: Political Map of Nigeria [6]

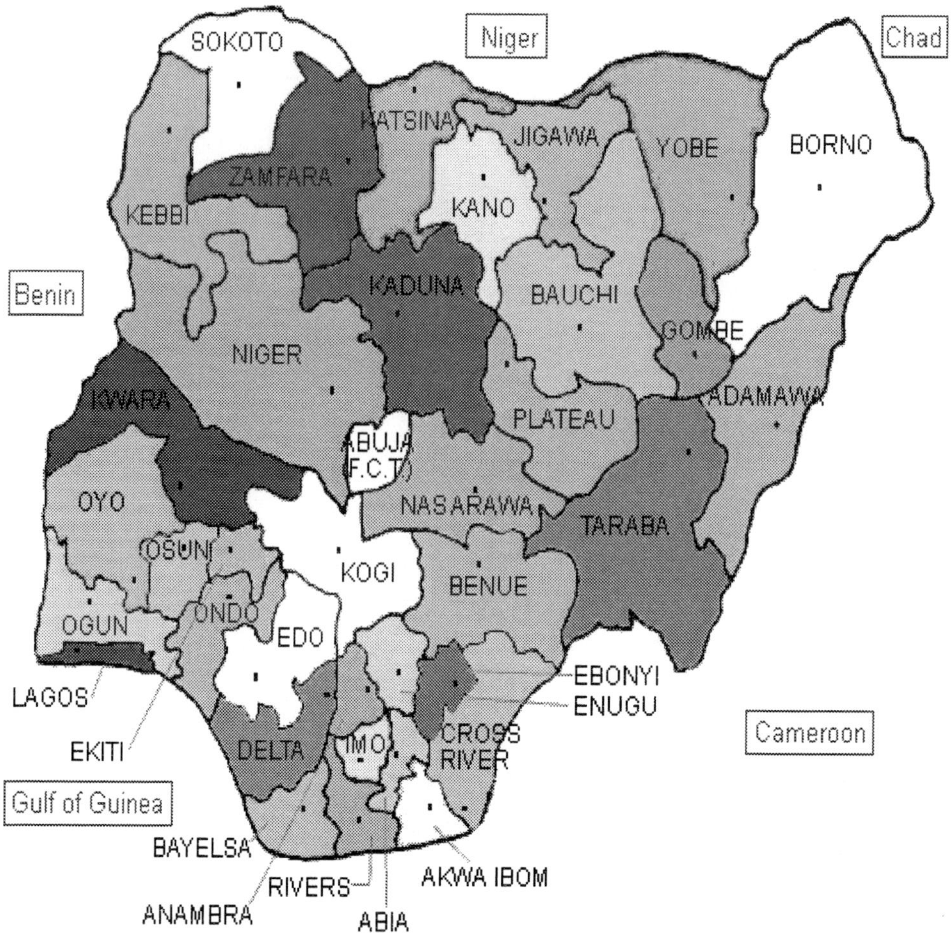

Figure 10-11: Nigeria's 36 States and the Federal Capital Territory (FCT) of Abuja [7]

The continent of Africa lies between longitudes 20^0 W and 50^0 E and between latitudes 37^0 N and 36^0 S (Figure 10-9). Africa consists of more than 40 countries [5]. The author's country Nigeria [6, 7] is Africa's most populated country; officially, its current estimated population is about 150 million. Nigeria is the most eastern country in the West African sub-region. It consists of 36 States and the centrally located Federal Capital Territory (FCT) of Abuja (Figures10-10 and 10-11). Readers should feel free to refer to these figures from time to time as they read this book.

The 2008 Nobel Prize for Medicine

As shown earlier in this chapter, a website [8] states emphatically that Chermann, Barre-Sinousse and Montagnier (Figure 10-12) co-discovered the AIDS virus at the Pasteur Institut in Paris in 1983.

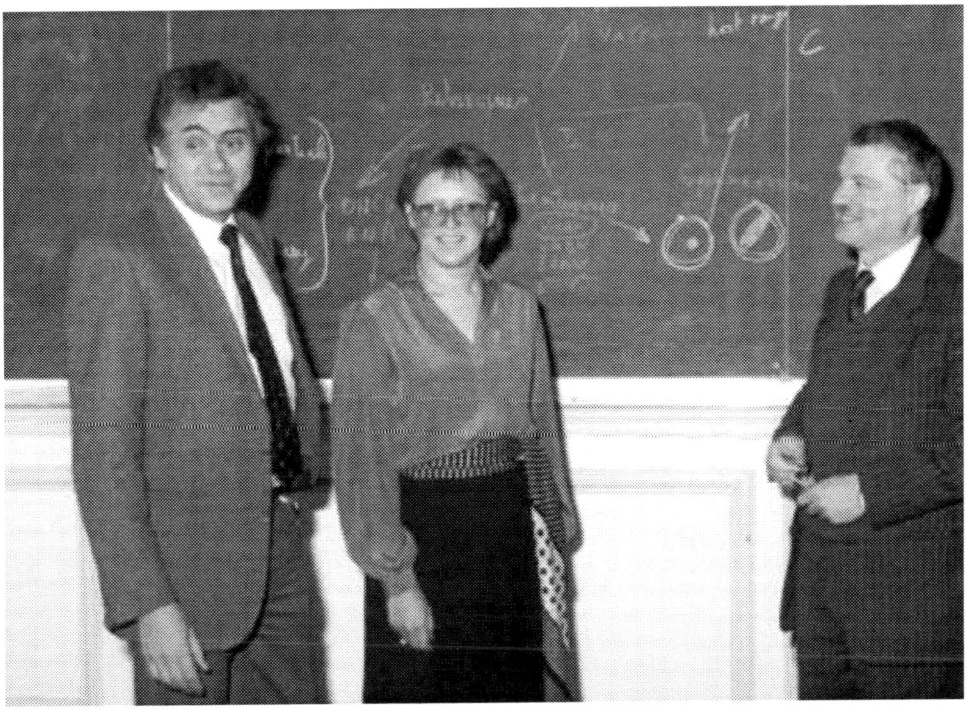

Figure 10-12: From L, Chermann, Barr-Sinoussi and Montagnier, the three discoverers of the AIDS virus in the office of Professor Chermann at Institut Pasteur in 1983. The notes on blackboard had been written by Chermann [5]

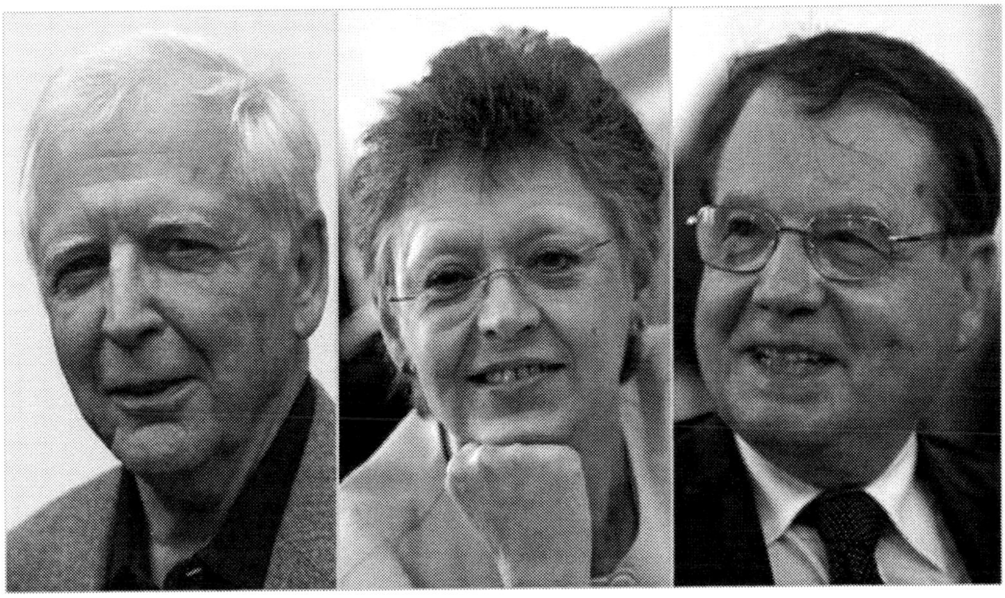

Figure10-13: The winners of the 2008 Nobel Prize for Medicine. From left: Dr. Harald zur Hausen, 72, of Germany, and French virologists Dr. Françoise Barré-Sinoussi, 61, and Dr. Luc Montagnier, 76 [6].

On October 6, 2008, the Nobel Prize for Medicine was announced. The following articles from the web give the details.

Discoverers of AIDS and Cancer Viruses Win Nobel
By Lawrence K. Altman
Published: October 7, 2008 (Tuesday)

The Nobel Prize in Medicine was awarded Monday (October 6, 2008) to three European scientists who had discovered viruses behind two devastating illnesses, AIDS and cervical cancer.

Half of the award will be shared by two French virologists, Françoise Barré-Sinoussi, 61, and Luc A. Montagnier, 76, for discovering H.I.V., the virus that causes AIDS (Figure 10-13). Conspicuously omitted was Dr. Robert C. Gallo, an American virologist who vied with the French team in a long, often acrimonious dispute over credit for the discovery of H.I.V.

The other half of the $1.4 million award will go to a German physician-scientist, Dr. Harald zur Hausen, 72, for his discovery of H.P.V., or the human papilloma virus. Dr. zur.Hausen (Figure 10-13) of the German Cancer Research Center in Heidelberg "went against current dogma" by postulating that the virus caused cervical cancer, said the Karolinska Institute in Stockholm, which selects the medical winners of the prize, formally called the Nobel Prize in Physiology or Medicine.

His discovery led to the development of two vaccines against cervical cancer, the second most common cancer among women. An estimated 250,000 women die of cervical cancer each year, mostly in poor countries.

This year's Nobel Prize-winning research focused on two viruses that take many years to cause damage. Much of the research was carried out a quarter of a century or more ago.

Since its discovery in 1981, AIDS has rivalled the worst epidemics in history. An estimated 25 million people have died, and 33 million more are living with H.I.V.

In 1983, Dr. Montagnier and Dr. Barré-Sinoussi, a member of his lab at the Pasteur Institute in Paris, published their report of a newly identified virus. The Karolinska Institute said that discovery led to blood tests to detect the infection and to anti-retroviral drugs that can prolong the lives of patients. The tests are now used to screen blood donations, making the blood supply safer for transfusions and blood products.

The viral discovery has also led to an understanding of the natural history of H.I.V. infection in people, which ultimately leads to AIDS and death unless treated.

H.I.V. is a member of the lentivirus family of viruses. The French scientists were cited for identifying a virus they called L.A.V. (now known as H.I.V.) in lymph nodes from early and late stages of the infection.

"Never before has science and medicine been so quick to discover, identify the origin and provide treatment for a new disease entity," the Karolinska Institute said.

Reached by the Nobel committee in Abidjan, Ivory Coast, where he is attending an international AIDS conference, Dr. Montagnier said, "The fight is not finished" and he was now working on a way to eradicate H.I.V. in those already infected. Dr. Montagnier now works at the World Foundation for AIDS Research and Prevention in Paris. For a brief time in the late 1990s, he worked at Queens College in New York City.

Nobel Foundation rules limit the number of recipients of its medical prizes to a maximum of three each year, and omissions often create controversy.

The dispute between Dr. Gallo and the French team spanned years and sprawled from the lab into the highest levels of government. Dr. Gallo, 71, now at the University of Maryland in Baltimore, worked for many years at the National Cancer Institute in Bethesda, Md.

While in Bethesda in 1984, a year after the French team's report, Dr. Gallo reported finding a virus that he called H.T.L.V.-3 and that was later shown to be nearly identical to the French L.A.V. After additional studies, Dr. Gallo said cultures in his laboratory had accidentally become contaminated with the French virus.

In 1986, Dr. Gallo and Dr. Montagnier shared a prestigious Lasker award, given in the United States; Dr. Montagnier was cited for discovering the virus and Dr. Gallo for determining that it caused AIDS.

In 1987, President Reagan and Prime Minister Jacques Chirac of France signed an agreement to share royalties and credit for the discovery.

But Maria Masucci, a member of the Nobel Assembly, told Reuters on Monday that "there was no doubt as to who made the fundamental discoveries."

Dr. Gallo told The Associated Press on Monday that it was "a disappointment" not to have been honoured with the French team. Later, Dr. Gallo issued a statement congratulating this year's Nobel Prize winners and said he "was gratified to read Dr. Montagnier's kind statement this morning expressing that I was equally deserving."

Dr. John E. Niederhuber, the director of the National Cancer Institute, said Monday that Dr. Gallo "was instrumental in every major aspect of the discovery of the AIDS virus. Dr. Gallo discovered interleukein-2 (Il-2), an immune system signaling molecule, which was necessary for the discovery of the AIDS virus, serving as a co-culture factor that allowed the virus to grow. Numerous scientific journal articles, many co-authored by Dr. Gallo and Dr. Montagnier, cite the two scientists as co-discoverers of the AIDS virus."

Dr. Anthony S. Fauci, a virologist and immunologist who directs the National Institute of Allergy and Infectious Diseases, said in an interview, "The committee has a long history of awarding the prize to the person or group that makes the first seminal observation or discovery, and they did that in this case." He added, "Nobel Prizes are always associated with great joy and great sadness, depending on who wins and who you are."

The link between human papilloma virus and cervical cancer took years to gain acceptance. When Dr. zur Hausen proposed the connection in the 1970s, infection with papilloma virus was thought to cause nothing more serious than common warts, and the prevailing scientific view was that herpes type 2 virus caused cervical cancer. But Dr. zur Hausen consistently failed to find herpes type 2 DNA in cervical cancer cells using the newer molecular biology laboratory techniques.

In the 1980s, an American researcher said that financing agencies in the United States had rejected as unpromising his grant proposals to study links between papilloma viruses and cancer. The National Institutes of Health did not reply on Monday to questions about such proposals.

In 1983, Dr. zur Hausen discovered the first H.P.V., type 16, among biopsies of women who had cervical cancer. He went on to show that more than one H.P.V. type could lead to cervical cancer, in part by cloning H.P.V. 16 and another type, 18. Further research has shown that the two H.P.V. types are consistently found in about 70 percent of cervical cancer biopsies throughout the world, the institute said.

Of the more than 100 human papilloma viruses now known, about 40 infect the genital tract and 15 of them put women at high risk for cervical cancer. But in a vast majority of cases, the body's immune system clears H.P.V. before the viruses cause harm. It is chronic infection that is dangerous.

H.P.V. viruses account for more than 5 percent of all cancers worldwide. Some types of H.P.V. are found in cancers of the vulva, penis, mouth and other areas. Other H.P.V. viruses cause warts on the foot and elsewhere.

Dr. zur Hausen's research has led to development of vaccines that protect against strains of H.P.V. that cause most cases of cervical cancers. However, controversy has arisen over who should get the vaccines.

The United States Food and Drug Administration has approved one papilloma virus vaccine, Gardasil, for girls and women ages 9 to 26 and with advice that they get immunized before sexual activity begins. Because the vaccine was developed recently, doctors do not know for how long it will last.

The Nobel Prizes were created in the will of Alfred Nobel, the Swedish explosives inventor and manufacturer, who died in 1896. The first prizes were awarded in 1901 [9].

Morning Edition, October 6, 2008:

The 2008 Nobel Prize for physiology or medicine goes to two French scientists for discovering the virus that causes AIDS. A German researcher shares the prize for discovering the viruses that cause cervical cancer.

Half the $1.4 million prize goes to Luc Montagnier and Francoise Barre-Sinoussi for their discovery of the AIDS virus. The other half goes to Harald zur Hausen, who established that most cervical cancer is caused by two types of human papilloma viruses.

In the case of HIV, or the human immunodeficiency virus that causes AIDS, the Nobel committee clearly waited until the dust settled over a bitter controversy over who really discovered the virus in the early 1980s - Americans or the French. The committee apparently accepts the results of an investigation done 15 years ago, which concluded that the American virus was actually a contaminant from the French lab.

Zur Hausen's work with HPV led to highly effective new vaccines - among the first to protect against cancer [10].

Interviews with the Winners of the 2008 Nobel Prize for Medicine

Luc Montagnier

The Nobel Prize in Physiology or Medicine 2008

Interview: "We are still fighting this virus, very strongly, and the AIDS epidemic"

Telephone interview with Luc Montagnier immediately following the announcement of the 2008 Nobel Prize in Physiology or Medicine, 6 October 2008

The interview was recorded while Luc Montagnier was attending a conference in the Ivory Coast, and the interviewer is Adam Smith, Editor-in-Chief of Nobelprize.org.

[Unknown] Hallo.

[Adam Smith] Hello, is it possible to speak to Professor Montagnier yet?

[Unknown] Yes, I'm going to bring him to you, okay?

[AS] Thank you very much indeed.

[Unknown] If you can hold on

[AS] Yes, of course.

[Unknown] Thank you.

[AS] Thank you.

[Unknown] Professor ... Professor ... Professor. Sorry, there's so many people around him right now.

[AS] I can imagine.

[Unknown] Can you hear me?

[AS] I can hear you very well, yes, thank you.

[Luc Montagnier] Hallo.

[AS] Hello, Professor Montagnier, can you hear me?

[LM] Yes, speaking.

[AS] My name is Adam Smith. I'm calling from the Nobel Foundation web site. Congratulations on the award of the prize.

[LM] Thank you. Thank you very much.

[AS] And I understand you are in the Ivory Coast at the moment?

[LM] Yes, I'm in a meeting of the ... Hello?

[AS] Hello, yes?

[LM] I'm in a meeting on AIDS, which will be chaired by the President of the Republic of Ivory Coast, and he's going to arrive at any time now – we are waiting for him.

[AS] Okay, I won't take very long. Your discovery for which you have been awarded the Nobel Prize was made in 1983, and this is 25 years later.

[LM] Yes.

[AS] What do you think is the main message that you would like to send out after this award?

[LM] Well, the main message I will convey that even after 20 years we are still fighting this virus, very strongly, and the AIDS epidemic – I am now in an African country – is still spreading in Africa in [inaudible], so the fight is not finished. And I appreciate that the Nobel Committee has put on the air this important disease which is not finished, and my message is that we should continue the research. And myself I'm working on a vaccine – not a preventive vaccine but on a therapeutic vaccine which is aimed at completing the antiretroviral therapy which is now given to many patients even in Africa, but which does not cure. So the idea is to eradicate the virus infection. I think this is the main step now.

[AS] Yes, and what is the most urgent research need, do you think, in AIDS nowadays?

[LM] Well, the important research should be done on completing the treatments which are given to patients, for life. And I know that in Africa it's not possible to give a treatment for life. Because we give up before. So the idea is to buy a treatment which, like for tuberculosis, could be given for a short period of time – 6 to 9 months – and then stopped. And then vaccinate the people by a combination of viral protein, which I'm working on, so that the immune system of the host, of the person which is infected, will defend himself. Nature has shown us a few percent of people which are in this stage. They are infected, they are not sick. So the idea is to make most of these people, infected people, never sick, for life. So I think this would be very important, but I've tried to quantify all the forms of the virus. So I'm also working on that. There are probably some very small forms of the virus which escape [inaudible] and the immune system. So we have to identify those foremost. I think the AIDS epidemic is caused by a very old virus. And probably the virus was in Africa for a long period of time, as shown in some recent papers.

[AS] Yes.

[LM] But, what is new in Africa, like in the North America, is the epidemic. The AIDS epidemic started about the same time in Africa, in big cities, in Africa and North America. And we have to explain why. I think there are factors; I've been promoting a virical cofactor for a long time. But I'm beginning now to think those cofactors may act indirectly by inducing mutations – oxidative stress, free radicals which can induce mutations in the virus. What they have shown the virus is the enormous potential to change all the time. This is new, quite new, and was the cause of the epidemic. So we have to put back the virus in this Pandora's box, you know. And for that we have to not only find physically treatments but also improve the hygiene conditions, especially in Africa, and these conditions are so very important so that the immune system will be very active.

[AS] Yes. So my last question. If you remember the day on which you first saw reverse transcriptase activity in the cultured cells from patients. Did you have any idea on that day in 1983 of the size of epidemic that you might be looking at?

[LM] Well not in the beginning of course, no. I was actually working on a possible viral cause of breast cancer. I'm still interested in cancer virus so I appreciate that the Nobel Committee also has awarded the Prize to Harald zur Hausen who has worked for a long time on this. But, when I realised that the virus could be the cause of AIDS and was present not only in gay men in France and the United States, and haemophiliacs, but also in African nations – so this was in September 1983 – I realised it could be big, okay?

[AS] Yes, yes.

[LM] Okay.

[AS] Okay, thank you.

[LM] Thank you.

[AS] It's been a pleasure to speak to you.

[LM] Good bye.

[AS] Good luck. Good bye [11].

Françoise Barré-Sinoussi

The Nobel Prize in Physiology or Medicine 2008

Interview

"This success in the discovery of the AIDS virus is really a success of a world team with different expertise."

Telephone interview with Françoise Barré-Sinoussi immediately following the announcement of the 2008 Nobel Prize in Physiology or Medicine, 6 October 2008

The interview was recorded while Françoise Barré-Sinoussi was visiting Cambodia, and the interviewer is Adam Smith, Editor-in-Chief of Nobelprize.org.

[Françoise Barré-Sinoussi] Hello.

[Adam Smith] Ah, hello, Professor Barré-Sinoussi.

[FB-S] Yes.
[AS] This is Adam Smith from the Nobel Foundation web site.
[FB-S] Okay.
[AS] We have a tradition of recording very short telephone interviews with new Nobel Laureates after the award, so would you mind if we spoke very briefly?
[FB-S] No, not at all, that's fine.
[AS] Thank you. Many congratulations, of course, on the award.
[FB-S] Thank you.
[AS] I gather that you are in Cambodia, and how did you hear the news?
[FB-S] I got the news indeed by a journalist from the French radio, the national radio, who called me in the afternoon in Cambodia for an interview, and I didn't know about the news before.
[AS] And...
[FB-S] It was a big surprise.
[AS] I can imagine. It's, indeed, it's 25 years after the publication of those two papers in which you describe the first lentivirus found in humans. Looking back at those experiments where you first identified retroviral activity in – coming from the cells of – cultured from patients, do you remember the sense of excitement when you found that result?
[FB-S] Ah, you know, the excitement was really in different phases, because first it was the isolation of the virus from a patient that was with symptoms associated with AIDS, but he had no AIDS yet. And regulate the virus on lymph node. And, of course it was the surface fragment to get this virus out of the cell culture. But at this time, it was the first isolate only, and secondly we had to compare if the virus had any relationship with HTLV-1, which was the second retrovirus known at that time. And, we obtained reagents from Gallo's lab to compare, and the second excitement was when we realised that the cross-activity, as we say, with HTLV-1 was negative. That was really for us, telling us that it's not a known virus up to now. Then we had electron microscopy pictures showing that the morphology was different, and so on. So, it was, I would say, a progressive excitement. Also the fact that each time that we make an hypothesis; for example, of course, we hypothesized that the virus was targeting CD4+ T cells, and then make the experiment, and the answer was, yes, this virus has a tropism mostly for CD4+ T cells, and also was killing the CD4+ T cells. So, you know, all the evidences were really in favour of the virus. Then, we developed diagnostic tests to make several epidemiological studies, and found out that only patients that were with AIDS or with pre-AIDS had antibodies against this virus, and not patients with other disease, or blood donors. So, all the evidence were going together to the role of this virus in this newly identified disease. So, again, it's a step-by-step excitement phase, I would say.
[AS] And what gave you the idea of looking for a retrovirus in the first place; the original hypothesis?
[FB-S] First thing is because most of the virus family were already explored. For example, some scientists thought that it could be viruses related to hepatitis virus, or to cytomegalovirus, and so on. The – almost the only family that was not explored was retrovirus. Secondly, as I mentioned before, the only known retrovirus at that time was HTLV-1, and it was reported that HTLV could infect T-lymphocytes. And, of course in this disease, in AIDS, we knew that T-lymphocytes were affected in the disease, characterized by immune deficiency in the patients. Thirdly, I will say that we knew also from the literature that cats, when they are infected by a retrovirus, called feline leukaemia virus, most of the cats are dying from immune deficiency before dying of leukaemia. So, it was several line of arguments telling us that we should look for

retrovirus really. So the reason, since we were working on mammalian retroviruses at Pasteur at that time, we said, okay, look, we have all the reagents, we have the technique, and so let's try.
[AS] Yes, and the award of the Nobel Prize will focus attention on the discovery, and on AIDS in general. What would you like the message of the Prize to be? Is there anything in particular you would like people to note at this point?
[FB-S] The main message I will say today is, first of all, that this success in the discovery of the AIDS virus is really a success of a world team with different expertise. And I think, for the future, it's also important, especially when working on infectious disease, to have a world network of clinicians, virologists and microbiologists, working in the hospitals and basic sciences. This was really essential for me in the discovery of the AIDS virus. And I think it's essential also for tomorrow for discovering new, emerging, or re-emerging agents responsible for infectious disease.
[AS] And, you find yourself now in Cambodia, so how do you intend to celebrate the award of this Prize?
[FB-S] Right now I must say I'm very, very busy by different phone calls from the media. I'm at the Pasteur Institute in Cambodia, and we try to answer as much as we can. Then, I will probably leave Cambodia earlier to go back to France tomorrow night. And we will certainly celebrate with my own laboratory. We have already started to celebrate with our collaborators here in Cambodia. For me it's important that the announcement was made at the moment that I was in a developing country because I've been working with developing countries since the mid-1980s and it's really working with those countries that gives me another view, or another way, of orienting my research after the discovery of HIV/AIDS, of the HIV virus. It's important to really know what's going on in those countries strongly affected by these kinds of disease.
[AS] Yes, and I know your laboratory has many, many links with developing countries. So ...
[FB-S] That's right.
[AS] ... When you come to Stockholm to receive the award in December, perhaps we can explore that in greater detail then. But for now I should let you get on. Thank you very much indeed for taking the time to speak to us.
[FB-S] Thank you, thank you very much.
[AS] Okay, and congratulations again.
[FB-S] Bye bye.
[AS] Bye bye.
[FB-S] Thank you. Bye [12]

Harald zur Hausen

The Nobel Prize in Physiology or Medicine 2008
Interview
"I hope indeed, that this Nobel Prize will of course create more awareness of the role of infectious agents in human cancer"

Telephone interview with Harald zur Hausen immediately following the announcement of the 2008 Nobel Prize in Physiology or Medicine, 6 October 2008
The interviewer is Adam Smith, Editor-in-Chief of Nobelprize.org.
[Harald zur Hausen] zur Hausen.
[Adam Smith] Oh hello, Professor zur Hausen.
[HzH] Yes.

[AS] This is Adam Smith from the web site of the Nobel Foundation ... Hello. Would you mind if we recorded a very brief telephone interview with you?
[HzH] No, it's fine.
[AS] Thank you.
[HzH] I was informed that this would come through.
[AS] Thank you very much. Well first of all, of course, many congratulations on the award of the Nobel Prize.
[HzH] Well, thank you very much. I'm of course totally surprised. And it's of course a great pleasure for me.
[AS] Where were you when you received the news?
[HzH] Here in the Institute, in my office.
[AS] This is in the DKFZ?
[HzH] In the DKFZ, indeed. Well I am an Emeritus as you may know, but I still kept my office. I'm still Editor-in-Chief of the *International Journal of Cancer*, and also keep a laboratory here.
[AS] Yes, yes indeed. So, if we may turn to the discovery. When you first suggested that human papilloma virus caused cervical cancer, the prevailing view was that it was herpes simplex virus.
[HzH] Yes.
[AS] So how was your suggestion at first received?
[HzH] Well it was not very welcome, let's say it this way. Because in the early phase indeed, quite a number of scientists believed that herpes simplex type 2 would do it. There were a number of reports which seemed to confirm that there are increased antibody titres to herpes simplex type 2 in cervical cancer patients. And I reported it for the first time in public in 1974 at a meeting in Key Biscayne in Florida, when there was a meeting which was specifically scheduled for herpes simplex type 2 in cervical cancer. And at that time I reported our negative results in trying to find herpes simplex type 2 DNA in cervical cancer cells. And at the same time I stated that it would be very worthwhile to look rather into genital papilloma viruses, because the reasoning for me was that I had surveyed the literature and found a number of anecdotal reports on malignant conversion of genital warts.
[AS] So I imagine, since the meeting was organised around herpes simplex virus, you were the unwelcome guest on that occasion.
[HzH] Almost. You are almost exactly stating it in the right way because my statements were not well received, and I felt as a lonely voice in that meeting.
[AS] And it took about 10 years before you discovered the main disease-causing genotypes, HPV16 and 18.
[HzH] Well it's true, let's say in the meantime, between – I started to work on papilloma viruses in 1972 myself – but in the meantime we could identify the, individual ... excuse me, I'm still a little bit nervous at the moment.
[AS] Understandable, yes.
[HzH] Well, we could demonstrate that there exists a plurality of papilloma virus types. So there was not, as initially assumed, only one single papilloma virus type, but a multitude of different types, which was also confirmed by the group of Gérard Orth in Paris. And, but we concentrated ourselves on trying to isolate the viruses from genital warts because initially we suspected that that virus may be responsible for cervical cancer development. In 1979/1980 we could finally – it was mainly in collaboration with my co-worker Lutz Gissmann – that we could identify HPV6, and Ethel-Michele de Villiers was cloning it subsequently, with Gissmann. And subsequently we could identify another one – that was HPV11, which was also in genital warts and laryngeal papillomatosis. In fact,

in the subsequent period, we were initially disappointed not to find HPV6 and 11 in cervical cancer, without one rare exception. But, the probes helped us to identify HPV16 and 18 subsequently. In 1983 and 1984 this was published, by two of my students, Mattias Dürst and Michael Boshart. And, so that was in a way for us a breakthrough because at that time period, of course, interest was awakening very substantially, and quite a large number of groups were collaborating there, and starting to work on papilloma viruses, and ask us for the probes, so we dispersed them very freely throughout the world.

[AS] Yes, I understand that you gave them to anybody who asked ...

[HzH] Right.

[AS] ... and indeed then others went on and claimed patents on some of them, but that's another story, perhaps.

[HzH] Alright.

[AS] It's perhaps surprising that vaccine development didn't immediately follow your discoveries.

[HzH] Well, I mentioned it some time ago – in Stockholm, even – that, I tried to contact very early the German, particularly German pharmaceutical companies. And one of the companies, the Behring company in Marburg, became quite interested in it initially, and so they even funded our research for a certain period of time, with the expectation that we could collaborate on the development of vaccines. But then they did, at the same time, a market analysis and according to this market analysis there would be no market for such a vaccine. And then they stopped the funding. And it stopped for a certain period of time, indeed, at our place, intention to work on vaccines.

[AS] It shows how wrong market analysis can be.

[HzH] Well, it was totally wrong of course, as seen today. But, I mean, there's a little bit of an excuse for these companies, because at that time the PCR technology was developed, and many people started to work with this technology, and there was – quite a wide variation in data had been obtained in this time period. And, so they ... from 0–100% in supposedly negative tissues turned out to be positive, and so on. So this confused industry too.

[AS] Right.

[HzH] And, in addition...

[AS] And, so what eventually changed?

[HzH] Well, eventually it changed basically as the continuation of some molecular studies, which demonstrated indeed that the virus must be closely involved, but also the epidemiology studies, which in the end clarified the situation in demonstrating that HPV16 and 18 were so-called high-risk viruses, and indeed major risk factors for the development of cervical cancer.

[AS] And the results of the vaccination trials that have so far been reported have been enormously promising. Do you think that vaccination programmes should be widened now?

[HzH] Yes. From my viewpoint, yes, clearly so. I think the vaccination is extremely successful. It is presently – the major disadvantage at this stage is that it is too expensive for those parts of the world which most badly need the vaccine; namely, the developing world. And so the prices have to go down in the future in order to enable those people to receive the vaccine. From my personal experience, what I hear is that, in Africa, for instance, and also other parts of the developing world, the willingness to be vaccinated is remarkably high, so it's more a question of how do we get it to those people and how do we get a drastic reduction of the present price.

[AS] One final scientific question. Do you think that in general we're going to see more link between infectious disease and cancer in the future?
[HzH] Well, if you ask me this way, yes. My personal feeling is, yes, we will see more links. One came up this year only – the so-called Merkel cell carcinoma polyoma virus, which – the virus is called Merkel cell polyoma virus – which has been found in Merkel cell carcinomas, and every evidence at this stage points to the fact that this is indeed aetiologically involved. I think it's, I hope indeed, that this Nobel Prize will of course create more awareness of the role of infectious agents in human cancer, and I'm so pleased that the HIV part is also awarded.
[AS] Yes, it's a fascinating linkage. What do you think gave you the dedication to stay with the studies of HPV's link with cervical cancer for so long?
[HzH] Well, my personal conviction that there must be ... first of all there must be an infectious aetiology of this type of malignant disease, but secondly also I was in-between always encouraged – in spite of the fact that we didn't find directly this virus – by the fact that I saw how many questions there remained open in the papilloma virus field. But, maybe I should mention it; I was not from the beginning mainly interested in papilloma virus, I was mainly interested in infectious agents in human cancer. So papilloma viruses came up as the most likely candidate from my viewpoint.
[AS] But yes, infectious agents had been the lifelong pursuit.
[HzH] Yes, indeed. Indeed.
[AS] So I shouldn't keep you on the telephone for too long, you have many other things to do, but may I just ask you if you have any plans for how you might celebrate this?
[HzH] I don't know yet. It was so surprising I really have to sleep about it for one night or so before I make any decisions.
[AS] I fear the chances of getting any sleep for the next little while may be rather small.
[HzH] Yes, there's a risk indeed. Alright ...
[AS] Anyway, my congratulations ...
[HzH] Thank you once again.
[AS] Thank you for talking to us.
[HzH] Thank you. Bye bye.
[AS] Bye bye [13].

Editorial in *Retrovirology* Journal on the 2008 Nobel Prize for Medicine

Editorial
2008 Nobel prize in Medicine for discoverers of HIV
Andrew ML Lever[1] and **Ben Berkhout**[2]
[1]University of Cambridge, Department of Medicine, Addenbrooke's Hospital, UK
[2]University of Amsterdam, Laboratory of Experimental Virology, Academic Medical Center, The Netherlands
Retrovirology 2008, **5:**91doi:10.1186/1742-4690-5-91

The electronic version of this article is the complete one and can be found online at:

http://www.retrovirology.com/content/5/1/91
Received: 13October 2008
Accepted: 14 October 2008

Published: 14 October 2008

Abstract

Françoise Barré-Sinoussi and Luc Montagnier, codiscoverers of HIV, the causative agent of AIDS, have been awarded the 2008 Nobel Prize in Physiology or Medicine. They share this prize with Harald zur Hausen who was responsible for establishing the link between human papilloma virus infection and cervical carcinoma.

Editorial

Nobel prizes have often attracted controversy and controversial figures. William Ramsay was awarded the Nobel prize in Chemistry for the discovery of inert gases and subsequently went on to claim chemical transmutation of elements. Individual, institutional and national pride are all at stake when they are announced. One small Cambridge college boasts unashamedly of having been the workplace of no less than four Nobel Laureates including Perutz, Kendrew and Klug. Their value is more than financial and the method of their choosing somewhat mysterious and, to some peoples' minds flawed. Arrhenius having won in 1903, reputedly then manipulated future choices in favour of his friends and attempted (unsuccessfully) to exclude some very significant scientific figures such as Paul Ehrlich.

This year virology has been honoured and three scientists chosen who worked with two very different viruses. Harald zur Hausen, professor emeritus of the German Cancer Research Center in Heidelberg (Germany) identified the link between human papilloma virus (HPV) infection and cervical cancer. It is timely that with the recent development of a safe and effective vaccine he should be recognised for first identification of this human pathogenic virus. He made several particularly noteworthy findings in papilloma virus research. The earliest was the recognition that there are multiple HPV genotypes, particularly that HPVs that cause non-genital warts are distinct from those that cause genital warts. His most important finding was the identification and molecular cloning of the HPV types 16 and 18 genomes, and that a majority of cervical cancers contained DNA from these two HPV types. A third critical finding was that the HPV DNA becomes integrated into the host genome in cervical cancer cell lines and that the viral E6 and E7 (onco)genes are preferentially retained and expressed in the tumors. His work is even more noteworthy because it was carried out in the 1980's when there was considerable scepticism whether viruses in general, and HPV in particular, caused any common cancers. Professor zur Hausen has continued to run a highly productive laboratory since these seminal early findings. No controversy thus far.

Retroviruses have generated more than their share of Nobel prizes. Peyton Rous for retroviral oncogenesis (1966), Temin and Baltimore for reverse transcriptase (1975) and Varmus and Bishop again for oncogenes that were originally described for retroviruses (1989). The human immunodeficiency virus (HIV) as the largest public health problem in the world was destined to follow sooner or later. The difference is that, unlike in papilloma viruses, and whilst antiviral treatment has made astonishing progress in 20 years, we are no nearer a cure and certainly years from a vaccine (should one ever be possible) against HIV. The Nobel committee have chosen to honour the scientists who most people agree were the first to actually isolate the virus at the Pasteur Institute in

Paris (France) in 1983: Françoise Barré-Sinoussi and Luc Montagnier. Following medical reports of a novel immunodeficiency syndrome in 1981, the search for a causative agent was on. The French researchers isolated and cultured cells from lymph nodes of patients with the lymphadenopathy characteristic of the early stage of acquired immune deficiency. They detected activity of the retroviral enzyme reverse transcriptase, a direct sign of retrovirus replication. They also observed retroviral particles budding from the infected cells. Isolated virus infected and killed lymphocytes from healthy donors and reacted with antibodies from infected patients. By 1984, Barré-Sinoussi and Montagnier had obtained several isolates of the novel human retrovirus from sexually infected individuals, haemophiliacs, mother to infant transmissions and transfused patients.

Nobel prizes can be split between a maximum of three individuals and sometimes a deserving fourth person has been omitted on what appear to be relatively tough pragmatic grounds. Had the Nobel committee decided this year that the prize was for the discovery of HIV alone there would have been only one possible third candidate. That they didn't may be perceived in some quarters as a more pointed statement. However the subjects into which the prize is divided may be very diverse. Peyton Rous shared his with Charles Huggins, honoured for his contribution to hormonal treatment of cancer. Luc Montagnier (perhaps with a winner's magnanimity) has said that the obvious third recipient should have been Robert Gallo. Others will quote Gallo's identification of HTLV-1 with Bernie Poiesz and the fact that many of the techniques used to grow viruses like HIV were dependent on discoveries from the Gallo lab as were some of the earliest blood tests for the virus. Had the Nobel committee honoured only those who contributed to the discovery of HIV rather than HPV as well the picture may have been different. Instead they chose to reward the two scientists most responsible for the first isolation of the virus. These two indeed deserve our congratulations. It would be churlish however not to acknowledge that the work of others, notably the Gallo lab – but also other scientists working at the time, and since – made very significant contributions without which it is likely that the unprecedented advances we have seen in our understanding and successful therapy of HIV might have been much slower in coming.

Competing interests

The authors declare that they have no competing interests.

Authors' contributions

Both authors contributed equally to the work [14].

Presentation Speech for the 2008 Nobel Prize for Medicine

Presentation Speech by Professor Jan Andersson (Figure 10:14), Member of the Nobel Assembly at Karolinska Institutet, Member of the Nobel Committee for Physiology or Medicine, 10 December 2008:

Your Majesties, Your Royal Highnesses, Ladies and Gentlemen,

This year's Nobel Prize in Physiology or Medicine rewards two discoveries of viruses that cause severe global diseases.

Human history has been subjected to and shaped by major epidemics, such as bubonic plague, cholera, tuberculosis, smallpox, measles and influenza. These communicable diseases have contributed to the downfall of peoples and cultures. They recognise no national boundaries, and when they first appear among a group of people they are often fatal. All new epidemics have generated anxiety and panic reactions due to uncertainty about how the infectious agent spreads. Our foremost antidote is and has been – knowledge.

One part of this year's Prize goes to Harald zur Hausen, who sought to understand what causes cervical cancer, the world's second most common cancer among women. Half a million are affected every year. When zur Hausen asserted that human papilloma virus – which was known to induce skin warts – caused this cancer, not many people believed him. He predicted that the virus existed in different types and changed shape in tumour cells. He realised that no virus was formed there, but that certain virus genes instead integrated into cervical cell genomes, thereby giving risc to the cancer over time.

It was not possible to culture the virus, but zur Hausen instead had to prove his hypothesis by using small bits of single-stranded DNA from the actual wart viruses. He used these bits of DNA as bait to be able to attract virus DNA copies, first from genital warts and later also from cervical cancer cells. After more than a decade of persistent work, he isolated different types of human papilloma virus that caused more than 70 per cent of all cervical cancer. Virus genes were present in the DNA of every cancer cell and re-programmed the cells to grow uncontrollably.

This discovery has led to vaccines against these viruses which provide protection against these infections. It has also lead to improved methods for predicting which women are in the risk zone.

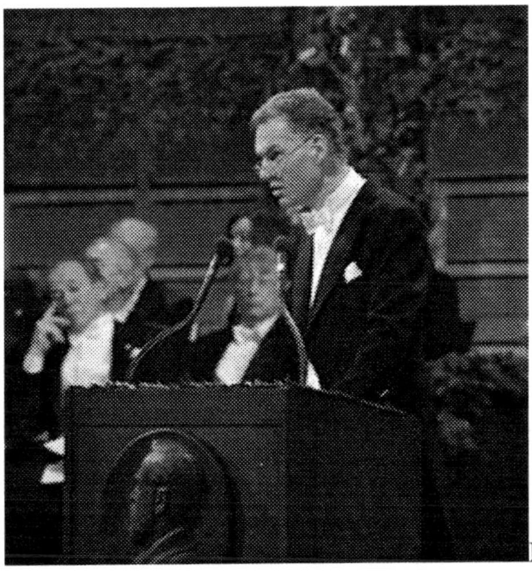

Figure 10-14: Professor Jan Andersson delivering the Presentation Speech for the 2008 Nobel Prize in Physiology or Medicine at the Stockholm ConcertHall, 10 Dec 2008 [12].

The other part of this year's Prize is related to the discovery of the human immunodeficiency virus (HIV). In 1981 there were a number of alarming reports that young, previously healthy people were dying of pneumonia or unusual tumours. This was the beginning of an epidemic whose enigmatic nature and impact on different cultures defied all previously described epidemics. It started during an era when we thought we had conquered all major infectious diseases. There were now antibiotics, vaccines, good hygiene and improved living conditions that would keep us immune. Institutes for infectious disease control would be shut down. But with everyone talking about AIDS, new concerns spread in many countries.

Françoise Barré-Sinoussi and Luc Montagnier speculated that AIDS was caused by an unknown retrovirus, a kind of tumour virus from the animal kingdom that had more recently also been found in humans. But how could a virus with a size of one ten thousandth of a millimetre trigger all these different manifestations of disease?

Barré-Sinoussi and Montagnier discovered HIV in the lymph nodes of recently infected patients. It was being produced in large quantities in white blood cells and it induced the death of cells of a kind that was missing in patients suffering from AIDS. HIV was like a chameleon. Each patient carried a unique virus variant, which could hide in the host cell genome. Barré-Sinoussi and Montagnier's discovery explained the progression of the disease and its communicability, enabling them to establish the connection between HIV and AIDS. Methods for discovering infected people and blood products were developed, and HIV/AIDS patients quickly gained access to effective anti-retroviral drugs that helped suppress their disease. So far 60 million people in the world have been infected with HIV, and a total of 25 million have died of AIDS. A growing number of people are receiving anti-retroviral drugs, even in developing countries. Another cause for celebration is that the epidemic is now declining among young people in the countries where it began. However, the best prophylactic against HIV/AIDS is and remains true love, generating longstanding relationships.

Sehr geehrter Herr Professor zur Hausen! Ihre Entdeckung hat zu der Erkenntnis geführt, daß Viren bei Menschen Krebs erregen können, und daß wir neue Möglichkeiten zur Vorbeugung von Krebs gefunden haben, der durch humane Papillomaviren hervorgerufen wird.

Professeurs Barré-Sinoussi et Montagnier! Votre découverte nous a révélé l'existence d'un nouveau virus, le VIH, et cette connaissance a ouvert la voie à de nouveaux traitements contre la maladie du VIH/SIDA.

On behalf of the Nobel Assembly at Karolinska Institutet it is my privilege and pleasure to express our warmest congratulations and our deepest admiration as I now ask you to step forward to receive the Nobel Prize from the hands of His Majesty the King [15].

Conclusion

The HIV/AIDS prevalence, morbidity and mortality rates are staggering especially in sub-Saharan Africa that is home to over 70 percent of the world's HIV/AIDS cases. Even though research has been able to elucidate quite a lot about the pathophysiological characteristics of HIV, the world is still said to be at least a decade away from the dawn of HIV vaccines.

In the author's opinion, this state of affairs is a great shame to HIV vaccine researchers and scientists of our era. Vaccines against smallpox and rabies for instance, were developed before anyone knew anything about the agents that caused them. We claim we have advanced scientifically beyond those eras. Yet, with all our pride and self approbation, for more than 20 years now, we have had this disease HIV/AIDS that has wreaked worldwide havoc that is worse than that caused worldwide by all cancers combined, but we still claim that it will take another decade for HIV vaccines to be developed if ever we will be able to develop any.

The author strongly believes that this is an appalling disgrace to our age and generation. If Edward Jenner and Louis Pasteur were somewhere watching us and our wayward search for HIV vaccines all these years, what do you think they would think of us? Will they commend us or rebuke us? The author thinks they are likely to be full of venomous reprobation for our failing humanity this much. 'To whom much is given, much is expected', says an adage. We claim we have developed much and are in the age of modern genetic engineering techniques or recombinant technology, human genome uncoding, space exploration, etc. But we have become empty barrels making so much loud noise praising ourselves but have virtually nothing to show for HIV vaccines? We should all bury our faces in shame.

Greater blame for this abysmal performance on HIV/AIDS vaccines goes naturally to those who have been trumpeting the arrogant and senseless posture that only the developed countries can conceive the idea of how to develop such vaccines. All their concepts have failed to date. It is far better for them to throw in the towel at this time and tell the world that in giving up, they are tendering their sincere apologies for the colossal havoc they have done to mankind since 1984. They should then declare an open field with everyone trying their hands at developing HIV vaccines without any preconditions or recipes. 'Pride goes before a fall', says another adage. The pride of claiming monopoly of knowledge about HIV vaccines development has indeed made the fall bigger and almost unpardonable.

Instead of following this path of honour, they are praising themselves on antiretroviral drug development that they describe as life-saving drugs to deceive the unwary. If they know these drugs are life-saving, why did they tell us since 1984 that HIV vaccines would be ready for testing in 2 years, and be on the market in 3 years? Why did they not talk about antiretrovirals then? While their arrogance has killed millions, they are criminally using their institutions of mass communications to shut up others so that their economies continue to grow on the sale of antiretrovirals to other countries? These are not the best of days for humanity at all, and it makes the author a very sad man indeed.

Half of the 2008 Nobel Prize for Medicine was awarded to two French researchers Françoise Barré-Sinoussi and Luc Montagnier for their 1983 discovery of the virus that causes AIDS. This laudable decision has again helped to highlight to the whole world the terrible disaster of HIV/AIDS.

The author developed safe and effective HIV vaccines since 1998/99, and informed the world, but the world, without carrying out any form of investigation whatsoever, prefers to shut him up and leave millions to die. Some are still keen on getting hold of the author, preferably dead, so that they can be left without any lone voice of opposition in the wilderness dedicated to their economic interests in antiretroviral drugs and condoms, waiting for the dawn of the day when HIV/AIDS would have opened desolate lands for them to occupy or colonize. HIV/AIDS continues to put the worst of human character on parade!

References

[1] Smith KA HIV Vaccine (2004). *Natl. J. Androl.* 10(10): 723-8.
[2] UNAIDS (2000). Report on the Global HIV/AIDS Epidemic. June 2000 Page 68
[3] http://csm.jmu.edu HIV/AIDS
[4] http://en.wikipedia.org/wiki/Robert_Gallo.
[5] http://www.waado.org/NigerDelta/Nigeria_Facts/NigerianMaps/Africa_PoliticalMap.html)
[6] http://images.google.co.uk/imgres?imgurl=http://www.sitesatlas.com/Maps/Maps/706.gif&imgrefurl=http://www.sitesatlas.com/Maps/Maps/706.htm&usg=__9bIkfaq_aJZSmryR7yfnvMw02_U=&h=625&w=746&sz=36&hl=en&start=26&um=1&tbnid=pt58UP57TSFo1M:&tbnh=118&tbnw=141&prev=/images%3Fq%3Dmap%2Bof%2Bnigeria%26start%3D18%26ndsp%3D18%26um%3D1%26hl%3Den%26rlz%3D1T4HPEB_en-GBGH277US279%26sa%3DN
[7] http://images.google.co.uk/imgres?imgurl=http://www.nigerians.biz/Image/Nigeria/nigeria.gif&imgrefurl=http://www.nigerians.biz/nigeria/_menu.html&usg=__kdpZ9XQOCjnhKkbe0gWvd7Ck9VU=&h=437&w=503&sz=31&hl=en&start=21&um=1&tbnid=LpD3zh76Qi6EiM:&tbnh=113&tbnw=130&prev=/images%3Fq%3Dmap%2Bof%2Bnigeria%26start%3D18%26ndsp%3D18%26um%3D1%26hl%3Den%26rlz%3D1T4HPEB_en-GBGH277US279%26sa%3DN
[8] http://www.nobelchermann.com/index_eng.html
[9] http://www.nytimes.com/2008/10/07/health/07nobel.html?hp
[10] http://www.npr.org/templates/story/story.php?storyId=95420499
[11] http://nobelprize.org/nobel_prizes/medicine/laureates/2008/montagnier-interview.html
[12] http://nobelprize.org/nobel_prizes/medicine/laureates/2008/barre-sinoussi-telephone.html
[13] http://nobelprize.org/nobel_prizes/medicine/laureates/2008/hausen-telephone.html
[14] http://www.retrovirology.com/content/5/1/91
[15] http://nobelprize.org/nobel_prizes/medicine/laureates/2008/presentation-speech.html.

Chapter XI

The HIV/AIDS Scourge

Abstract

The HIV/AIDS scourge has come to the world, not just killing and destroying human lives but exposing the wickedness and murderous irrationality of our species, the Homo sapiens. The West has literally been looking the other way while its cleverly schemed strategy of leaving HIV/AIDS to devastate sub-Saharan Africa continues to work wonders. They have silenced everybody and prevented them from delving into HIV vaccine development. Any rebel that dares to delve into the field are mercilessly shot down with laser guided technology so that nothing interferes with the great job the HIV/AIDS scourge is doing for them in sub-Saharan Africa. The imposition of antiretrovirals on the whole world completes the onslaught. An American writer has succinctly put it in these words "If one in four adults in the United States were infected by HIV, I am confident that such a critical rethinking of the scientific community's battle plan already would have happened." This chapter is about these and other related issues.

Introduction

The author does not wish to involve himself in the many theories that abound regarding the possible origin of AIDS since they are nothing more than theories. At best, only one of them may be correct; all of them may be wrong! The author does not see anything tangible to be gained from the distraction of this controversy of theories. We are most unlikely to ever know for sure where the virus originated just as we have never known for sure where other viruses, bacteria, protozoa and other living creatures originated. And even if we were to know the origin of HIV for sure, how would that help us deal with the pandemic on our hands? However, we know for sure that the first cases of AIDS reported by man were found by USA doctors on USA gay citizens living in the USA in 1981. We also now know for sure that sub-Saharan Africa has been ruined by the HIV/AIDS pandemic; about 70 percent of the world's cases of the disease occur in that region, which accounts for just about 10 percent of the world's population. That region, therefore, suffers more than any other region over the failure to develop HIV vaccines.

If he who wears the shoe knows best where it pinches, this region of the world should be the most desperate about developing HIV vaccines. Unfortunately, the American Gallo ordained in 1984 that only the developed countries can conceive how HIV vaccines can be developed. The UN, other developed countries, other nations and the African sub-region all fell behind Gallo. If it were just the simple fact that the world has failed to develop any HIV vaccines since 1984, there would be little cause for condemnation and alarm.

However, during the years that the world failed to develop HIV vaccines, HIV/AIDS did not just stay waiting and watching! It has killed tens of millions, created several million orphans, and ruined the socio-economic fabric of sub-Saharan Africa in particular. And the pandemic continues its carnage even as the author is writing this book. HIV/AIDS has not promised or accepted any ceasefire!

Under these circumstances, would any reasonable human being blame anybody from the sub-Saharan sub region for attempting to develop HIV vaccines in order to retard or halt the human genocide being perpetrated by HIV/AIDS? The rest of humanity has not only heaped opprobrium on the author for developing HIV vaccines, but has gone ahead to ensure that his remedy is not put to use by any HIV-infected persons. Could this stance ever be justified? The more the author studies the situation, the more he is drawn to the conclusion that the West may indeed have another HIV/AIDS agenda, namely, to do everything within their collective power to leave the HIV/AIDS scourge to depopulate Africa, in other words, using HIV/AIDS for biological warfare against sub-Saharan Africa.

The Americans went further! For over 20 years, they have forcefully been subjecting US visa applicants from the author's country to HIV screening. All those who test positive receive the cruel treatment of denial of US visa! These practices run counter to what the same Americans have been preaching to the world all these 20 or more years. The same Americans have done nothing to restrict their own HIV-positive citizens within the shores of the US! HIV/AIDS has come not only to kill and to destroy, but to expose the worst aspects of man's inhumanity to man, to expose the depth of depravity to which some people and nations have fallen while pretending to be beacons of hope for other parts of the world, and to expose the devils that pose as angels of light among Homo sapiens.

The Shock and Awe of the HIV/AIDS Scourge

The data on HIV/AIDS infection are frightening indeed. Cohen [1] writes thus:

"More than one in every three adults who live in Botswana or Zimbabwe is infected with HIV. Let that number sink in: 35.8% of the schoolteachers, doctors, cement mixers, mothers, engineers, truck drivers, seamstresses, and politicians are infected with a lethal virus that, in most cases, will cut their lives short by decades. Lesotho, Namibia, South Africa, Swaziland, Zambia, and Zimbabwe are only slightly better off, where the number is one in five adults. In five other countries in sub-Saharan Africa, it is more than one in ten. All told, sub-Saharan Africa now accounts for two-thirds of the estimated 40 million HIV-infected people in the world, and AIDS on that continent is the leading cause of death for adults. Hundreds of thousands of children are infected, and even more have been orphaned. Life expectancy, which steadily had been climbing during the past several decades, is rapidly declining: In

Botswana, for example, the World Health Organization (WHO) says the average child born today will live to be about 40; the same child could have expected to live to 70 in the absence of HIV.

While HIV crumbles sub-Saharan Africa, shaking it like an earthquake that will not stop, Americans largely have lost interest in AIDS. With the advent of powerful cocktails of anti-HIV drugs in the late 1990s, journalists began trumpeting the idea that AIDS was history, which the American public readily accepted. Death rates from AIDS plummeted for a time, furthering the notion that the epidemic has abated and will soon disappear altogether. AIDS activists, politically savvy and effective rabble-rousers who for a decade drew attention to the disease and sped development of treatments, have become as anachronistic as hippies.

Most of the world cannot afford the wonder drugs that have staved off disease and death for infected people in wealthier countries. And even in the United States, the advances celebrated a few short years ago are slipping, in no small part because the virus eventually develops resistance to every drug thrown at it. Look at AIDS deaths alone. In 1997, the year after the advent of the powerful drug cocktails, the U.S. death rate from AIDS plunged by 42%. The next year, the drop was only 20%, and the number of new AIDS cases had also nearly doubled from 1997. This is, in short, no time for any country to let down its guard against HIV, especially the United States, which spends more money on AIDS research than all other countries combined.

There are many ways to slow the spread of HIV. Using condoms and clean needles, abstaining from sex, treating other sexually transmitted diseases, male circumcision, and screening blood products all have proved effective — to a point. But the best hope the world has to thwart this virus is the same weapon effectively used against smallpox, polio, hepatitis B, rabies, and other devastating viruses: a vaccine.

Much effort indeed has gone into finding an AIDS vaccine, and the scientific problems are staggering. Yet there are problems that supersede science. This book describes in detail how scientists came to the impasse they are facing, explaining plainly the complicated mixture of scientific, business, political, and ethical forces that haphazardly steer the enterprise. I also offer a solution to the non-scientific problems that, I believe, ultimately would speed the search for a vaccine, possibly shaving years off the time it takes to slow HIV. My proposal is neither revolutionary nor unique: I argue that scientists should approach the problem in a logical, stepwise fashion, testing vaccines in meaningful animal experiments and following up on all promising leads. This book documents how, amazingly, this has not happened to date, and shows the strong forces in the U.S. scientific culture that resist such an approach. And I am convinced that similar problems dog the search for vaccines against malaria, tuberculosis, and hepatitis C—and will hamper vaccine research for new diseases that in the future will suddenly assault populations the way AIDS did in the 1980s.

I doubt that my book, which I began researching in 1989 and completed with help from a Sloan Foundation grant, will single-handedly change the U.S. scientific culture. But maybe, when the public and scientists alike take a careful look at the shortcomings of the AIDS vaccine research effort, a momentum will build to attack the problem with all of the might the world can muster. If one in four adults in the United States were infected by HIV, I am confident that such a critical rethinking of the scientific community's battle plan already would have happened." [1]

It is not just the loss of interest in HIV/AIDS by the Americans. The US and other developed countries may be more concerned with protecting the huge investments that their multinational pharmaceutical companies have made in antiretroviral drugs (ARVs) than in genuinely researching for HIV vaccines. They call the toxic and costly ARVs 'wonder drugs' or 'life-saving drugs' even though these drugs do not cure HIV/AIDS.

In 1916, when there were just 27,000 cases of polio in the US with 7,179 deaths, there was national panic and fear. In New York where over 2,000 died from the disease, some people went as far as using ox blood, frog blood and radium water for a remedy! Is it morally or scientifically justified for the same US to be involved in deliberate efforts to deprive others from using safe and effective HIV vaccines (just a human blood product) that have been available since 1998/89 even when they have continued to use human blood products /extracts for other ailments?

Many readers may be severely shocked by the HIV prevalence rate of 35.8 percent that Jon Cohen wrote about. Such readers should please tighten their seat belts because about twice that HIV prevalence rate exists in some regions of sub-Saharan Africa even in the year 2008. The author is not joking. UNAIDS has been telling the world that their prevention efforts especially the 'ABC' slogan have slowed down the prevalence rates of HIV in many countries in sub-Saharan Africa. UNAIDS figures are based on the data given to it by the governments of these countries.

But UNAIDS knows, or ought to know, that these Governments are dishonest; they have no culture of scientific data and investigation; they are only interested in hoodwinking the developed world into believing that the grants they receive from them to fight HIV/AIDS are being invested prudently whereas the truth is that the grants actually end up in the bank accounts of the corrupt officers that are in positions of power in these countries. The true facts are that the HIV prevalence rates in these countries are increasing daily, not falling!

The following article appeared on page 7 in the *Sunday Vanguard* newspaper in Nigeria on August 17, 2008:

> '7 out of every 10 Akwa Ibom girls HIV positive
> *Council boss' wife charges women to fight scourge
>
> THE wife of the chairman of Eket LGA, Mrs. Emem Emmanuel Udoh, has urged women particularly wives of councillors in the eleven political wards in Eket to lead the fight against HIV in their various communities.
>
> She stated that the scourge is real, as investigation shows that seven out of every ten girls in Akwa Ibom are HIV positive. The same result, according to her, is obtainable in the case of pregnant women in the state. "This is a sad and dangerous development in our society which must not be tolerated," she added. Mrs. Udoh made these comments during an interactive session with Eket legislators' wives and female councillors in Eket Local Government secretariat. "As women at the grassroots, I charge you all to intensify your efforts in spreading the message of total abstinence from casual sex even as reliance on condom has proved unreliable.
>
> "In as much as times are difficult, we should not relent in our determination to save this generation from the HIV doom by guiding and encouraging our people to utilize the services of hospitals and or any approved medical centres for regular test and check-up to confirm their HIV status. We should do away completely with stigmatization but show love and understanding with the unfortunate victims of the dreaded disease", she added.
>
> The chairman's wife, a teacher by profession, responding to questions at the forum, explained that HIV could also be contacted not only through sex but the use of unsterilized tools and transfusion of infected blood. She used the forum to speak on social and moral uprightness of women in the council, demanding that they lead by example, showing love, respect and great understanding with their spouses who as politicians are exposed to all forms of pressures.
>
> Mrs. Udoh admonished the councillors' wives to comport themselves with dignity, be seen'

(Perhaps, it was the printer's devil but that is how the article in the newspaper ended!)

For the benefit of readers who do not know much about Nigeria, Nigeria is a country that consists of 36 States and the Federal Capital Territory of Abuja. Akwa Ibom State is one of the southeastern coastal States in Nigeria (Figures 10-10 and 10-11 in Chapter 10). According to HIV prevalence rates released to the world by Nigeria's Federal Ministry of Health, there is hardly any State with a prevalence rate of over ten percent. Here we are with a far different prevalence figure of 70 percent. From the author's experience of his country and the HIV screening tests he has performed, the Eket Local Government HIV prevalence figure is far more accurate and realistic that what the country's Health Ministry and other Agencies have been turning out to the world.

The author would not be surprised at all if he hears later that the security agencies of Nigeria's Federal Government descended on either the newspaper or the Mrs. Udoh credited with revealing the HIV prevalence figure in her Local Government, accusing either or both of them of all sorts of crimes ranging from dissemination of false news to actions detrimental to the national interest!

Then US President Bill Clinton in his Commencement address at Morgan State University in Baltimore, Maryland, on May 18, 1997 declared:

> "...science is about more than material wealth or the acquisition of knowledge. Fundamentally, it is about our dreams. America is a nation always becoming, always defined by the great goals we set, the great dreams we dream. We are restless, questing people. We have always believed, with President Thomas Jefferson that 'freedom is the first-born daughter of science.' With that belief and with willpower, resources and great national effort, we have always reached our far horizons and set out for new ones. ...
>
> Today let us look within and step up to the challenge of our time, a challenge with consequences far more immediate for the life and death of millions around the world. AIDS will soon overtake tuberculosis and malaria as the leading infectious killer in the world. More than 29 million people have been infected, 3 million in the last year alone, 95 percent of them in the poorest parts of our globe.
>
> Here at home, we are grateful that new and effective anti-HIV strategies are available and bringing longer and better lives to those who are infected, but we dare not be complacent. HIV is capable of mutating and becoming resistant to therapies, and could well become even more dangerous. Only a truly effective, preventive HIV vaccine can limit and eventually eliminate the threat of AIDS.
>
> This year's budget contains increased funding of a third over two years ago to search for this vaccine. In the first four years, we have increased funding for AIDS research, prevention, and care by 50 percent, but it is not enough. So let us today set a new national goal for science in the age of biology. Today, let us commit ourselves to developing an AIDS vaccine within the next decade. (Applause)
>
> There are no guarantees. It will take energy and focus and demand great effort from our greatest minds. But with the strides of recent years it is no longer a question of whether we can develop an AIDS vaccine; it is simply a question of when. And it cannot come a day too soon.
>
> If America commits to finding an AIDS vaccine and we enlist others in our cause, we will do it. I am prepared to do all I can to make it happen. Our scientists at the National Institutes of Health and our research universities have been at the forefront of this battle.
>
> Today, I'm pleased to announce the National Institutes of Health will establish a new AIDS vaccine research centre dedicated to this crusade. And next month at the Summit of the Industrialized Nations in Denver, I will enlist other nations to join us in a worldwide effort to find a vaccine to stop one of the world's greatest killers. We will challenge America's pharmaceutical industry, which leads the world in innovative research and development, to work with us and to make the successful development of an AIDS vaccine part of its basic mission.
>
> My fellow Americans, if the 21st century is to be the century of biology, let us make an AIDS vaccine its first great triumph. (Applause)" [1].

There was no ambiguity in President Clinton's 1997 message. He said the American pharmaceutical industry leads the world in innovative research and development *(like most people, the author agrees with him)*, and therefore should be the first *(not necessarily, in the author's view)* to develop an AIDS vaccine! He said that America should commit itself to developing an AIDS vaccine by 2007, a decade from 1997. 2007 has come and gone but the US and other countries are yet to produce an AIDS vaccine. In fact, USA researchers and vaccine developers now tell us that if ever HIV vaccines would be developed at all, we are still a decade away at least.

Meanwhile, some developed countries like the US, France and Great Britain, as well as the UN and its institutions such as the WHO and UNAIDS, have continued to actively suppress the news of the development of safe and effective HIV vaccines since 1998/99 even after the scientific publications of the work in reputable international medical journals [2-8]! It is most probable that all their HIV vaccine 'experts', developers, scientists and researchers have read these publications of and about the author's HIV vaccines work, but they decided to bomb it with shock and awe into oblivion. One can only reach the inescapable conclusion that it is just HIV vaccines developed by them in compliance with their guidelines that interests them!

One just has to wonder if the millions that have been dying annually of HIV/AIDS ever bothers them at all. If some Americans used frog blood, ox blood and radium water as a remedy for polio when faced with a polio epidemic that killed over 2,000 in New York in 1916, why should any American think/consider it wrong, scientifically, ethically or otherwise, when pure human blood extract is used as a remedy for HIV in an era where human blood and its various components continue to be used worldwide, the US included, for various medical reasons. The author hopes, apparently against reasonable hope, that all this posturing is not a decoy to shield what some have said is the real aim of the West, namely, using the HIV/AIDS that was first discovered in man in the US as a handy weapon of biological warfare against sub-Saharan Africa in order to create a desolate land for their occupation.

HIV/AIDS in the Author's Country Nigeria

Here is the official information about HIV/AIDS in the author's country [9]:

"Nigeria's HIV/AIDS prevalence rate of 5.8% may seem small in comparison to some Southern African nations with seropositivity rates of over 30% of the adult population.

However, the West African nation is home to nearly one-tenth of the world's HIV/AIDS-infected persons with 3.5 million infected people (UNAIDS 2001 estimate), the largest HIV-positive population in Africa after South Africa. Nigeria's population is expected to double by the year 2025, which will multiply the spread of the HIV virus astronomically. In addition to the devastation HIV/AIDS has caused and continues to cause among Nigeria's adult population, half of the current population is under the age of 15. With only 55% of primary school-aged children in school and the high HIV/AIDS prevalence rates among adults, Nigeria faces serious challenges and significant obstacles in the education and health care sectors (USAID Congressional Budget Justification, 2004). In late July 2001, the government of Nigeria announced a major AIDS treatment program. President Obasanjo declared that his government would provide cheap generic drugs to AIDS patients beginning September 2001. Patients are expected to pay about $7 a month for the treatment. The government of Nigeria plans to distribute anti-retroviral drugs to an estimated 10,000 patients, but numerous obstacles have inhibited the implementation of this program."

The author has always maintained that the official Nigerian Government HIV prevalence figures are grossly and deliberately scaled down in order to give the Western aid donors and the rest of the world the incorrect impression that they are achieving some success in fighting the scourge. In that way, they justify all the HIV aid from the developed countries even though all the aid ends up in the private accounts of the government officials and their cronies in the pervading crime of embezzlement of public funds at all levels of government in Nigeria and most likely, in other sub-Saharan countries.

In any case, the author personally wrote many times between 1999 and 2007 when President Obasanjo was in power and informed him on each occasion about the development of safe and effective HIV vaccines in Nigeria, and asked him for his directives. The author received no response at all, not even an acknowledgement. More than two years after the author first wrote to inform him, "In late July 2001, the government of Nigeria announced a major AIDS treatment program. President Obasanjo declared that his government would provide cheap generic drugs to AIDS patients beginning September 2001. Patients are expected to pay about $7 a month for the treatment."

What a devilish leader! With peanuts, he could have readily harnessed resources and treated all the HIV-infected citizens in his country with the therapeutic vaccine, and also treated all other citizens with the HIV preventive vaccine that the author had developed since 1999. But not the devil incarnate called Olusegun Obasanjo! Instead, he decided to waste scarce resources to purchase antiretrovirals to treat just 10,000 out of the official figure of 3.5 million infected with the virus in his country! And there was no chance that any of those he placed on the antiretrovirals would ever be cured of the virus! It is more than wickedness. It is sadism at its worst.

Sub-Saharan African countries and their governments in particular, have no culture of scientific research, development and discovery. Accordingly, President Obasanjo's administration must have outrightly dismissed the author's letters to him as '419', Nigeria's popular slang for criminal deceit or fraud.

After all, there is no individual or Institution in Nigeria that is involved in any attempt to delve into HIV vaccine development, as far as Olusegun Obasanjo knows. Besides, which Nigerian has ever been involved in any medical scientific breakthroughs in the country's history? None as far he knows. In countries that value their scientists, such an action as Obasanjo's by their leader would likely bring the leader down whenever the public knows the facts. But in Nigeria where there is no culture of scientific research and development, some of the populace adore Obasanjo for his decision because whatever the white man produces is always the best that humans can produce. If the white man says there is no cure for HIV/AIDS and that antiretrovirals are the best for treating the infection, that's it; it is final because only God can do better! Of course, the author does not subscribe to these primordial and incorrect instincts.

In the author's country as in other sub-Saharan African countries, the problem is far more than just the pervading disinterest in scientific issues. There is no premium placed on hard work or merit. Posts and positions are filled, not by the best-qualified candidates but by people who have the strongest "connections" with those in authority, while better-qualified persons are just ignored. In Nigeria, the Constitution states that posts should be filled based on 'federal character'. This has been taken to mean that whatever job is available, merit is thrown to the dogs. One of the first important issues to be addressed is to zone the post to the South or North, then to a geopolitical region, then to a State in that zone, then to a Senatorial zone, a local Government etc. Additionally, the determination of whether one comes from the North or South, his geo-political region, State, Senatorial zone or Local Government Council is his origin, not his place of domicile /residence or birth even if the person had been born and resident in any place other than his place of origin in the country all his life. In Nigeria therefore, citizens cannot aspire to any post, elective or professional unless they are indigenes of such a Local Government Council, State or geo-political region. Citizens are stuck to their father's ancestral origin for life!

More retrogressive matters abound. It is a fundamental practice that one would not be considered for any government job at any level unless such a person belongs to the ruling political party. Any one who ignores this practice does so at the risk of his life. There is also the national practice of tribal or religious consideration. For any job, one of the factors considered is one's religion. From the onset, it is usually decided that the job must be given to a Moslem and not to a Christian or vice versa. A decision would also have been taken about the tribe of the occupier of any office even before applications are invited form the general public. In a country with over 200 tribes, the reader may well imagine the intrigues involved especially when there has never been much love lost between the various tribes and with each tribe continuing to harbour intense suspicion and xenophobia for other tribes as their ancestors had done before them. This intense suspicion and xenophobia extends to religious beliefs and politics in Nigeria, thereby inserting more cruel nails into the coffin of merit in the country.

When the author announced his successful development of safe and effective HIV vaccines, the first questions or remarks from other Nigerians are one or more of the following:

> Which part of the country does he come from? Which is his political party?
> What is his tribe?
> Where is his State of Origin?
> From his name of Jeremiah, he must be a Christian. So forget about him! If he had been a Moslem, I would have considered his claim, but not any claim from a Christian.
> From his name of Jeremiah, I presume he is a Christian. Is he a Roman Catholic, Pentecostal, Baptist, Anglican, Redeemed, Jehovah's Witness, Celestial or Christ Apostolic? For me, I will only support such a claim if it comes from my own Christian denomination!
> Nigerians are not interested in the merits or lack of merits of the claim!

In the history of mankind, no country has achieved greatness or development on these primordial considerations, but Nigerians are not interested in the lessons of history. Research and development especially in the sciences are a sine qua non for development in any society but not in Nigeria, a country that continues to deride itself in the delusion that technology is to be transferred from the developed to the developing countries. Any Nigerian that attempts to ignore these entrenched positions in Nigeria is immediately forced to graduate with the Nigerian 'PHD', 'pull him/her down' degree, meaning that the graduate should be pulled down from his Olympian height to the reality of the Nigerian culture, practices and position!

One then has to superimpose on these retrogressive culture and practices the other pervading national monsters of corruption and insatiable avarice. An official entrusted with responsibility for handling any matter would first of all ensure he has his own deal settled before he acts. Failure to meet his demands means the end of the road on the matter. Embezzlement of public funds in Nigeria and fraudulent activities continue to be practised almost everywhere by everyone that must have continued to keep the devil shuddering in shock, awe and unbelief!

Consequently, many unfortunate and avoidable oddities abound in Nigeria and other countries with similar national practices. In the author's view, one of the worst of such oddities in his country is the Niger-Delta crisis. Nigeria's main source of foreign exchange earnings since the 1970s is the crude oil. Nigeria is the world's 7th biggest crude oil exporter in the Organization of Petroleum Exporting Countries, OPEC. Virtually all the crude oil produced in Nigeria comes from the southern part of the country especially the coastal States of Bayelsa, Rivers, Delta, Akwa Ibom, Cross River and Ondo States. The ecology and socio-economic activities of these areas have been terribly devastated by the oil exploration and mining but the country has callously abandoned these communities as if they are not part of Nigeria.

The revenue from the crude oil is used to provide infrastructure in other parts of the country especially the Northern States. In a country where 'the concept of indigeneship or place of origin' as opposed to place of domicile /residence or birth reigns supreme, one can imagine the degree of agony that has been the lot of the communities in the oil producing States since the 1970s. The injustice has resulted in armed struggle and unrest by some of the youth from these areas, popularly called the Niger Delta crisis, in some of the oil producing States. The truth however is that this development was literally forced on the indigenes of these States by the callousness of the rest of the country. It can never be justified or proper to muzzle, ignore or destroy the communities from which the main foreign exchange earning for the country is derived.

In the author's view, the solution is glaringly simple and straightforward. The country should immediately apologize to the affected States for the inhuman treatment meted out to them all these years. Pari passu with the public apology and as a bona fide demonstration of that apology, at least 50 per cent of the revenue from Nigeria's crude oil for an interim period of 12 months should be given to the States that lay the golden egg of crude oil for the urgent rehabilitation of their destroyed infrastructure and socio-economic activities. During the 12 months interim period, the Nigerian authorities should enter into serious dialogue with the representatives of these States. Further advantage should be taken during the negotiations to get the country to abandon indigeneship or place of origin for place of domicile /residence. If the people from the oil producing States had been allowed to claim the States they reside in, the inhumanity to them would have been severely downgraded.

Unfortunately for Nigeria, Obasanjo personified, and continues to personify these primordial features of the Nigerian society. Obasanjo like most Nigerians is so deeply atavistic that he is mentally and intellectually incapable of even imagining that some of the citizens in his country, even if they are few, could delve into any scientific field, work hard and make new discoveries that would help the Nigerian society and humanity at large. After all, he is very conscious of the fact that he himself has never tried to do any scientific research and develop anything for his country all the years of his life so far. He has projected his own inadequacies, atavism and conservatism to the author and his HIV vaccines research.

Readers may ask why the author bothered to inform President Obasanjo about his HIV vaccines when the author had reason to know that it would likely be ignored based on the culture in his country and on the man's antecedents. The author was already a doctor for more than 4 years at the time of Obasanjo's tenure as Military Head of State from 1976 to 1979, and he knew Olusegun Obasanjo had no respect whatsoever for scientific matters then. However, at his inauguration as civilian President in May 1999, Olusegun Obasanjo had announced that his Government would not only encourage scientific research, but would recognize and reward such effort. The author decided to write and inform him about his HIV vaccines development to give him the benefit of the doubt, hoping that as President, he would avail himself of the development and use it for the greater interest of the citizens of his country and humanity at large. The man had actually not changed from what he was as Military Head of State; in truth and fact, he had become worse and more callous. The author has found out since that the adage "A leopard hardly changes its spots" aptly describes Olusegun Obasanjo.

In contrast to Olusegun Obasanjo, let me recall that the French and US Presidents intervened to settle the bitter 3-year dispute between their scientists Luc Montagnier and Robert Gallo respectively over the first scientist to isolate the virus that causes AIDS. If one of the two scientists involved had been a Nigerian, one can be absolutely certain that his country and government, particularly under Obasanjo's presidency, would not only abandon him, but would do everything to make sure he is disgraced, criminalized and jailed for daring to involve himself with a white man over an issue about which the Nigerian scientist ought to know he could not have discovered anything. In fact, the Nigerian Government would have gone ahead to apologize publicly to the government of the country of the other scientist over the matter. The author will reveal worse actions by the Nigerian Government over his HIV vaccines in Chapter 49 dealing with Nigeria's Presidency.

Suffice it to say for now that President Obasanjo's declaration in 2001 that opted for anti-retroviral drugs and jettisoned the HIV vaccine developed in his country without the expenditure of a dime of government funds casts him exactly as he is, a treacherous, sadistic and atrocious leader ready to sacrifice the lives of its citizens, mortgage their economic future to antiretrovirals and disgrace the efforts of his country's scientists. The present and future generations of Nigerians may never forgive President Obasanjo, a self–declared 'Mr. Know All' but in reality, an empty, pompous, sadistic and wicked leader that would not even investigate the claim of a purported major scientific discovery by his own country's researcher before he throws it out as dangerous garbage!

Matters are even worse because, as stated earlier in this chapter, there was an August 2008 Nigerian newspaper report of 70 percent HIV prevalence rate in a Local Government Area (the equivalent of a county in some countries) in the country! From the author's experience of his country and the HIV screening tests he has performed, the Eket Local Government HIV prevalence figure of 70 percent is far more accurate and realistic that what the country's Health Ministry and other agencies have been turning out to the world.

The US and Forced HIV Testing of Some of Its Visa Applicants

Universally, HIV infection is diagnosed through the detection of anti-HIV antibodies in the blood. Those immunized with HIV envelope proteins would test positive on screening for HIV antibodies even though they are not HIV-infected. Some of the HIV-infected persons that have come to the author for treatment informed him that they knew for the first time that they were HIV-positive when they went for a US visa interview. Bewildered, the author asked the first person to tell him this information, 'How?' According to them, all Nigerian applicants for a US visa are subjected willy-nilly to HIV screening by the US Embassy in Nigeria, and any applicant who tests positive is denied a US visa! The author was dumbfounded!

The author has only recently confirmed from the horse's mouth, so to say, that what his patients told him some years ago was indeed the gospel truth. The author saw the following account on the Internet recently [10]:

> "Senate agrees to triple anti-AIDS funding
>
> By JIM ABRAMS, Associated Press Writer *1 hour, 19 minutes ago*
>
> WASHINGTON - The (US) Senate voted Wednesday (July 16, 2008) to triple spending for a much-acclaimed program that has treated and protected millions in Africa and elsewhere from the scourges of AIDS, malaria and tuberculosis.
> The 80-16 vote committed the United States to spending up to $48 billion over the next five years for the most ambitious foreign public health program ever launched by the United States. ...
>
> Senate changes will have to be worked out with the House. Those include a measure added to the Senate bill by Sens. John Kerry, D-Mass., and Gordon Smith, R-Ore., that would reverse a policy that has made it difficult for HIV-positive foreigners to visit or seek residency in the United States.
>
> 'For 20 years the United States has barred HIV-positive travellers from entering the country even for one day,' said Rachel B. Tiven, executive director of Immigration Equality. 'Today the Senate said loud and clear that AIDS exceptionalism must come to an end. ...
>
> The bill is S. 2731"

Oh dear! The report started with a deliberate falsehood when it said, "The (US) Senate voted Wednesday (July 16, 2008) to triple spending for a much-acclaimed program that has treated and protected millions in Africa and elsewhere from the scourges of AIDS, malaria and tuberculosis." Where are the treatment and protection from AIDS that the US claims here? After using all sorts of false propaganda to prevent Africans and others elsewhere from taking safe and effective HIV vaccines that were developed since 1998/99, the USA is now pretending to have a much-acclaimed program that has treated and protected millions in Africa and elsewhere from the scourges of AIDS even though the US has been indirectly responsible for the death of millions in Africa and elsewhere! Yet, there is no doubt that it was the same US that gave the world the first cases of AIDS!

The whole world, including the US, has been advocating voluntary HIV screening. And the same US, one of the most vocal countries that preach against any form of discrimination against HIV-infected persons, have had this policy for the past 20 years?! God's own country has a policy of open, shameless and unethical but legal discrimination of HIV-infected persons since 1988 and forcefully subjects US visa applicants to HIV screening!

For the past 20 years, the US, which has been advocating that HIV screening should be voluntary and that there should be no form of discrimination against HIV-infected persons, has only been pretending and talking with its tongue in the cheek? So, for the past 20 years, the US has been guilty of 'Do what I say about voluntary HIV screening and non-discrimination of HIV-infected persons but, for the US, it is our policy to forcefully carry out HIV screening tests on all US visa applicants and to discriminate against those of them that are HIV-positive'!? The author needs urgent help because the ground is giving way under his feet!

So, one should no longer trust the words emanating from even the very top US government officials and US Embassies/Consulates on HIV/AIDS? Is it not possible that the US has other obnoxious policies on HIV/AIDS? Is it not possible that the US has a policy or policies concerning the development of HIV vaccines by non-US citizens? In particular, is it not possible that the US has a policy or policies for non-US citizens that develop safe and effective HIV vaccines before the US? Oh dear! The questions go on and on ad infinitum.

After weeping uncontrollably for several hours, the author thereafter has been left utterly flabbergasted, shocked, devastated, disgusted and battered since he read about the Senate vote last Thursday July 17, 2008 and came across this 20-year old US policy. How many other countries are in tandem with the US on similar obnoxious and inhuman policies on any aspect of HIV/AIDS? Let them tell us now. What has the world turned into, dear brothers and sisters that are reading this?

The HIV screening method used by the US Embassy does not differentiate between anti-HIV antibodies resulting from HIV infection and antibodies caused by HIV candidate vaccine trials championed by the same US. Before the US and other countries test their candidate HIV vaccines on nationals of other countries, they do not inform them about this policy of the US! Is that ethically proper, justified or defensible?

The author decided to search for more information on this US policy on the web. Here is what he got:

> In June 1987, the U.S. Public Health Service added AIDS to its list of diseases for which people on public health grounds could be excluded from the USA [11].
>
> Subsequently in July, the "Helms amendment" created by Senator Jesse Helms added HIV infection to the exclusion list [12]. Few foresaw the implications of the addition and it went virtually unnoticed [13].
>
> On April 2, 1989, Hans Verhoef, a Dutch man with AIDS, was jailed in Minnesota under the federal law banning travellers with HIV from entering the USA [14].
>
> In March 1993, the House of Representatives in the USA voted overwhelmingly to retain the ban on the entry into the country of HIV positive people [15].

The author is surprised that the US has done nothing to bar or discourage its own HIV-positive citizens from travelling to other countries. If the fear of the US is that non-US HIV-infected persons visiting the US may spread the virus to some US citizens, then by the same token the US should have been forcefully screening its own citizens that apply for US passports for HIV and denying all its own HIV-positive citizens the US passport so as to prevent such US citizens from travelling to other countries and having the opportunity of infecting some citizens of those countries.

As far as the author has been made to understand, international relations are based on mutual respect. He has also been made to understand that in international relations, there are no permanent friends or enemies; what is permanent is the economic interest of every country. When he looks back over his comments about his country's Presidency under Olusegun Obasanjo, some might have thought that the author was too harsh. Now see this development. Obasanjo must have known as Nigeria's President for 8 years that his country's citizens were being subjected by force to undergo HIV screening when they apply for a US visa. If he took it up and was told it was US policy, why did he not put a similar policy in place for US applicants for Nigeria's visa? His failure to do that vindicates the author's earlier description of him and his leadership of Nigeria. Since the US has practised that policy all these years, the author believes if other countries had been treating US citizens that apply for other countries' visas in the same way, the US would have reconsidered and likely reversed that obnoxious policy a long time ago.

In the author's view, this 20-year old US policy is evil incarnate, a monster of man's inhumanity to man. Where was the US Judiciary these past 20 years that the policy was in place? Is this 20-year old policy of the US not enough to sustain a charge against the US for crimes against humanity before the International Criminal Court?

The author wonders as a layman whether all the US leaders in the Executive, Legislature and Judiciary who have upheld this obnoxious policy for 20 years do not qualify to be charged *en mass* before that Court for trial! The minimum alternative, in the author's view is a public US apology to all other countries that have been subjected for 20 years to this evil US policy that has done tremendous damage to the way other countries may now start viewing the words and actions of the US: we urge you to do what we say but remember we are doing the opposite!

Conclusion

The toll of HIV/AIDS in sub-Saharan Africa is not just incredible; it is mind boggling. For the past 20 years, the US has virtually driven a cruel nail into the HIV/AIDS coffin that has been the lot of sub-Saharan Africa to bear by forcefully forcing them to undergo HIV screening whenever they apply for US visa, and then heartlessly discriminating against them by denying them entry into the US. This, in the author's view, is one of the pinnacles of man's inhumanity to man, of crimes against humanity. After all, it is an unchangeable fact of history that the first cases of AIDS known to man were reported in 1981 by US doctors who found the disease in US gay citizens living in the US! The author would echo the US Supreme Court's judgment on the disputed 2000 Presidential election results in Florida by saying "We may never know for sure where the disease AIDS started from, but we know for sure where it was first discovered".

References

[1] Cohen J (2001). Shots in the dark: the wayward search for an AIDS vaccine. W.W. Norton and Company, New York. The quotations are from the author's copy that Cohen kindly emailed to him in 2004 after *Vaccine* published his report.

[2] Spier RE (2004). Jerimiah Abalaka and HIV in Nigeria. *Vaccine* 22, 3817-3818.

[3] Abalaka JOA (2004). Attempts to cure and prevent HIV/AIDS in central Nigeria between 1997 and 2002: opening a way to a vaccine-based solution to the problem? *Vaccine* 22, 3819-3828.

[4] Lehner T (2005). Letter to the Editor: Editorial and Report by J.O.A. Abalaka. "Attempts to cure and prevent HIV/AIDS in Central Nigeria between 1997 and 2002: opening a way to a vaccine-based solution to the problem". *Vaccine* 23, 1093-1094.

[5] Abalaka J (2005). Letter to the Editor: Reply to Thomas Lehner's Letter to the Editor. *Vaccine* 23, 1095-1096.

[6] Abalaka JOA (2007). Preliminary evidence of efficacy from an open label trial of a therapeutic AIDS vaccine derived from the blood of HIV-positive donors. *Int. J. Biotechnology* 9(3/4):236-245

[7] Huang YF, Lu NQ (2005). Jeremiah Abalaka and His HIV Vaccine. *Natl. J. Androl.* 11(1): 7-8.

[8] Abalaka JOA (2005). Design, Development and Successful Application of Safe and Effective HIV Therapeutic and Prophylactic Vaccines. *Natl. J. Androl.* 11(1): 8-16.

[9] http://www.fas.org/sgp/crs/row/IB98046.pdf

[10] Downloaded from Yahoo! News on Thursday. July 17, 2008

[11] Jambs J.S. (1991), 'HIV travel/immigration ban: background, documentation' in www.aids.org

[12] Senate Record Vote Analysis (1987) 'Supplemental appropriations/AIDS testing for immigrants', 100th Congress, 1st session, June 2, Vote No. 142 in www.senate.gov

[13] Wachter R.M. (1991) *The Fragile Coalition*, St. Martin's Press, New York, p.29

[14] Olszewski L. (1989) 'S.F. Protest planned over INS detaining of Dutch man with AIDS', *San Francisco Chronicle*, April 6

[15] Cooper K.J. (1993) 'House backs HIV immigration ban nonbinding resolution at odds with Clinton's campaign pledge', *The Washington Post*, March 12

Section III:
Colossal Global Efforts to Develop Safe, Effective HIV Vaccines

Chapter XII

Margaret Heckler's 1984 Press Conference

Abstract

This Chapter recounts from records at the author's disposal the bare facts of the events that transpired at Margaret Heckler's 1984 press conference. Readers may want to know why the author is occupying their time with the details of that press conference. That concern is well taken. The author is convinced that when the reader goes through the press conference, the answer to the question would be very obvious. Most of what the rest of this book deals with would find their roots in that press conference. The author believes that the best way to tackle any problem is to get at the root of the problem; pecking at the stem, branches or the leaves of the problem will not solve the problem. Let us get to the root of the problem of the universal failure to develop HIV vaccines since 1984; let us know the details of Margaret Heckler's 1984 press conference.

Introduction

We saw in Chapter 11 that following the CDC alert on GRID (gay-related immune deficiency) in 1981, researchers in several laboratories mobilized to try to find the cause of the disease. This included Robert Gallo's lab C at the National Institutes of Health (NIH), and Luc Montagnier's lab at the Pasteur Institute in Paris, France [1].

In a *New York Times,* April 22, 1984 article *'Federal official says he believes cause of AIDS has been found',* Altman L.K. wrote that Dr. Mason of the CDC had said, "I believe we have the cause of AIDS." He was referring to the French virus, LAV, and he was basing his opinion on the findings made in the preceding weeks by the researchers at the Pasteur Institute who had discovered the virus the previous year.

That article was the impetus that compelled the United States Health and Human Services Secretary Margaret Heckler to announce at a press conference the following day, April 23rd, that Dr. Robert Gallo of the National Cancer Institute had isolated the virus which caused AIDS, that it was named HTLV-III, and that there would soon be a commercially available test able to detect the virus with "essentially 100 percent certainty". It was a dramatic and optimistic announcement that also included:

> "We hope to have a vaccine [against AIDS] ready for testing in about two years."
> And it concluded with:
> "Yet another terrible disease is about to yield to patience, persistence and outright genius".

The same day patent applications were filed covering Gallo's work, but there was clearly a possibility that LAV and HTLV-III were the same virus. The scientific papers regarding Gallo's discovery of HTLV-III were published on 4th May, 1984, eleven clear days after Margaret Heckler's press conference. By May17th, private companies were already applying to the Department of Health and Human Services for licenses to develop a commercial test, which would detect evidence of the virus in blood, a test which it had already been said would be used to screen the entire supply of donated blood in the USA [2].

On the 31st of March, 1987, at a ceremony at the White House attended by President Reagan, it was announced that an agreement had been reached regarding ownership of the HIV antibody test patent. The Pasteur Institute agreed that it would end its legal challenge, and would share the profits from the test with the U.S. Department of Health and Human Services. Although the agreement officially resolved the question of who had invented the HIV antibody test, it did not address the question of who had discovered HIV and identified it as the cause of AIDS. It was generally agreed that "historians can decide who found the AIDS virus first." But to many people it appears clear that HIV was isolated in Paris a year before it was isolated in the USA [3].

Let us also recall the following:

> "Today it is generally agreed that Montagnier's group first identified HIV, although Gallo's group is credited with much of the science that made the discovery possible, and to demonstrating that it causes AIDS. Gallo's group also was the first to grow the virus in an immortalized cell line, leading to the development of blood tests for HIV and the ability to screen donated blood for this virus. Also, Gallo insisted the work of Montagnier had relied on a technique previously developed by Gallo for growing T cells in the laboratory by supplementing interleukin-2. *The two scientists continued to be at the centre of a bitter dispute between the United States and France over royalties from the blood test patent until 1987, when they agreed to share credit for the discovery of HIV.* In the November 29, 2002, issue of *Science*, Gallo and Montagnier published a series of articles, one of which was co-written by both scientists, in which they acknowledged the pivotal roles that each had played in the discovery of HIV" [4].

The Available Details of Margaret Heckler's 1984 Press Conference

What led to the bitter dispute between France and the US over royalties from the blood test patent until 1987? Of course, it was Margaret Heckler's 1984 Press Conference that caused the bitter dispute. The most comprehensive account of Margaret Heckler's 1984 landmark press conference that the author can lay his hands on is the one written by Jon Cohen [5]. Readers should please note that it was the author who produced and inserted the sub-headings in the following account.

Reagan's Press Secretary jokes publicly about the "gay plague":

THE WHITE HOUSE
Office of the Press Secretary

PRESS BRIEFING BY
LARRY SPEAKES
October 15, 1982
The Briefing Room
12:45 P.M. EDT

Q: Larry, does the President have any reaction to the announcement - the Centres for Disease Control in Atlanta, that AIDS is now an epidemic and have over 600 cases?

MR. SPEAKES: What's AIDS?

Q: Over a third of them have died. It's known as "gay plague." (Laughter.)
No, it is. I mean it's a pretty serious thing that one in every three people that get this have died. And I wondered if the President is aware of it?
MR. SPEAKES: I don't have it. Do you? (Laughter.)
Q: No, I don't.
MR. SPEAKES: You didn't answer my question.
Q: Well, I just wondered, does the President—
MR. SPEAKES: How do you know? (Laughter.)
Q: In other words, the White House looks on this as a great joke?
MR. SPEAKES: No, I don't know anything about it, Lester.
Q: Does the President, does anybody in the White House know about this epidemic, Larry?
MR. SPEAKES: I don't think so. I don't think there's been any—
Q: Nobody knows?
MR. SPEAKES: There has been no personal experience here, Lester.
Q: No, I mean, I thought you were keeping—
MR. SPEAKES: I checked thoroughly with Dr. Ruge this morning and he's had no—(laughter)—no patients suffering from AIDS or whatever it is.
Q: The President doesn't have gay plague, is that what you're saying or what?
MR. SPEAKES: No, I didn't say that.
Q: Didn't say that?
MR. SPEAKES: I thought I heard you on the State Department over there. Why didn't you stay there? (Laughter.)
Q: Because I love you, Larry, that's why. (Laughter.)
MR. SPEAKES: Oh, I see. Just don't put it in those terms, Lester. (Laughter.)
Q: Oh, I retract that.
MR. SPEAKES: I hope so.
Q: It's too late.

On October 15, 1982, Larry Speakes, then the spokesperson for President Ronald Reagan, like most people in the world, had no idea that a new epidemic disease, acquired immunodeficiency syndrome, was racing around the United States, Europe, and Africa.

... The sexual promiscuity of gay men in these liberated years, where it was not uncommon for people to have 50 partners in a year, offered the disease a chance to firmly establish itself on these more developed continents. And these were places where doctors had been trained to take note of odd cases, such as young men dying from Pneumocystis carinii pneumonia, a normally wimpy disease.[1*]

[1*] Standards of training for any profession in any country are not stagnant. Curricula are always being reviewed in all countries in order to update them. In the author's view, it is imprudent to make this sweeping statement "and these more developed continents are places where doctors had been trained to take note of odd cases, such as young men dying from Pneumocystis carinii pneumonia, a normally wimpy disease." This statement implies that doctors trained in less developed continents are not trained to make such observations. In the author's opinion, one should not make such statements until one has done extensive comparative studies of the

Five cases of this rarely fatal disease in gay men indeed caught the attention of a Los Angeles physician in 1981, and he reported his findings on June 5, 1981, in the Morbidity and Mortality Weekly Report (MMWR), a no-frills, but widely read publication issued by the U.S. Centres for Disease Control (CDC) to alert the medical community to public health issues. By October 1982, when Speakes joked about the emerging epidemic, MMWR had published 11 reports on AIDS. Articles had appeared in the major medical journals. True, the popular media had been shy about covering the story, but even by that point it had appeared on the network news and on front pages of major daily newspapers. Larry Speakes, in short, should at least have known that AIDS existed. And his ignorance highlighted the Reagan Administration's indifference—and even outright hostility—toward homosexuals. It also foreshadowed how unprepared the people at the top were to lead the battle against this burgeoning epidemic, especially when it came to organizing the search for a vaccine.

The Influence of USA Presidents on Conquering Disease

Presidents can make enormous differences when it comes to conquering disease. Fifty years earlier (1932), when thousands of children in the United States were being crippled each year by polio, President Franklin Delano Roosevelt organized charity balls on his birthday "to dance so others may walk." These balls evolved into the National Foundation for Infantile Paralysis, colloquially known as the March of Dimes, which would successfully lead the campaign to research and develop the first polio vaccines. But then, FDR had polio himself. He also appointed his former law partner, Basil O'Connor, to run the March of Dimes.

Ronald Reagan for many years refused even to say the word "AIDS" in public. And Reagan's top aides had as difficult a time with AIDS as he did. Consider this exchange between Speakes and journalists at a White House Press briefing on June 13, 1983:

> Q: Larry, does the President think that it might help if he suggested that the gays cut down on their "cruising"? (Laughter.) What? I didn't hear your answer, Larry.
>
> MR. SPEAKES: I just was acknowledging your interest—
>
> Q: You were acknowledging but—
>
> MR. SPEAKES:—interest in this subject.
>
> Q: —you don't think that it would help if the gays cut down on their cruising—it would help AIDS?
>
> MR. SPEAKES: We are researching it. If we come up with any research that sheds some light on whether gays should cruise or not cruise, we'll make it available to you. (Laughter.)
>
> Q: Back to fairy tales.

---

training of doctors with regards to observations in the more developed countries and in the less developed countries. The data on such comparative studies should then be presented so that others may be able to see the rational for the conclusion. Besides, in this case, how do we know that there were no other cases of Pneumocystis carinii pneumonia that had gone unnoticed by doctors in these more developed countries? In the same more developed countries with the presumed (but unconfirmed and possibly untrue) better training of doctors about observing odd cases, are all the doctors in those countries of the same acumen in observation? The author doubts if they are.

Could the person who handled the press for FDR publicly have made jokes about polio and lived to see the inside of the White House again?

Barrister Margaret Heckler takes the driver's seat at HHS

At the Time (June 13, 1983) Larry Speakes was making fun of gay cruising, Margaret Heckler had been the Administration's top health official for three months and was preparing for a speech the next day to the U.S. Conference of Mayors, at which she would declare that AIDS was the "number one health priority."

A lawyer by training, Heckler had represented Massachusetts in the Congress for 16 years before Reagan appointed her to head the Department of Health and Human Services (HHS), a mammoth agency tasked with overseeing both the National Institutes of Health (NIH) and the CDC. Heckler's chief of staff, C. McClain "Mac" Haddow, recalled that his boss knew little about AIDS when she took the HHS post. So Haddow, a former Utah state representative, and other staffers scheduled a briefing for her.

To educate Heckler about the disease, they brought in James Mason, head of the CDC in Atlanta, Georgia. Edward Brandt Jr., the assistant secretary for Health, also came to the gathering in her office, as did a gay man who had been a close aide to Heckler since her time on Capitol Hill. Mason walked Heckler through the basics of how AIDS appeared to be transmitted, explaining that it focused on homosexuals and why that might be. "He was talking about anal intercourse and Heckler got this shocked look on her face and said, 'What?'" recalled Haddow. "Jim Mason, who's a very straight-laced Mormon and was having a little difficulty with this, said the rectal wall was more fragile than the vaginal wall."

> "Anal intercourse?" said Heckler, looking at her trusted, gay staffer. "You do that?"
>
> Ed Brandt looked at Haddow. "I think we better come back and discuss this a little later," said Brandt.
> Haddow said that everybody in the room was stunned. "Mrs. Heckler didn't understand that homosexuals engaged in anal intercourse."

Pre-Press Conference Discussions

ON APRIL 23, 1984, MARGARET HECKLER summoned Robert Gallo into her office at the Hubert H. Humphrey Building in Washington, D.C. A prominent and controversial researcher at the National Cancer Institute (NCI), Gallo had just raced home from a scientific conference in Italy to attend what would turn out to be one of the most awkward, confused—and talked about—scientific press conferences in history: in a few hours' time, Heckler would announce that Gallo's lab had found the cause of AIDS, firing the starting gun for the vaccine search. But before she made this grand declaration, she wanted Gallo's input about the amount of time it would take to translate his laboratory's discovery into an AIDS vaccine.

Scientists who make discoveries in basic research long have shied away from offering predictions about practical outcomes, and reporters long have hounded scientists to offer just such predictions. Mac Haddow wanted Heckler to be able to address this question head on, and for days he had been pressuring the NIH to give him a time line. "The NIH public affairs office was asked, and they came up with a whole list of possible answers," said Haddow. "The bottom line was it was going to have to be Gallo's call. And he would have to be comfortable with it."

When Haddow first began seeking an answer to this question, he thought he would have several weeks to find an answer. Plans called for announcing the explosive news of the Gallo lab's discovery in concert with the May 4 issue of Science, which would contain four back-to-back papers describing how the lab had fingered a new virus as the culprit and grown large quantities of it. But Haddow's PR plans became fouled up when news stories hinting at the discovery began to dribble out during the second week of April. Creating further grief for HHS, the White House had high hopes of using the news during this election year to confront criticisms about the Reagan Administration's AIDS record. At Ed Brandt's urging, Gallo and NIH director James Wyngaarden, who had travelled together to the conference in Italy, both hastily returned home to attend this Monday afternoon press conference.

When Gallo, Wyngaarden, and NCI director Vincent DeVita Jr. arrived at Heckler's office that morning, Haddow quickly dressed them down for a story that had appeared the day before on page 1 of the New York Times. Headlined "Federal Official Says He Believes Cause of AIDS Has Been Found," the article was not about the findings in Gallo's lab. Rather, it quoted James Mason, head of the CDC, describing the work of researchers at the Pasteur Institute in France, and Mason said he had not yet seen the papers from Gallo's lab. Haddow was livid about the perception that the CDC and the NIH—both of which are part of HHS—were at odds with each other, and contended that the NIH was to blame for some of the tension between the institutes. After the bickering about who was at fault died down, Haddow asked how long it would take to develop a vaccine. The question caught Gallo unawares. "I hadn't thought about it before we went in there," said Gallo. "I didn't even anticipate the question."

DeVita and Wyngaarden attempted to convince Haddow that the idea of offering a time line was a mistake. "People have tried to make vaccines against all sorts of things, and the record is generally one of failure," Wyngaarden said. Wyngaarden had little respect for Haddow, who he thought was "authoritarian" and "gave the scientific point of view no shrift." The NIH director, who personally oversaw a $4.5 billion budget (1% of which went to AIDS) and had extensive clout on Capitol Hill, also had little respect for Heckler. "The woman was one of the worst listeners I've ever encountered in any capacity," he said. "She'd listen to one sentence or two, and then her mouth wouldn't close again."

By all accounts, Gallo came up with the official line: within two years, an AIDS vaccine would be ready for human testing. "I assume as much credit or blame for that as anyone," Gallo later acknowledged. Haddow recalled having "a lengthy discussion about why it was defensible." Said Haddow: "I wanted to be sure before Heckler said it and was brought into it that there was a reasonable expectation that we could accomplish that goal."

Brandt, who was also part of these discussions, put great faith in Gallo's enthusiasm. "He was convinced that he had all the makings of a vaccine, that he was fully prepared to move on that very quickly, as a matter of fact," said Brandt. "I really had great confidence in Gallo's ability to pull that off."

Gallo and Heckler's tete-a-tete before the Press Conference

Heckler, who had a severe case of laryngitis that day, invited Gallo into her office for a one-on-one chat.

> "Will we be able to get a vaccine?" she asked in her scratchy voice.
>
> Gallo said he believed so. "I just said, 'I think, you know, due to the fact we have an unlimited amount of virus now and we're sure it causes the disease, I can't think that this should take that long.' I didn't perceive the difficulties."

The Press Conference proper

Hundreds of Journalists jammed into the first-floor auditorium of the Hubert H. Humphrey Building for the 1:15 P.M. press conference. Heckler stepped up to the lectern first. She had a dyed blonde head of helmet hair, and its cartoonish effect was exaggerated by her bright red dress, which sported a high white collar. Behind her, a dramatic, 20-foot-high blue curtain served as a backdrop. Flanking Heckler were Gallo and the agency's top brass: HHS assistant secretary Brandt, NIH director Wyngaarden, CDC director Mason, and NCI director DeVita.

Heckler opened the proceedings with a joke. "As I believe you anticipate, this press conference will be devoted to the subject of AIDS, in which area there is, of course, important news," she said from behind the thicket of microphones sprouting from the lectern. "But, unfortunately, we have not made similar breakthroughs in the field of laryngitis. So I apologize for the state of my voice today."

Heckler continued in an increasingly faltering voice. "Today, I am pleased to whisper"—the reporters laughed—"that the arrow of funds, medical expertise, research, and experimentation with the Department of Health and Human Services, and its allies around the world, have [sic] aimed and fired at the disease AIDS, and has hit the target only two or three rings from the bulls eye itself."

It would be quickly forgotten, but at the time of this announcement, several far-flung theories about the cause of AIDS still competed with each other. Some researchers recently had argued that a fungus caused AIDS. Others maintained that AIDS was the result of using amyl nitrate inhalants, called poppers that many gay men snorted to strengthen the power of orgasm. The list of suspected causes also included cytomegalovirus, Epstein-Barr virus, swine flu virus, herpes virus, and the fanciful idea that several of these possible causes were assaulting the immune system in concert. Gallo himself for a time tried to pin the disease on one of the two known human T-cell leukaemia viruses, HTLVs, obscure pathogens recently discovered by his lab.

Only a year before, Gallo and his co-workers had thrust HTLV-I and HTLV-II into the spotlight when they published, again in Science, two papers arguing that these viruses were the possible cause of the then two-year-old AIDS epidemic. Another paper in that 1983 issue from a group headed by Luc Montagnier—a researcher at the Pasteur Institute in Paris,

France, who would later enter a protracted battle with Gallo about who deserved credit for discovering the cause of AIDS—bolstered the case. In the subsequent year, Gallo and his colleagues refined their argument, and now they were contending that the cause was a new member of this viral family, HTLV-III.

The Gallo lab's four 1984 Science papers showed that they had isolated HTLV-III from 48 patients with the disease and spelled out how to grow the virus continually in laboratory cultures, a critical feat because it routinely killed the cells it infected. Heckler emphasized to the journalists that the ability to grow the virus in mass quantities would allow scientists to characterize the agent in detail, understand its behaviour, and develop a blood test in as little as six months. "Finally, we also believe that the new process will enable us to develop a vaccine to prevent AIDS in the future," she said. "We hope to have such a vaccine ready for testing in approximately two years."

Heckler proceeded to apportion credit for this discovery to the people sitting behind her. The next paragraph in her prepared statement, which had been distributed to the press, praised the work of researchers at the Pasteur Institute. But Heckler, her voice jumping into what sounded like a helium-induced register, abruptly abandoned the prepared statement, asking Gallo and Brandt to come forward. (Margaret Heckler's prepared text explicitly acknowledged the advances made by the Pasteur Institute researchers. It read: "They have previously identified a virus which they have linked to AIDS patients, and within the next few weeks we will know with certainty whether that virus is the same one identified through the NCI's work. We believe it will prove to be the same.")

Gallo's contributions at the Press Conference

A hunch-shouldered Gallo moved into the spotlight. With his perpetually unkempt steel-wool hair, a too-casual camel-coloured sport coat, and a slightly crooked tie, Gallo looked every bit the academic, which was in keeping with the NIH style. He proceeded to explain himself in tortured English. "Many of you, or all of you, have seen discussions about work in Paris," he said. "There was. There is not. There has never been any fights or controversies between us and a group in France. . . . We have active collaboration in the coming month. If what they identified in Science a year ago is the same as what we now have produced more than 50 isolates of and in mass production, and in detailed characterization, if it turns out to be the same, I certainly will say so, and I will say so with them in collaboration."

Gallo fielded several questions, finally passing on this one: "How many years will it be before there is a marketable vaccine, based on previous experience?" Brandt, at Gallo's urging, came forward. "We're estimating a minimum of two years, probably more like three years," Brandt said. "In two years, we think it's possible to begin to start human trials. But I think we have a—one of the first steps that has to be accomplished is to mass-produce this virus in sufficient quantity to accomplish that. So I think we're talking about probably three years. We're going to hustle." There. Brandt had said it. Three years until a vaccine was on the market.

"Excuse me," the reporter said. "The French told me this morning that they would predict at least five years. And Luc Montagnier"—this was the first mention of Montagnier's name at the press conference by anyone—"said he thought it might be five to 10 years. Why are you more optimistic than the French are?"

> "I'm more optimistic, I guess," said Brandt. "I don't know. I'm more optimistic. Except that I believe it can be done, that's all."

An astute reporter pointed out that there were a number of viruses, "known for as long as two decades," that scientists had yet to defeat with vaccines. "Why are you confident that you can get one for AIDS in two years?"

Gallo finally spoke his mind on the question, backpedalling mightily and, in effect, undermining what he had told Heckler and Haddow earlier. "I believe that the reason that there's a wide difference in what time it takes, you know, it obviously is not in the interest of the scientist to give a fast prediction," he said. "You'll only press us all, say, 'Remember what you said eight months ago, four months ago?' You'll be giving us a clockwatch, … Now your question gets tricky. How do you know you'll have one that really works in AIDS patients? Of course, the prediction for that is impossible. You have no hundred per cent proof that it will be two years, a hundred years, or it may never come from vaccination. It depends on the subtleties of biology. But the principles are there. The likelihood, the best we can say in science, with the technology available, we should have things ready to be able to be tried by then."

Brandt and Gallo traded off answering questions, which ranged from uninformed to insightful, a reflection that the conference had attracted both general assignment reporters and those who regularly covered the science beat. The smartest questioners kept returning to the subject of vaccines. "Dr. Brandt," asked one, "in talking about approval of a vaccine, aren't you sort of blithely leaping over what could be a very difficult ethical problem, namely, the testing of this for safety and efficacy on healthy individuals?"

Brandt misunderstood the clairvoyant question. "Absolutely not. I mean, we would certainly test any vaccine," he said.

Another sharp reporter asked whether they intended to test a live- or a killed-virus vaccine. These are the traditional methods of making a viral vaccine: either killing the virus or weakening a live version of it. These modified versions of the virus then safely can teach the immune system how to defend itself should the real thing ever invade. "Can you comment on the difficulty of human clinical trials of such a vaccine?"

Brandt, an earnest and well-meaning man, did not seem to understand this question either. "Well, we're going to develop the vaccine first," he said. "Then we'll be able—it depends entirely on what kind of vaccine comes out of it. So we certainly are not going to test in humans any vaccine that would put those people at risk of the disease."

The reporter, obviously baffled, kept pressing Brandt, who accused the journalist of "presupposing the kind of vaccine" they intended to develop. "I'm not presupposing anything," the journalist snapped back.

> "We don't have a vaccine at the moment," said Brandt. "And we would certainly take all . . ."
>
> "You're talking about having one in a couple of years," the journalist interrupted, raising the question again about how they planned to stage tests of the vaccine in healthy volunteers.
>
> "Well, as soon as we see the vaccine, then I'll be able to answer that question."

Had Brandt understood vaccine development better, this testy exchange need not have happened. Long before AIDS came around, scientists well recognized that the testing of a vaccine against a lethal disease raises difficult ethical questions. Inevitably, the issue comes down to weighing risks against benefits—and carefully describing the two sides of the scale to anyone who volunteers for the trial. What is more, Brandt's charge that the journalist was "presupposing" the type of AIDS vaccine that would be developed was particularly off-base because if anyone was presupposing anything about the formula for an AIDS vaccine, it was Gallo, as he revealed in a subsequent answer.

Gallo's formula for HIV preventive vaccines

> "You keep asking about the vaccine, when it comes up, what's going to be available in two years," Gallo said to a reporter who had not asked about the vaccine. "As best as a scientist can calculate. We can't predict anything 100%. But you've got to give some answers."

Gallo, who had never made a vaccine against anything, went on to detail a recipe for an AIDS vaccine that, instead of relying on the entire virus like the traditional live and killed approaches, only called for using a piece of the agent that had been produced with genetic engineering techniques. Just such a hepatitis B vaccine was then being engineered that contained the surface protein, or envelope, of that virus. When it came to AIDS, said Gallo, the same logic would apply. "In my view, you'd vaccinate with the envelope protein of the virus," said Gallo. "We'll go to recombinant technology, we are doing that now, and we will produce the protein that way. That protein, I would certainly be willing to take if I were a high-risk person, and I'd do it voluntarily. . . . That's the direction we're kind of thinking about."

48 hours after the Conference

A Couple of days after the Press Conference, June Osborn, then a University of Wisconsin virologist who headed the NIH's AIDS Advisory Committee, received a phone call from an outraged gay researcher she knew in Los Angeles. The researcher explained to her how hard he and his colleagues had been working to convince the gay community in Los Angeles that sex clubs and bathhouses were spreading AIDS. Before the press conference, the researcher said these businesses were empty. But Heckler's enthusiasm about the development of a vaccine had created a euphoric sense that the end of the epidemic was near. Last night, he complained, he saw a bathhouse with a four-hour waiting line.

Media reports from the press conference did dutifully report Heckler's comment that an AIDS vaccine would be ready for testing in about two years. They also by and large left out Brandt's more declarative statement that, by three years, a vaccine probably would be on the market. Still, regardless of the specific language used in the distilled and packaged versions of what was said in the Hubert H. Humphrey auditorium on April 23, 1984, the public heard a simple message: An AIDS vaccine was just around the corner.

Looking back at the conference 14 years later

Looking back on the press conference nearly 14 years later, many of the participants had serious regrets about the vaccine predictions. Brandt said he still "winced" every time he heard reference to an AIDS vaccine being tested in two years, and he had completely forgotten about his own declaration of a marketed vaccine in three. "Certainly there wasn't much experience with the whole idea of a vaccine," acknowledged Brandt. "There was a general belief moving about at the time that this was really going to be a fairly easy nut to crack. It was just a matter of time until some quick breakthrough, or whatever the word is, until that happened. I suspect if we really understood the complexity of the organism at that time, things might have happened differently."

Gallo acknowledged that, at the time, he had "zero previous experience in my life on a vaccine" and only the crudest understanding of the basic immune mechanisms that protect people from infectious diseases. "You can't imagine the level of my own feeling of confidence at that time," he said, by way of explaining his role in the optimistic predictions. His lab had just played major roles in the discoveries of HTLV-I and HTLV-II, as well as uncovering a critical immune system messenger, interleukin-2 that tells cells to grow. With AIDS, they had convincing evidence for the first time that a virus isolated from ailing people caused the disease. Their ability to mass-produce this so-called HTLV-III—which later became known as human immunodeficiency virus, HIV, when it proved to have no relationship to the other HTLVs—laid the groundwork for a blood test, treatment, and a vaccine. They were hot on the trail of discovering which cells the AIDS virus preferred, the various ways it was transmitted, and what genes it had. "There was so much data pouring in that I, too, thought—probably believed—we could have solved the whole bloody thing, you know?"

Gallo's greatest regret is that the press conference was held at all, as it violated an agreement he had made with Montagnier and the other Pasteur researchers earlier that month—and seriously incensed them. "I was terribly, terribly nervous," remembered Gallo. "I had massive conflicting emotions. I felt this shouldn't have been done. I didn't act strong enough that we should have waited until we compared the virus with the French and made a joint announcement." The perception that Gallo made a credit grab was compounded by Heckler's laryngitis, which forced her to skip the parts of her prepared statement that acknowledged the Pasteur's contributions.

There is, of course, no way of knowing for certain whether an HIV vaccine would be any closer to market had the announcement of the discovery of the cause of AIDS been handled differently. But the April 23, 1984, press conference and the attendant backroom imbroglios communicated in bold type that the search for an AIDS vaccine was off to a bad start.

Reagan's Press Secretary makes public jokes about AIDS again

THE WHITE HOUSE
Office of the Press Secretary

PRESS BRIEFING BY
LARRY SPEAKES
December 11, 1984

The Briefing Room
12:03 P.M. EST

MR. SPEAKES: Lester's beginning to circle now. He's moving in front. (Laughter.) Go ahead.

Q: Since the Centre for Disease Control in Atlanta—(laughter)—reports—
MR. SPEAKES: This is going to be an AIDS question.
Q: —that an estimated—
MR. SPEAKES: You were close.
Q: Well, look, could I ask the question, Larry?
MR. SPEAKES: You were close.
Q: An estimated 300,000 people have been exposed to AIDS, which can be transmitted through saliva. Will the President, as Commander-in-Chief, take steps to protect Armed Forces food and medical services from AIDS patients or those who run the risk of spreading AIDS in the same manner that they forbid typhoid fever people from being involved in the health or food services?
MR. SPEAKES: I don't know.
Q: Could you— is the President concerned about this subject, Larry—
MR. SPEAKES: I haven't heard him express—
Q: —that seems to have evoked so much jocular—
MR. SPEAKES:—concern.
Q: —reaction here? I—you know—
Q: It isn't only the jocks, Lester.
Q: Has he sworn off water faucets—
Q: No, but, I mean, is he going to do anything, Larry?
MR. SPEAKES: Lester, I have not heard him express anything on it. Sorry.
Q: You mean he has no—expressed no opinion about this epidemic?
MR. SPEAKES: No, but I must confess I haven't asked him about it. (Laughter.)
Q: Would you ask him Larry?
MR. SPEAKES: Have you been checked? (Laughter.)" [5]

Credit hogging by scientists in the USA is legal

By 1986 the struggles of Jonas Salk had become legend, while Gallo's troubles were escalating. The outrage felt by Luc Montagnier and his colleagues at the Pasteur Institute two years before, when Gallo and the U.S. government officials stood before TV cameras and slighted the French contribution to the discovery of the AIDS virus had led to a lawsuit.

The law does not have a mechanism to punish a scientist for hogging credit, nor does it offer compensatory damages to the aggrieved party. But scientific credit feuds often end up in court under the guise of patent disputes. In this case, the Pasteur Institute sued the U.S. Department of Health and Human Services (HHS) over its patent claims for an AIDS blood test. The technical charge was that Gallo's lab had "misappropriated" from the Montagnier group the specific isolate of AIDS virus used to make the U.S. test.

The legal action by the French

The Pasteur suit rested on a question that surfaced at the 1984 Heckler press conference: how similar was the virus that Montagnier's lab had promoted as the cause of

AIDS to the one spotlighted by Gallo's group? As had become clear in late 1984, not only were the viruses they had isolated similar; they were indistinguishable from each other.

This was as unfathomable as the same person winning the lottery in Paris and Washington, D.C., on the same day. Like all viruses, HIV mutates when it copies itself. But it differs from many viruses because it replicates at a blinding speed, meaning the world is filled with an incredibly diverse array of HIV strains. So there were three main explanations for the similarity between the French and American viral isolates. The first, and least likely, was that the French and American isolates of the virus came from people who were having sex with each other. The Pasteur suit ignored this possibility.

The charge of misappropriation focused on a sample of the putative AIDS virus that Montagnier's lab had shared with Gallo's group during the summer of 1983. The French gave the Americans the virus, which they called LAV, to study it. But following the realization that the two labs had "discovered" identical viruses, the French arrived at the other two most plausible explanations: Gallo and his co-workers had either contaminated their own viral cultures with the French sample, or outright stolen LAV and renamed it HTLV-III [6].

(Italics is for clarity to highlight the excerpts that would be used in the next chapter.)

Conclusion

The author would like readers to note that in 1984, Gallo was a researcher in the National Cancer Institutes (NCI) whose Director was De Vita. We are told, "Flanking Heckler (at the Press Conference) were Gallo and the agency's top brass: HHS assistant Secretary Brandt, NIH director Wyngaarden, CDC director Mason, and NCI director DeVita." The author has reproduced in this Chapter the drama called Margaret Heckler's 1984 Press Conference, the drama that led to a 3-year bitter dispute between two super powers, the US and France. That bitter dispute is child's play when compared to the other fall outs of that conference. We will take a closer look at the drama in the next chapter. Read on.

References

[1] http://en.wikipedia.org/wiki/Robert_Gallo.

[2] http://www.avert.org/his81_86.htm

[3] http://www.avert.org/his87_92.htm

[4] http://csm.jmu.edu HIV/AIDS

[5] Cohen J (2001). Chapter 1 Fast Predictions in Shots in the dark: the wayward search for an AIDS vaccine. W.W. Norton and Company, New York. The quotations are from the author's copy that he kindly emailed to me in 2004 after *Vaccine* published my report.

[6] Cohen J (2001). Chapter 2 The Next Breakthrough in Shots in the dark: the wayward search for an AIDS vaccine. W.W. Norton and Company, New York. The quotations are from the author's copy that he kindly emailed to me in 2004 after *Vaccine* published my report.

Chapter XIII

1984 Mirage of a Formula for Safe, Effective HIV Vaccine Development

Abstract

Gallo knew it was not proper for him to attend the April 1984 Press Conference called by HHS Secretary Margaret Heckler, but he was not strong enough to do so. He attended and participated. One would have thought that Gallo who had great reservations about attending that Conference would talk as little as possible, and that whenever he had to talk he would limit himself to the isolation of the virus that he had done. That was wishful thinking. When he was called upon to talk at the conference, his lips literally refused to close again. He happily but recklessly went into issues about which no one had asked anything. He posed as a vaccine development expert even though he had no such experience at all before he attended that conference. He made himself the pace setter for HIV vaccine development. He affirmed that a vaccine to prevent AIDS would be ready for testing within two years and for the market just another year on. As a result, HIV vaccine research and development came under the reign of waywardness, pride, vanity and prejudice since 1984. The harvest has been the loss of millions of lives with serious socio-economic disruptions in many nations from HIV/AIDS, which continues to infect hundreds of people every day on our planet.

Introduction

This is an interesting and true story about a man called Robert Gallo, a great scientist employed by his country's National Cancer Institutes under the country's Health Department. But at the beginning of the story the author is about to narrate, this great scientist admitted that he not only had zero previous experience in his life on a vaccine, but he had only the crudest understanding of the basic immune mechanisms that protect people from infectious diseases.

While attending a scientific conference in Europe in April 1984, he probably received an urgent Sunday afternoon trans-Atlantic phone call from the lady in charge of his country's Health Department directing him to hurry back home immediately. She explained that there was need in the national interest for him to attend a press conference with her the following day to announce that his lab had isolated the virus that caused AIDS. The Secretary further explained to the great scientist that the Press back home had just carried the news that the French had isolated the virus a year earlier, but since they were lucky that the French had not announced it, it was urgent for them to beat the French to the announcement. The great scientist hurriedly took the next available trans-Atlantic flight back home. During the flight back home, the scientist probably debated with himself throughout.

He weighed the pros and cons of the problem confronting him. A year earlier, his scientist cum researcher colleagues in France had, on their own initiative, given him a viral sample labelled 'LAV' for him to study; they had told him then that they believed it was the virus that causes AIDS. AIDS had been described for the first time in 1981, and everyone was in a race to try and identify what caused the disease. Like his colleagues in France, he too was involved in the race to identify the cause of AIDS. Besides, he had agreed with the French earlier in the month of April 1984 that both teams of researchers on both sides of the North Atlantic ocean would address a press conference on the matter at a date mutually agreeable to both sides.

As the great scientist wrestled with himself over the matter during his westward flight to God's own country, sorry, to his own country, he had no doubt in his mind that his best option was not to attend the press conference. That would mean that the conference would be called off. But then, how would the Health Secretary feel about having to cancel the conference that she had already arranged just to give official stamp to the rumours the Health Department had already passed to the Press that Gallo's lab had isolated the virus that cased AIDS? Of course, she could not call such a press conference without Gallo in attendance to confirm the Secretary's assertions, and answer questions from the Press.

It would cause him a lot of problems back home if he refused to attend the Health Secretary's press conference the next day. He had just recalled that a big chunk of his funds for his research on the cause of AIDS had been coming from the Health Department. He was employed by the Health Department, too. Would he not be called 'unpatriotic' by his country if he failed to perform this national duty? The Secretary had clearly told him on the phone that it was in the national interest for them to call that press conference that Monday. What would happen to him and his job if he failed to attend that conference? He was back to the starting point.

By the time he checked out of the airport, he had made up his mind. Continue to read on for this rapidly unfolding and breaking news drama.

Gallo Eventually Decided to Attend Heckler's 1984 Press Conference

In the last chapter, we saw Margaret Heckler's 1984 Press Conference in detail. Here are relevant excerpts from it.

At the time Larry Speakes was making fun of gay cruising, Margaret Heckler had been the Administration's top health official for three months and was preparing for a speech the next day to the U.S. Conference of Mayors, at which she would declare that AIDS was the "number one health priority."

A lawyer by training, Heckler had represented Massachusetts in the Congress for 16 years before Reagan appointed her to head the Department of Health and Human Services (HHS), a mammoth agency tasked with overseeing both the National Institutes of Health (NIH) and the CDC. Heckler's chief of staff, C. McClain "Mac" Haddow, recalled that his boss knew little about AIDS when she took the HHS post. So Haddow, a former Utah state representative, and other staffers scheduled a briefing for her.

On April 23, 1984, Margaret Heckler summoned Robert Gallo into her office at the Hubert H. Humphrey Building in Washington, D.C.

Scientists who make discoveries in basic research long have shied away from offering predictions about practical outcomes, and reporters long have hounded scientists to offer just such predictions.

After the bickering about who was at fault died down, Haddow asked how long it would take to develop a vaccine. The question caught Gallo unawares. "I hadn't thought about it before we went in there," said Gallo. "I didn't even anticipate the question."

Hundreds of Journalists jammed into the first-floor auditorium of the Hubert H. Humphrey Building for the 1:15 P.M. press conference. Heckler stepped up to the lectern first. She had a dyed blonde head of helmet hair, and its cartoonish effect was exaggerated by her bright red dress, which sported a high white collar. Behind her, a dramatic, 20-foot-high blue curtain served as a backdrop. Flanking Heckler were Gallo and the agency's top brass: HHS assistant secretary Brandt, NIH director Wyngaarden, CDC director Mason, and NCI director DeVita.

Heckler emphasized to the journalists that the ability to grow the virus in mass quantities would allow scientists to characterize the agent in detail, understand its behaviour, and develop a blood test in as little as six months. "Finally, we also believe that the new process will enable us to develop a vaccine to prevent AIDS in the future," she said. "We hope to have such a vaccine ready for testing in approximately two years."

A hunch-shouldered Gallo moved into the spotlight. With his perpetually unkempt steel-wool hair, a too-casual camel-coloured sport coat, and a slightly crooked tie, Gallo looked every bit the academic, which was in keeping with the NIH style. He proceeded to explain himself in tortured English. "Many of you, or all of you, have seen discussions about work in Paris," he said. "There was. There is not. There has never been any fights or controversies between us and a group in France. . . . We have active collaboration in the coming month. If what they identified in Science a year ago is the same as what we now have produced more than 50 isolates of and in mass production, and in detailed characterization, if it turns out to be the same, I certainly will say so, and I will say so with them in collaboration."

Gallo fielded several questions, finally passing on this one: "How many years will it be before there is a marketable vaccine, based on previous experience?" Brandt, at Gallo's urging, came forward. "We're estimating a minimum of two years, probably more like three years," Brandt said. "In two years, we think it's possible to begin to start human trials. But I think we have a—one of the first steps that has to be accomplished is to mass-produce this virus in sufficient quantity to accomplish that. So I think we're talking about probably three years. We're going to hustle." There. Brandt had said it. Three years until a vaccine was on the market.

"Excuse me," the reporter said. "The French told me this morning that they would predict at least five years. And Luc Montagnier"—this was the first mention of Montagnier's name at the press conference by anyone—"said he thought it might be five to 10 years. Why are you more optimistic than the French are?"

An astute reporter pointed out that there were a number of viruses, "known for as long as two decades," that scientists had yet to defeat with vaccines. "Why are you confident that you can get one for AIDS in two years?"

What is more, Brandt's charge that the journalist was "presupposing" the type of AIDS vaccine that would be developed was particularly off-base because if anyone was presupposing anything about the formula for an AIDS vaccine, it was Gallo, as he revealed in a subsequent answer.

"You keep asking about the vaccine, when it comes up, what's going to be available in two years," Gallo said to a reporter who had not asked about the vaccine. "As best as a scientist can calculate. We can't predict anything 100%. But you've got to give some answers."

Gallo, who had never made a vaccine against anything, went on to detail a recipe for an AIDS vaccine that, instead of relying on the entire virus like the traditional live and killed approaches, only called for using a piece of the agent that had been produced with genetic engineering techniques. Just such a hepatitis B vaccine was then being engineered that contained the surface protein, or envelope, of that virus. When it came to AIDS, said Gallo, the same logic would apply. "In my view, you'd vaccinate with the envelope protein of the virus," said Gallo. "We'll go to recombinant technology, we are doing that now, and we will produce the protein that way. That protein, I would certainly be willing to take if I were a high-risk person, and I'd do it voluntarily. . . . That's the direction we're kind of thinking about."

Still, regardless of the specific language used in the distilled and packaged versions of what was said in the Hubert H. Humphrey auditorium on April 23, 1984, the public heard a simple message: An AIDS vaccine was just around the corner.

Looking back on the press conference nearly 14 years later, many of the participants had serious regrets about the vaccine predictions. Brandt said he still "winced" every time he heard reference to an AIDS vaccine being tested in two years, and he had completely forgotten about his own declaration of a marketed vaccine in three.

Gallo acknowledged that, at the time, he had "zero previous experience in my life on a vaccine" and only the crudest understanding of the basic immune mechanisms that protect people from infectious diseases."

Gallo's greatest regret is that the press conference was held at all, as it violated an agreement he had made with Montagnier and the other Pasteur researchers earlier that month—and seriously incensed them. "I was terribly, terribly nervous," remembered Gallo. "I had massive conflicting emotions. I felt this shouldn't have been done. I didn't act strong enough that we should have waited until we compared the virus with the French and made a joint announcement." The perception that Gallo made a credit grab was compounded by

Heckler's laryngitis, which forced her to skip the parts of her prepared statement that acknowledged the Pasteur's contributions. ... [1]

The outrage felt by Luc Montagnier and his colleagues at the Pasteur Institute two years before, when Gallo and the U.S. government officials stood before TV cameras and slighted the French contribution to the discovery of the AIDS virus had led to a lawsuit.

The law does not have a mechanism to punish a scientist for hogging credit, nor does it offer compensatory damages to the aggrieved party. But scientific credit feuds often end up in court under the guise of patent disputes. In this case, the Pasteur Institute sued the U.S. Department of Health and Human Services (HHS) over its patent claims for an AIDS blood test. The technical charge was that Gallo's lab had "misappropriated" from the Montagnier group the specific isolate of AIDS virus used to make the U.S. test.

The French gave the Americans the virus, which they called LAV, to study it. But following the realization that the two labs had "discovered" identical viruses, the French arrived at the other two most plausible explanations: Gallo and his co-workers had either contaminated their own viral cultures with the French sample, or outright stolen LAV and renamed it HTLV-III [2]

Gallo, Being Gallo, ...

(Donald) Francis also collaborated with Montagnier and his Pasteur colleagues, helping them in their unsuccessful race against Gallo's lab to be the first to prove that HIV causes AIDS. And along the way, Francis, who had once given a pint of his own blood to Gallo for an experiment, became Gallo's arch enemy. "The ethics of science are that you've got to build on the shoulders of predecessors," said Francis. "You've got to give credit where credit is due. Here's a man who's powerful and receives major funding. This guy violated all the standards of virology I know. I had to watch this man for two years after the press conference [announcing that HIV causes AIDS] never mentioning the French. What 'I, I, I did.' " [2]

On July 2, 1998, after a remarkable showdown between Farthing and Ruprecht over the pros and cons of the attenuated vaccine approach at a packed scientific session during the World AIDS Conference in Geneva, the following account was recorded:

When the microphones opened to the audience, Gallo came out swinging. Unlike attenuated vaccines made against viruses like polio or smallpox, "a retrovirus is forever," Gallo said. "How long would you be prepared in a pilot study to wait before you thought it was safe?"

Before Farthing could answer the question, Gallo, being Gallo, went on the offensive. Every single retrovirus in every single species, from chicken to man, causes disease, Gallo declared. "Every. Single. One." This is not strictly true, as SIV does not cause disease in African monkeys, but Farthing failed to point this out. Instead, he countered that Ruprecht's monkey data seemed inconsistent with data from humans who had weakened strains of HIV. "We'll never know unless we do an experiment in humans," said Farthing.

Gallo allowed that Farthing made some good points, but he appealed to his common sense.

"Let's just talk facts like we were in a barroom, instead of posturing in front of a big audience," Gallo said. "I don't know when you'd be able to tell in a pilot study that it was safe. It's going to be after your lifetime. That's the problem. And it's going to take a lot of people, too." Retroviruses, said Gallo, can take 30 years to cause disease [3].

In 2005, the following interview of Gallo was broadcast on December 1, 2005 in Israel to mark World AIDS Day [4]:

WORLD AIDS DAY – 2005

In Israel, Prof. Robert Gallo is optimistic about finding an HIV vaccine
'It is feasible that we'll get a successful vaccine against HIV'
'This will be a milestone, not just for AIDS but for other viruses as well'
Broadcast December 1st, 2005 on IsraCast.com

The American scientist who discovered AIDS, Prof. Robert Gallo, said on his visit to Israel that there has been great progress in developing a vaccine against the disease, which kills millions of people every year. Since discovered in 1981, the virus has taken the lives of more than 25 million people around the world. At present, the vaccine is effective for three to four months, and has been tested successfully on mice, dogs and rabbits, and lately on monkeys. The results, according to Prof. Gallo, are promising. Prof. Gallo, who will receive an honorary award from Bar-Ilan University, was interviewed on Israel's Channel 2.

Question: Professor Gallo, you have set a milestone in understanding AIDS back in 1983 by defining the HIV. What has happened since, any breakthrough?

Prof. Gallo: Well, as you know, we don't like to use the word breakthrough because it sounds like everything is finished but there have been scientific milestones. Certainly since the period of 83'-85' when the virus was clearly shown to be the cause of the AIDS and a blood test was developed, so the first milestone I guess, was the blood test and it allowed us to be able to protect the blood supply for blood transfusions for medical purposes. It also allowed us to have a test that followed the epidemic from the time of infection throughout the disease and we didn't have to wait until the clinical signs of AIDS appeared. Following that, the next practical milestone was of course the beginning of therapy. Since this is a virus that stays with you, it's a virus of the type we call retrovirus, that once you are infected you are infected forever, unlike the vast majority of viruses which come and go, therefore we really needed treatment, and treatment began in 1986 and culminated in the mid 90's.

Question: And 20 years later we have no vaccine yet. How close are we?

Prof. Gallo: Vaccine has been the most significant failure of the scientific quest. In our institute there has been some important progress. I don't want to say breakthrough, I don't even want to say yet milestone, but the progress that has been made is proving that you can get a vaccine candidate that will make an immune response of the type we believe to be what's needed to block HIV from entering the cell. A type which raises neutralizing antibodies and can do it against the majority of strains of HIV. But we don't have other technical problems solved yet; we can't make that vaccine last a long time. We want to get it to the right levels; those are problems we are still working on with collaborators. While I'm here in Israel it's important for me to point out that intellectually the contributions for this vaccine came from one of my colleagues Dr. Devito, but also from an Israeli scientist, a young guy from the Weizmann institute then, he's now in Tel-Aviv, John Gershoni, who made important intellectual contributions to this pathway.

Question: So finally Prof. Gallo I would like to ask you if today in the year 2005 you can see the day when we will be able to declare we won the battle on AIDS?

Prof. Gallo: Yeah, I do, personally I have to believe, you lose your spirit and your drive if you don't. Intellectually I think it is feasible that we'll get a successful vaccine against HIV and I think like therapy if we get the vaccine against HIV it will be something important for biology in general; it will be that kind of milestone, not just against that disease and that virus. But remember, it has already proven that you can treat a viral disease and the vaccine against HIV, if successful, will give courage against any kind of virus, I believe, and I think the progress made is giving us encouragement [4].

Zooming in on Gallo

Even though the author has neither met Robert Gallo nor been in any form of communication with him, the author has heard and read about him and his work. Like many others, the author holds him in his highest esteem and he has great respect for this great biologist, senior colleague in medicine, researcher and retrovirologist.

On April 23, 1984 when Margaret Heckler called her Press Conference, Robert Gallo (DOB 23.3.1937) had just clocked 47 years of age. The author has the following nagging reservations about Gallo's involvement, participation and utterances at that Conference and thereafter:

> Gallo's greatest regret is that the press conference was held at all, as it violated an agreement he had made with Montagnier and the other Pasteur researchers earlier that month—and seriously incensed them. "I was terribly, terribly nervous," remembered Gallo. "I had massive conflicting emotions. I felt this shouldn't have been done. I didn't act strong enough that we should have waited until we compared the virus with the French and made a joint announcement."

These were said to be Gallo's words 14 years after the Conference. At the age of 47 in 1984, Gallo could not act strong enough to keep to the agreement he had made with Montagnier and his group earlier that month? Why could Gallo not act strong enough and keep away from that Press Conference? If Gallo had acted properly - by being strong enough, by keeping to the agreement he willingly entered with his colleagues in France - and avoided that Conference in April 1984, perhaps the world might have been spared the tragic consequences that have followed his participation at that Conference.

> "Many of you, or all of you, have seen discussions about work in Paris," he said. "There was. There is not. There has never been any fights or controversies between us and a group in France. . . . We have active collaboration in the coming month. If what they identified in Science a year ago is the same as what we now have produced more than 50 isolates of and in mass production, and in detailed characterization, if it turns out to be the same, I certainly will say so, and I will say so with them in collaboration."
>
> The ethics of science are that you've got to build on the shoulders of predecessors," said Francis. "You've got to give credit where credit is due. Here's a man who's powerful and receives major funding. This guy violated all the standards of virology I know. I had to watch this man for two years after the press conference [announcing that HIV causes AIDS] never mentioning the French. What 'I, I, I did.' "

The first words from Gallo at the Press Conference were lies about the French. In the light of the issue just treated, was Gallo honest in his assertions especially when it was the French that sent him a sample of their virus a year earlier for him to study? Why did Gallo not tell everyone at the Conference that he was already in collaboration with the French who had, a year earlier, sent him a sample of their virus for him to study? Even when some journalists at that Conference kept talking about the French with one of them mentioning Luc Montagnier by name, Gallo still refused to open up about the French. If one is to call a spade a spade, Gallo was not honest enough on this at all. The average man on the Street in the USA or elsewhere is likely to be far more honest than Gallo was that Monday afternoon. It is more condemnable that a renowned biologist, medical doctor, researcher and retrovirologist displayed such paucity of basic honesty.

The observations of Francis over two years after the press conference are a terrible indictment of Gallo. Francis tells us that for two years after the Press Conference, Gallo never mentioned the French! It is getting clearer that Gallo's back stabbing and betrayal of the French at the press conference was pre-meditated. He went all out for credit grabbing knowing fully well that there is no law against such unethical conduct in his country, God's own country. His behaviour at that Conference and thereafter is a terrible disgrace to his reputation and to scientists.

> After the bickering about who was at fault died down, Haddow asked how long it would take to develop a vaccine. The question caught Gallo unawares. "I hadn't thought about it befote we went in there," said Gallo. "I didn't even anticipate the question."

Scientists who make discoveries in basic research long have shied away from offering predictions about practical outcomes, and reporters long have hounded scientists to offer just such predictions.

DeVita and Wyngaarden attempted to convince Haddow that the idea of offering a time line was a mistake. "People have tried to make vaccines against all sorts of things, and the record is generally one of failure," Wyngaarden said. …

By all accounts, Gallo came up with the official line: within two years, an AIDS vaccine would be ready for human testing. …

You keep asking about the vaccine, when it comes up, what's going to be available in two years," Gallo said to a reporter who had not asked about the vaccine. "As best as a scientist can calculate. We can't predict anything 100%. But you've got to give some answers."

Gallo, who had never made a vaccine against anything, went on to detail a recipe for an AIDS vaccine that, instead of relying on the entire virus like the traditional live and killed approaches, only called for using a piece of the agent that had been produced with genetic engineering techniques. Just such a hepatitis B vaccine was then being engineered that contained the surface protein, or envelope, of that virus. When it came to AIDS, said Gallo, the same logic would apply. "In my view, you'd vaccinate with the envelope protein of the virus," said Gallo. "We'll go to recombinant technology, we are doing that now, and we will produce the protein that way. That protein, I would certainly be willing to take if I were a high-risk person, and I'd do it voluntarily…That's the direction we're kind of thinking about."

Let the reader please recollect that during the pre-Conference discussions, Gallo admitted he hadn't thought about how long it would take to develop a vaccine and that he hadn't anticipated the question. Both Gallo's own boss, NCI Director De Vita and NIH Director Wyngaarden were also there; both Directors, we are told, attempted to convince Haddow, Heckler's Chief of Staff that the idea of offering a timeline was a mistake. Wyngaarden said, "People have tried to make vaccines against all sorts of things, and the record is generally one of failure." After witnessing the contributions of the two directors, one of whom was his boss, Gallo, being Gallo, came up with the official line: within two years, an AIDS vaccine would be ready for human testing. The author finds this very educative in a bizarre way.

Is this typical of official relationships in the USA? The author wonders why Gallo came up with anything at all after his own boss and Director De Vita had answered the question. Should Gallo not have kept quiet on the issue just out of respect not only for his boss and Director De Vita but also for NIH Director Wyngaarden? Why did he publicly oppose his own Director's opinion when he was just a researcher at the NCI? In the end, Gallo's boss De Vita and NIH Director Wyngaarden were correct, and Gallo who showed no respect for these two Directors was very wrong. Gallo's mouth had already said too much without thinking even about basic respect for his own boss, and the same mouth, refusing to close at the Press Conference, poured out more garbage!

During the Conference, we were told: Gallo fielded several questions, finally passing on this one: "How many years will it be before there is a marketable vaccine, based on previous experience?" Brandt, at Gallo's urging, came forward. "We're estimating a minimum of two years, probably more like three years," Brandt said. "In two years, we think it's possible to begin to start human trials. But I think we have a—one of the first steps that has to be accomplished is to mass-produce this virus in sufficient quantity to accomplish that. So I think we're talking about probably three years. We're going to hustle." There. Brandt had said it. Three years until a vaccine was on the market.

Gallo had realised that he was not qualified to answer this question that was 'based on previous experience'. Unfortunately, he had no such experience. So, Gallo rightly passed on the question to Brandt. However, a few minutes later, the same Gallo made a U-turn, changed his mind and decided to answer the question that had already been answered by Brandt. The author finds it difficult to understand this great retrovirologist and researcher Robert Gallo!

Anyway, in answering the question, Gallo went on an unscientific and reckless voyage of his own — he did not only go on to outline a recipe for the vaccine but he lied and told the journalists at that conference, "We'll go to recombinant technology, we are doing that now, and we will produce the protein that way. That protein, I would certainly be willing to take if I were a high-risk person, and I'd do it voluntarily.... That's the direction we're kind of thinking about." Gallo concocted all this falsehood within the few minutes that had elapsed since he passed the question on to Brandt who had answered the question. Good gracious!

The truth was that Gallo had not thought about when an HIV vaccine would be available until he was asked just before the conference. He was doing nothing at that time about HIV vaccines but told the conference 'We are doing that now.... That's the direction we're kind of thinking about'. Gallo was doing nothing about HIV vaccines when he made these assertions. He was not involved in any HIV vaccine development with anyone at the time he dishonestly and repeatedly used the word 'we'. Gallo concocted all these false assertions to give the impression that he had both previous and current experience in vaccine production at the time of the Press Conference!

The questioner expected an answer that was 'based on previous experience' and so Gallo tailored his answer, building it on false foundation just to meet that condition. Gallo had no such experience at all. So why did he decide to attempt to answer the question? Therefore, the formula or recipe for an AIDS vaccine that Gallo detailed was not in response to any question. It would appear that Gallo deliberately planned to float that recipe for reasons he did not tell the Conference. Gallo acknowledged that, at the time, he had "zero previous experience in my life on a vaccine and only the crudest understanding of the basic immune mechanisms that protect people from infectious diseases." Besides, journalists had reminded him that the French were not as optimistic as Gallo and the other top-ranking officers of the Department of HHS in their estimate of when a vaccine would be available for testing.

The journalists had also reminded Gallo that there were a number of viruses known to man for over two decades and man was yet to conquer them with vaccines, so why such optimistic from him and the DHHS about the new causative agent of AIDS? Despite these circumstances, Gallo went ahead to detail his recipe for an HIV vaccine. Why? Why? Why? He had never had any experience in vaccine production in his life at that time! And why has no scientist in the entire USA or elsewhere taken up these issues with Gallo since 1984? The author is very perplexed.

Gallo's 1984 HIV vaccines recipe, a concocted potpourri of unpardonable, unprovoked and deliberate falsehood, should have been dumped and buried in a rubbish bin as soon as the Conference closed. Instead, Gallo's garbage of a recipe for HIV vaccine preparation has enslaved the whole world since 1984! Why has basic questioning and rational thinking taken flight for so long from scientists worldwide?

The consequences of thoughtlessly and recklessly following Gallo's recipe have been very clear to everyone since 1984 – the number of deaths from HIV/AIDS, the failure by researchers worldwide to develop HIV vaccines because of blindly following Gallo's recipe, the socio-economical wreck the HIV/AIDS pandemic has caused humanity, the billions of dollars wasted in the recurring failure worldwide to develop HIV vaccines along Gallo's worthless recipe, etc. Gallo himself admitted in 2005 during his interview in Israel that over 25 million people had died from HIV/AIDS since 1984! Pheu! Gallo's hands are indeed dripping with the blood of millions of people just because he engaged falsehood dressed brilliantly with pride, vanity and recklessness to float his recipe for HIV vaccines development in April 1984and thereby prevented the use of other approaches for the development of such vaccines up till today.

> When the microphones opened to the audience, Gallo came out swinging. Unlike attenuated vaccines made against viruses like polio or smallpox, "a retrovirus is forever," Gallo said. "How long would you be prepared in a pilot study to wait before you thought it was safe?" Before Farthing could answer the question, Gallo, being Gallo, went on the offensive. Every single retrovirus in every single species, from chicken to man, causes disease, Gallo declared. "Every. Single. One." This is not strictly true, as SIV does not cause disease in African monkeys, but Farthing failed to point this out (1998 in Geneva).
>
> Since this is a virus that stays with you, it's a virus of the type we call retrovirus, that once you are infected you are infected forever, unlike the vast majority of viruses which come and go (2005 in Israel)

Gallo, being Gallo indeed, came out four years later in Geneva, not at a Press Conference this time but at a scientific Conference swinging as he did when he belched out his concocted HIV vaccine recipe in 1984. He emphasized that a retrovirus is for ever, that once you are infected with a retrovirus, you are infected for ever. It baffles the author that a scientist who is mortal man like the author can utter such words persistently and with emphasis. The author does not think it is proper for any human to habitually make such statements; to say it once may be taken as a slip of tongue, but to persist with it beats the author hollow. Is Gallo God, the omniscient? The best any human should say is something like this, "With our present knowledge and experience, I think it is very or extremely difficult to get rid of a retrovirus once you are infected with it".

In the author's view, the hallmark of a scientist should be the avoidance of extreme dogmatic statements or unyielding positions. In the past, diseases like tuberculosis, leprosy and syphilis (the 'great pox' or 'big pox', to differentiate it from smallpox) were labelled 'incurable', but we all now know uncountable number of people that were infected with those micro-organisms but have been cured. Just as Gallo appealed to Farthing's common sense in Geneva in 1998, the author wishes to appeal to Gallo's common sense to please learn to bridle his tongue and utterances as a researcher, a doctor and a scientist.

> (HIV) Vaccine has been the most significant failure of the scientific quest. In our institute there has been some important progress. I don't want to say breakthrough, I don't even want to say yet milestone, but the progress that has been made is proving that you can get a vaccine candidate that will make an immune response of the type we believe to be what's needed to block HIV from entering the cell. A type which raises neutralizing antibodies and can do it against the majority of strains of HIV.

Gallo made this statement in 2005, 21 years after his bizarre recipe for making such a vaccine. For 21 years, he had laboured to produce just such a vaccine that raises neutralizing antibodies to prevent HIV infection and had not succeeded, but he is not prepared to review his approach. In 1998 in Geneva, Gallo told Farthing, *"Let's just talk facts like we were in a barroom, instead of posturing in front of a big audience. I don't know when you'd be able to tell in a pilot study that it was safe. It's going to be after your lifetime. That's the problem. And it's going to take a lot of people, too."* Would some people please help the author drum it into Gallo's ears that he has followed his bizarre 1984 recipe for 21 years; he has failed persistently. Won't he have a rethink? The problem is that it's not only going to be after his lifetime; already tens of millions of people have been taken to the great beyond by the HIV/AIDS while he is chasing the shadows of his concocted and impetuous 1984 recipe!

It therefore saddens the author profoundly that at Margaret Heckler's 1984 Press Conference and thereafter, the great Robert Gallo jettisoned his own standards and achievements as a biologist, doctor, researcher and retrovirologist. Many would like to be euphemistic by calling Margaret Heckler's 1984 Press Conference 'controversial' and/or 'unfortunate'. The author would go farther and further by saying emphatically that Gallo's utterances at that Conference and thereafter have caused unmitigated disaster for humanity, for HIV vaccine research and development, for science, and for proper scientific principles or approach. Here are my other reasons for saying so.

> Ostensibly, Gallo was at that Press Conference for the sole purpose of informing the world that his laboratory had identified the virus responsible for the disease AIDS. He should have limited himself as much as

possible to that purpose. He should have demonstrated cautious scientific approach to issues like when a vaccine for the virus would be available, just as the other big wigs from the NCI, CDC and NIH did during the pre-conference discussions. After all, he had not done any work on producing a vaccine against the virus or against any other micro-organism at the time he attended that Press Conference.

In attending that Conference, he should have been honest enough to admit at that Press Conference that he had never produced a vaccine against anything and as such, he was not in a good position to speculate about when the vaccine against the virus would be available. Instead, he went into details of how a vaccine against the virus should be developed. He even went further to state that a vaccine would certainly be available for testing in two years. Over 20 years after his utterances, he has still not got the vaccine. If the author were to find himself in Gallo's position, the author would have called another Press Conference soon after the 2 years expired, and publicly apologized profusely for the dogmatic statements he had made at that Press Conference, for the false recipe he had enunciated, for his false statements, etc. Of course, the author would have apologized publicly to the French several months earlier. He would then end that Press Conference by withdrawing his 1984 utterances.

The author expects that Gallo knew before that Press Conference that over 90 percent of all the successful viral vaccines in human medical use today were not first developed by those that isolated the causative agents of the diseases. Just recalling that historical fact would have been enough to check his utterances and limit himself to the isolation of the virus – he had a less than 10 per cent chance of being the first one to develop safe and effective vaccines against the virus he had isolated. Perhaps, he also got carried away by the euphoria and publicity of the moment!

Gallo rightly said at that 1984 Press Conference that modern genetic engineering techniques for vaccine production had become the third method of developing vaccines. Hitherto, viral vaccines were developed in two ways: live attenuated or inactivated (killed) whole virus vaccines. The new generation modern vaccines are prepared by this third method that uses just protein(s) from the viral surface proteins (envelope) or even portion(s) of the protein(s). According to protagonists (and they constitute an overwhelming majority) of this modern (third) method of vaccine preparation, its great advantage is that such vaccines can never cause an infection since they are devoid of viral RNA or DNA, the crucial infective substance in viruses. With the dawn of this modern method of vaccine preparation, researchers and scientists like Gallo began referring derogatorily to the first two methods as 'old-fashioned' or 'traditional'. The derogation, it should be noted, does not change the fact that most of the vaccines in use even now are still produced with the 'old-fashioned' or 'traditional' methods, and they are safe and effective. There was no scientific basis for Gallo to declare at that Press Conference that genetic engineering techniques would be used to develop HIV vaccines. He should have left the field open especially when the biological characteristics of the virus he had just isolated were not known. In 2005, Gallo still maintained his position even after over twenty years of failure. Meanwhile, millions have perished from the HIV/AIDS pandemic while several millions have become infected since 1984, a great tragedy for humanity.

Immunology Heresy!?

Gallo narrowed the options to only an HIV preventive vaccine. Without much thought, most people would agree with him on this because the overwhelming majority of vaccines known to medicine are preventive vaccines. Just as Gallo implied at the press conference, it is true that many deny the existence of any therapeutic vaccine; many indeed ridicule the idea.

In the author's country, there is this prolific newspaper writer Professor Tam David-West who, in his own words in one of his newspaper write-ups, said he is 'an internationally and WHO-recognized' Professor of Virology. He was a Minister of Petroleum Resources and of Mines, Power and Steel during General Ibrahim Babangida's Military dictatorship in the 1980s. Even though he has never communicated directly with the author, he has launched several attacks on the author and his HIV vaccines on the pages of several Nigerian newspapers. Here are some excerpts:

To be fair to Augustine also, he never was adventurous (as Abalaka) to use humans as experimental guinea pigs; which is roundly unethical professionally [5].

Abalaka's scientific (medical) adventurism can only occur in Nigeria – Nowhere else in the whole civilized world. In fact, he cannot even contemplate the saga of his so-called "HIV/AIDS vaccine" treatment." If he dares, he will be picked up and sentenced for medical recklessness. This is without prejudice to the merits (or otherwise) of his claims. It is because he has been rather reckless with the fundamentals.

Do vaccine (sic) *cure?* The answer is of course No. Even a first year microbiology undergraduate knows this.

My object therefore, is to subject his claims to time-honoured fundamentals in the field. In this, Abalaka can be seriously strictured in terms of modus operandi (methodology) and ethical imperatives. It is most unfortunate that the whole matter has been overdosed with politics and personalization. This has therefore, blurred the serious professional questions that we should be asking.

It is germane to reiterate that my object is to raise issues (alarm!) over the claims and methods used by Dr. Abalaka in his said breakthrough with HIV/AIDS therapy. I am not a clinician, so I find myself inadequate to make comprehensive valued judgement on Abalaka's claims on his patients; or the testimonies of the "cured." However, I feel that I can safely make the point that mere weight gain or an unmonitored (long duration) sero-positive (HIV) to sero-negative (N HIV) are hardly adequate to establish the said efficacy of his "vaccines"; especially for a deadly disease like AIDS. There are carefully worked out International Standards for this. I had argued earlier that Science is international (Never local) [6].

Perhaps Dr. Abalaka was overzealous when he was reported to have also claimed that his vaccine also cures. This is immunology heresy. Vaccines don't cure, they prevent [7].

Readers may be interested in knowing the author's response, if any. At an International AIDS Forum organized by the then reigning Miss Nigeria 2000, Vien Bemigho Tetsola at the Sheraton Hotel And Towers, Ikeja, Lagos, Nigeria on August 15, 2000, the author was invited to deliver, and he delivered a guest lecture on the topic 'The facts about my HIV adventures and all the various responses so far to my discoveries'. In that guest lecture, he answered the renowned Professor of virology in these words:

> **"A renowned Professor of Virology has been serializing his article in the last two editions of** *The Weekend Concord* **under the caption** *AIDS VACCINE: Blame Nigeria, Not Abalaka.* **His article is to be continued next Saturday. It is possible that the internationally recognized virologist may be present here with us. Permit me, ladies and gentlemen, to reproduce excerpts of his article so far that I consider germane to our discourse (the same excerpts reproduced above). ...**

With the greatest respect, I sympathize with the Professor of international repute because, as he himself admitted, he is not a medical practitioner. HIV infection and AIDS produce serious symptoms and signs in those afflicted. Many seek medical attention in the first place because of their troublesome symptoms. My HIV vaccines ameliorate such symptoms with the sort of rapidity that dwarfs the clinical improvement attributed to the antiretroviral drugs that are very costly and toxic.

In rabid animal bites, the victim is infected with the rabies virus the moment the animal bites him/her. The rabies vaccine that is given to such a victim enables the body to get rid of the wild rabies virus already present in the victim, i.e., the victim is cured of the rabies virus already in him. To the virologists and microbiologists, vaccines may not cure as the Professor said emphatically, but to those of us who are clinicians, vaccines may either be preventive or curative. My highly effective and safe HIV vaccines are both preventive and curative. The vaccine gets rid of the virus in those already infected, but in those not yet infected with the virus, the vaccine protects the person from acquiring the infection.

The carefully worked out International Standards mentioned by the erudite and learned Professor have not been published yet. Fortunately, I have dealt with the United Nations guidance document already. I have also discussed the Physician's oath in detail. I have not used any human being as guinea pig so far except myself. I am almost certain the Professor of Virology would apologize to me for claiming that I have used humans as guinea pigs. (He has not apologized in any way up till now, 2008.) In any case, the United Nations has agreed that human guinea pigs are allowed in HIV vaccine research and development, as I showed earlier.

The Professor, with due respect, did not define the word "cure", and so I am at a loss as to what that word means to him. In the context of HIV infection, I define cure as reversion to sero- and vironegativity in a person previously positive. It is clear to me that the learned Professor of Virology has placed International Standards, scientific language, ethical considerations, methodology and the like as the issues at stake, but has neglected the health of the HIV-infected patient, which is my first consideration as a clinician. I understand his handicap in that he is not a clinician but a virologist.

I would like to remind the Professor and others that any statutory bodies or agencies anywhere in the world do not certify blood transfusions. Yet, doctors throughout the world carry out blood transfusions everyday. My HIV curative and preventive vaccines consist of human blood processed without adding any chemicals whatsoever to the blood that is collected in standard blood bags. At the end of my innovative treatment of such blood, I add just about 0.4 mg per ml of Gentamycin to the vaccine I obtain. Each patient receives 1 ml of the curative vaccine at every visit. The curative vaccine is given at weekly intervals during the first month followed by monthly booster doses of 1 ml until cure is achieved. A bag of whole blood transfusion is about 500 ml.

Doctors all over the world may decide to transfuse either whole blood or portions of such blood, e.g. packed red cells, platelets, leucocytes or plasma may be transfused at the doctor's discretion and without certification by anybody or agency. I give 1 ml of a part of human blood by intramuscular injection and people are howling, saying it has not been registered or certified. *In any case, my HIV preventive and curative vaccines are covered by Federal Government of Nigeria Patent No. RP 13567 dated July 22, 1999 and sealed on January 21, 2000.*

I hope with these clarifications, they would be satisfied.

Time would not permit me to read out to you the different testimonies from the various patients that have benefited from my HIV vaccines. I have made my vaccines available to many doctors across the country for their use on their patients. They have all attested to the efficacy and safety of my HIV vaccines. I have not yet seen or heard about any serious or significant adverse effect arising from the use of my HIV vaccines.

I have not said I have AIDS vaccines. I make no such claim. What I have developed are effective and safe HIV preventive and curative vaccines. AIDS simply means HIV infection complicated by something else called opportunistic infections and/or cancers. My HIV vaccines are ineffective against the "something else" in AIDS."

Readers may likely observe that in spite of this public response the author gave to the Professor's newspaper articles, the same Professor stood on his ground like the Rock of Gibraltar; he came out again after 10 months in another newspaper in June 2001 and wrote, "Perhaps Dr. Abalaka was overzealous when he was reported to have also claimed that his vaccine also cures. This is immunology heresy. Vaccines don't cure, they prevent."

Sorry for the digression; let us continue our discussion on Gallo please. In the author's view, a renowned scientist and researcher of Gallo's status should have kept a more open scientific mind since Gallo knew, or ought to have known that therapeutic vaccines have been in existence in human medical practice for long. In man, rabies vaccine since it was first developed by Pasteur over 100 years ago has remained a therapeutic vaccine when administered to a person bitten by a rabid animal; the person bitten became infected with the virus at the time he was bitten. Also, a therapeutic hepatitis B vaccine is used to abort infections in newborns of mothers who carry that virus.

Let me say one more word about this bizarre 'immunology heresy' of vaccines preventing and not curing. We saw in Chapter 10 that Prof. Luc Montagnier of France was one of the three researchers that were awarded the 2008 Nobel Prize for Medicine for his work on the discovery of the AIDS virus. Here are relevant excerpts from Chapter 10:

> "Telephone interview with Luc Montagnier immediately following the announcement of the 2008 Nobel Prize in Physiology or Medicine, 6 October 2008
>
> The interview was recorded while Luc Montagnier was attending a conference in the Ivory Coast, and the interviewer is Adam Smith, Editor-in-Chief of Nobelprize.org.
>
> ....
>
> [LM] Well, the main message I will convey that even after 20 years we are still fighting this virus, very strongly, and the AIDS epidemic – I am now in an African country – is still spreading in Africa in [inaudible], so the fight is not finished. And I appreciate that the Nobel Committee has put on the air this important disease which is not finished, and my message is that we should continue the research. And myself I'm working on a vaccine – not a preventive vaccine but on a therapeutic vaccine which is aimed at completing the antiretroviral therapy which is now given to many patients even in Africa, but which does not cure. So the idea is to eradicate the virus infection. I think this is the main step now.
>
> ...."

At the end of the day therefore, the author is not the only immunology heretic as Prof Tam David-West authoritatively declared in his newspaper exposition. One of 2008 Nobel Laureates for Medicine recognized in 2008 the existence of preventive and therapeutic vaccines also. If one were to applying Prof. Tam David-West's standards to Nobel Laureate Dr. Luc Montagnier, then one would have to say that the 2008 Nobel Laureate for Medicine, the retrovirologist Dr. Luc Montagnier is not just guilty of immunology heresy but that Luc Montagnier does not know what Prof. Tam David West's undergraduate students in Microbiology know; those students know that vaccines are for prevention, not for therapy!

Why Should HIV Viral Envelope Proteins and/or Genes Be the Only Recognized Immunogens for HIV Vaccine Development?

Gallo literally ruled out other methods of HIV preventive vaccine development when he announced at his press conference that the 'same logic' of using genetic engineering techniques and recombinant technology that utilized the viral envelope protein for vaccine preparation would be employed to develop an HIV preventive vaccine. He underscored that view by declaring that he would voluntarily take such a vaccine if he were a high-risk person. When faced with any viral epidemic or disease, it is, in the author's opinion, unscientific to exclude from the very beginning, the use of other known and effective methods for its vaccine development just because the causative agent was isolated at a time genetic engineering techniques were being used to develop a hepatitis B vaccine.

Still basking in the euphoria and limelight of being the first to announce at any country's press conference the isolation of the virus that caused AIDS – when the chips are down, that was the aim of the Press Conference that had to be brought forward to under cut the French who were actually the first to isolate the virus, Gallo went further to say that an HIV vaccine would be ready for testing in 2 years! Some would say it was very premature, heady and unscientific for him to have gone that far. As it has turned out, that prediction was very wrong.

What Gallo, in 1984, called the 'same logic' of HBV vaccine preparation using modern genetic engineering techniques for preparing an HIV preventive vaccine has, for over 20 years, turned out to be very illogical indeed - so far, no logic has been established between HBV vaccine production using genetic engineering techniques and HIV vaccine production. The HBV is not the HIV! The HBV and the HIV are not identical twins at all; in fact, they are not even distant relations as far as vaccines against the causative viruses are concerned!

When Gallo stated that he would use the same logic of genetic engineering techniques employing the HIV envelope protein to produce an HIV preventive vaccine, he had willy-nilly implied that an effective HIV preventive vaccine must result in the production of anti-HIV antibodies since protein immunogens (antigens) act mainly by stimulating specific antibody production.

In his interview in Israel in 2005, he maintained that stand very clearly when he said:

> "(HIV preventive) Vaccine has been the most significant failure of the scientific quest (for over 20 years). In our institute there has been some important progress. I don't want to say breakthrough, I don't even want to say yet milestone, but the progress that has been made is proving that you can get a vaccine candidate that will make an immune response of the type we believe to be what's needed to block HIV from entering the cell. A type which raises neutralizing antibodies and can do it against the majority of strains of HIV."

This dogmatism is beyond the author's comprehension. Gallo and the overwhelming majority, if not all, of the HIV vaccine researchers worldwide are still groping for candidate HIV vaccines that raise neutralizing anti-HIV antibodies even after over 20 years of failure with that approach. Would they not look back critically at their failed efforts spanning over 20 years and start afresh with open scientific minds and approaches?

In the author's view, this is the most significant damage Gallo bestowed on humanity, science, scientific approach and HIV vaccine research during Margaret Heckler's 1984 Press Conference. His declarations then and thereafter have been swallowed hook, line and sinker by the scientific world. All of them are following the pace-setter Robert Gallo, searching frantically for the elusive golden treasure from the viral envelope protein or another part of the HIV virion that would raise anti-HIV neutralizing antibodies. Did Gallo get a divine revelation on this? The answer is 'No'. It is just his belief. Having unquestioningly tried that belief for over 20 years without success, would the scientific community not stop, take deep breaths, take stock, and start afresh?

They have not, and there is no indication that they intend to ever do so. Instead, they have persisted that the immunogen of any candidate HIV vaccine must be either a part of the envelope protein of the virus or some of the genes of the HIV virion, and must stimulate the production of anti-HIV neutralizing /binding antibodies in experimental animal models and in human trials. Unfortunately and very surprisingly, these researchers have refused to even notice that the persistent failure with this approach since 1984 indicates there is most probably a fundamental flaw with the 'same logic' recipe initiated by Gallo.

Worldwide, HIV vaccine researchers have been carried away by Gallo's idea of developing an HIV preventive vaccine, as if Gallo's idea in 1984 and thereafter is infallible. Invariably, they are all involved in an unsuccessful race to use modern genetic engineering techniques to develop the vaccine using one or more HIV viral proteins or genes. After all, did Gallo not mention genetic engineering techniques in his 1984 recipe? If that approach is flawed, and it is definitely flawed, recurrent failures would continue to be the dividend.

Researchers, as they have done and are still doing without critically looking back, would continue to follow a blind pompous leader along a blind alley, looking for the elusive viral protein(s), part(s) of such protein(s) or viral genes with which to develop the vaccine. In any case, they all forget that when the chips are down, out of the many human viral vaccines in use today, it is an overwhelming minority that were developed with modern genetic engineering techniques. Most of them are the product of 'old-fashioned' or 'traditional' techniques.

The use of viral envelope proteins, part of such proteins or viral genes results in the production of antibodies against such proteins in the recipient. HIV infection generates high titres of binding and effective anti-HIV antibodies in those infected with the virus, but despite this, HIV infection progresses relentlessly to AIDS and death. The author does not think it is difficult for the average person to see the incongruity and unreasonableness in an approach that insists that HIV preventive vaccine candidates must generate anti-HIV antibodies when we all know that our immune responses do not depend on antibodies alone.

In 2002, Swiss researchers reported the first fully documented case of an HIV-positive man who was additionally infected with a second strain of HIV through unprotected sex more than two years after he was first infected [8]. In other words, anti-HIV antibodies do not protect HIV-infected persons against HIV infection by another strain despite the fact that such people already have high titres of binding and effective anti-HIV antibodies. Also, anti-HIV antibodies do not prevent the relentless progression of HIV infection to AIDS and death. The author must admit that he just cannot see any scientific basis for following Gallo's worthless 1984 recipe at all. The author is more perplexed that after following that recipe for over 20 years and achieving nothing but failure, the scientific community worldwide is still shopping for candidate HIV vaccines that generate "neutralizing antibodies and can do it against the majority of strains of HIV."

Retroviral Infection in Man Is No Longer Forever

At the 2005 interview in Israel, Gallo said the HIV is "a virus of the type we call retrovirus, that once you are infected you are infected forever, unlike the vast majority of viruses which come and go, therefore we really needed treatment, and treatment began in 1986 and culminated in the mid 90's". The author must confess again that he is completely at a loss here. Who told Gallo that once you are infected with a retrovirus, you are infected forever? Does Gallo really mean that? This is beyond the author's understanding of science.

Gallo did not support his assertion with any scientific evidence or data. The fact that Gallo and others have tried to develop an HIV preventive vaccine along Gallo's lines of proposals and failed for over twenty years does not eliminate the possibility that others, applying recipes that are different from Gallo's recipe, may succeed in curing HIV infection, as has been happening with the author's HIV therapeutic vaccine since 1998.

The author is not aware Gallo has done any work on attempting to develop HIV therapeutic vaccines. How could he when he himself has said that once you are infected with the HIV or any other retrovirus, you are infected forever?

What Is Cure of HIV Infection?

Let the author digress a little here to sort out this recurring but important problem. In practical terms, what does Gallo mean by 'once you are infected (with the HIV) you are infected forever'? Gallo did not elaborate for us to get him clearly. Like many others, the author's understanding of what Gallo said is that once you are infected with the HIV, you remain infected for life; in other words, that HIV infection is incurable. Many others have used the same or similar words as Gallo did. For instance, statements such as 'HIV infection is incurable' or 'once you are infected with the HIV you are infected for life or forever' or 'there is no cure for HIV infection' are ubiquitous. What exactly do these statements mean and how does one establish that someone infected with the HIV has been cured?

The world has indeed been bombarded with the slogan 'HIV infection is incurable' but there is no matching slogan telling us the definition of 'incurable', 'curable' or even 'cure'. According to the March 2000 prepublication version of UNAIDS guidance document on HIV preventive vaccine research (we will carry out a surgical operation on that document later in Chapter 16), 'currently available treatments (for HIV infection) are inadequate because they do not lead to cure'. Unfortunately also, that document does not define 'cure'. And as we all know, many English words do not only have more than one meaning, but the meaning of words in any language including the English language may change or be modified with time.

What then does one mean by 'cure' of HIV infection in our days or era?

An English Dictionary [9] defines 'cure' thus: *'To make somebody healthy again. To treat an illness, etc successfully'*

Another English Dictionary [10] defines 'cure' in these words: *'A method or course of remedial treatment, as for disease. Successful remedial treatment; restoration to health. A means of healing or restoring to health; remedy.'*

A Medical Dictionary [11] defines 'cure' as *'the course of treatment of any disease, or of a special case. The successful treatment of a disease or wound. A system of treating diseases. A medicine effective in treating a disease.'*

Regarding 'cure of HIV infection', the author was, and is still not satisfied with any of the above definitions. And he has not been able to see or clearly infer the definition of 'cure' for HIV infection wherever he has come across the term.

The author thinks it is essential that we all agree on the definition of 'cure of HIV infection' in the interest of scientific and social consistence or uniformity. Since he is unaware of any universal definition of 'cure of HIV infection', he suggests that its meaning should be intimately related to how we diagnose HIV infection.

The universally accepted method of diagnosing HIV infection is by the screening for, and /or the confirmation of the presence of anti-HIV antibodies in the blood. Accordingly, in the author's opinion, 'cure' of HIV infection ought conversely to be the serodeconversion to anti-HIV antibody negative status in a person previously seropositive for such antibodies. And this has always been his working definition of 'cure' of HIV infection.

If it is indeed true, as researchers have told us, that antibodies to the HIV viral envelope proteins such as gp120 and gp41 persist for life [12], then any treatment that results in the elimination of anti-gp120 and anti-gp41 antibodies in a person previously confirmed positive for these antibodies is effective therapeutically and has resulted in cure of the infection.

It is easy to test for anti-gp120 and anti gp41 antibodies since most screening or confirmation tests for HIV including the Western Blot detect these antibodies. In other words, it should be easy, convenient and cheap to confirm or refute the efficacy of any therapy that claims 'cure' for HIV infection. Even when those on HAART (highly active antiretroviral therapy) have persistent undetectable virus in their blood, they remain positive for anti-gp120 and anti-gp41 antibodies; they are therefore not cured of their HIV infection, and as we saw earlier, if they stop their HAART, the viral load becomes detectable in a few days.

Any Need for Controls in HIV Therapeutic Vaccine Efficacy Trials?

It has been established worldwide that HIV infection is incurable and that it progresses relentlessly to AIDS and death. Therefore, anyone who conceives a candidate HIV therapeutic vaccine has actually only one river to cross before human trials; he must establish the safety of his candidate vaccine. Once the safety of the vaccine is established, the researcher only needs to test for the efficacy of the vaccine in willing HIV-infected patients – the author insists on such patients reducing their consent into writing. There would be no need for controls. The infection is incurable. If the safe candidate vaccine cures even one person of HIV infection, it would be a remarkable achievement since the disease would no longer be tagged 'incurable'.

An analogy may make this point clearer. A person's death is irreversible. If someone claims he has discovered a therapy that brings the dead back to life, we should just give him corpses to treat. If any of the corpses wakes up and continues his /her life as a human being, the person has confirmed his claim. There would be no need at all for any controls of any sort or description.

Safety and Efficacy

Only two factors are crucial to everyone including the physician and the patient when we are dealing with any remedy for human diseases - safety and efficacy.

A safe candidate remedy for an incurable pandemic like HIV/AIDS automatically qualifies for efficacy trials in man, and there would not be any need for controls or meeting any imposed ethical considerations at all since it is safe.

Any drug, vaccine or remedy that is both safe and efficacious qualifies automatically for clinical use even if such a remedy has not followed any laid down procedure or protocol, even if no one understands or knows how it works, even if there are no preceding scientific publications by the researcher on the remedy involved. In other words, when it comes to a candidate therapeutic remedy for a deadly and incurable pandemic like HIV/AIDS, protocols, ethical considerations and scientific publications take the back seat since they exist just to ensure that the candidate remedy is safe when administered to HIV-infected persons. Therefore they become irrelevant and unnecessary if the safety of the candidate remedy is established beyond reasonable doubt.

The author apologizes for the digression. Let us please continue.

Should Scientists Disregard New Discoveries Published in Reputable Scientific Medical Journals?

The author has many confirmed HIV-infected patients that have been cured of HIV infection with the author's HIV therapeutic vaccine. It follows therefore that Gallo's statement that once you are infected with the HIV you are infected forever is completely untrue.

The author believes that Gallo and his team must have come across the publication of the author's work in reputable scientific Journals like the *Vaccine* in 2004. In the published report in the *Vaccine* Journal, the author provided readers with his telephone number and email address. The author does not know Gallo's telephone number or email address. The reader may wish to see References 2 - 8 in Chapter 11 for publications of and about the author's HIV vaccines.

One wonders why Gallo has not made any contact with the author since 2004, four years ago. Is that the way of science? The author is of the opinion that Gallo has not made any effort to get in touch with him because he rigidly believes that the only way to get safe and effective HIV preventive vaccines is through his own approach.

Of course, the author now knows that for Gallo, therapeutic HIV vaccines are a myth since Gallo himself has said that once you are infected with the HIV you are infected forever! If only he had got in touch with the author as other researchers have done, he would have had the golden opportunity of obtaining blood samples of those who have been cured of HIV infection so that he can use all the modern facilities at his disposal to elucidate how these people have overcome HIV. Such knowledge would then have assisted him in his own effort to develop his own HIV preventive vaccine using his own recipe, modified as and if he wishes.

Similarly, he would have gotten blood samples of human beings who have received the author's HIV preventive vaccine for whatever tests he likes. He would also have gotten samples of the author's HIV vaccines to study as he wishes. The editorial preceding the author's report in the *Vaccine* Journal in 2004 informed readers that the author was willing to provide samples of blood for anyone that might wish to have them. It also asked for further investigations into the author's work, but no scientist has taken up the challenges. What else does the scientific world want the author to do? The author is convinced that the it is au unfortunate tragedy that this planet's scientific community is not interested in investigating the author's claims of developing safe and effective HIV vaccines since 1998/99!

One other point — it is even possible that there are other methods of developing safe and effective HIV vaccines other than the three methods recognized by vaccine researchers of our generation! What is the scientific basis for saying or thinking that other methods do not exist? The author knows of none. There is therefore need, in the author's view, for HIV vaccine development researchers especially to always keep very open and receptive scientific minds, otherwise all their shots in the dark would not only continue to be a wayward search for an AIDS vaccine, but would also continue to result in HIV/AIDS sending many more millions to the world beyond.

Conclusion

Looking back on Margaret Heckler's 1984 PCess conference nearly 14 years later (that is, in 1997/98), many of the participants had serious regrets about the vaccine predictions. Brandt said he still "winced" every time he heard reference to an AIDS vaccine being tested in two years, and he had completely forgotten about his own declaration of a marketed vaccine in three years.

Gallo acknowledged that, at the time, he had "zero previous experience in my life on a vaccine" and "only the crudest understanding of the basic immune mechanisms that protect people from infectious diseases."

Gallo's greatest regret is that the press conference was held at all, as it violated an agreement he had made with Montagnier and the other Pasteur researchers earlier that month—and seriously incensed them. "I was terribly, terribly nervous," remembered Gallo.

"I had massive conflicting emotions. I felt this shouldn't have been done. I didn't act strongly enough that we should have waited until we compared the virus with the French and made a joint announcement."

The author would have loved to confront them in a barroom situation to ask them one by one how each one feels now as they look back on that press conference they held more than 25 years ago. The author would appeal to their common sense and attempt to use reason and facts to let them see that their attendance and utterances at that press conference were an unmitigated disaster for mankind, for science, for HIV vaccine research and development, for HIV-infected persons, etc. The author would not be surprised if, by the time he finished his discussion with them, some of them ended up weeping profusely like babies because they would have realized that their hands are deeply soiled with the blood of millions as a result of that press conference. The author doubts if the greatest culprit, Gallo, would show remorse!

References

[1] Cohen J (2001). Chapter 1 Fast Predictions in Shots in the dark: the wayward search for an AIDS vaccine. W.W. Norton and Company, New York. The quotations are from the author's copy that he kindly emailed to me in 2004 after *Vaccine* published my report.

[2] Cohen J (2001). Chapter 3 Empiricists Versus Reductionists in Shots in the dark: the wayward search for an AIDS vaccine. W.W. Norton and Company, New York. The quotations are from the author's copy that he kindly emailed to me in 2004 after *Vaccine* published my report.

[3] Cohen J (2001). Chapter 15 Disparate Measures in Shots in the dark: the wayward search for an AIDS vaccine. W.W. Norton and Company, New York. The quotations are from the author's copy that he kindly emailed to me in 2004 after *Vaccine* published my report.

[4] http://www.isracast.com/transcrips/011205a-trans.htm

[5] AIDS VACCINE: Blame Nigeria, Not Abalaka, in Nigeria's *The Weekend Concord* newspaper, August 5, 2000, page 8

[6] Tam David-West: AIDS VACCINE: Blame Nigeria, Not Abalaka, in Nigeria's *The Weekend Concord* newspaper, August 12, 2000, page 8

[7] 'PTF spent N800m on expired AIDS kits, says David-West', an article in the Nigerian *Comet* newspaper, Tuesday, June 12, 2001

[8] Goulder P.J.R. and Walker B.D. (2002) 'HIV-1 super infection - a word of caution', The *New England Journal of Medicine* 347:756-758

[9] Hornby AS (1998). *Oxford Advanced Learner's Dictionary of Current English.* 5th Edition. Oxford: Oxford University Press.

[10] *Webster's Encyclopaedic Unabridged Dictionary of the English Language*. New York: Gramercy Books; 1989.

[11] *Dorland's Illustrated Medical Dictionary*. 24th Edition. Philadelphia and London: W B Saunders Company; 1965

[12] Broder S, Merigan TC, Bolognesi D (2000). *Textbook of AIDS Medicine.* Baltimore: Williams and Wilkins 4:47.

Chapter XIV

Factors Militating Against Safe, Effective HIV Vaccine Development

Abstract

The world's HIV vaccine experts, developers and researchers have been telling us for decades why it is difficult, perhaps impossible to ever develop HIV vaccines. Their excuses have become irritating because they all claim they must understand or know this, and that, and that and this before they can develop HIV vaccines. History tells us clearly that one does not need to understand or know much before developing safe and effective vaccines against infectious disease agents. Have they not heard or read about Edward Jenner, Louis Pasteur and many others who successfully developed vaccines? What did they know or understand? Humanity is looking for safe and effective vaccines against the HIV/AIDS pandemic. Those who should be working hard to get the vaccines are still enjoying their parties of knowing this or understanding that. They should all be ashamed. Even when they knew nothing about the HIV, they had already announced the recipe for its vaccine preparation. It has become an eyesore. And when a non-entity abandoned their recipe and successfully developed HIV vaccines, their response is to dismiss him offhand, discredit him, disgrace him, disown him and collectively attempt to bury his effort. When it comes to HIV vaccine development, the certified repeated failures of HIV vaccine development since 1984 are appointed as members of a jury by their powerful and vociferous governments, institutions of mass communications, multinational pharmaceutical companies, the UN, etc., to decide whether the world should accept the work of someone who has succeeded in developing those vaccines. The same jury members and the powers who applaud, approbate and appoint them called Merck's V520 candidate HIV preventive vaccine 'the most advanced vaccine ever developed', 'the vaccine of vaccines', and with lightening speed mobilised the world to rally behind V520. With all the optimism one can imagine, they were going to announce the results of the large field trials of V520 in 2009. Preparations for celebrations, hand pumping, back slapping and partying have been in top gear since 2006 or thereabouts. The higher they lift themselves, the worse the fall! More than a year to the D-day, V520 had not only failed to prevent HIV infection; it made HIV infection worse in recipients of the vaccine who became infected with the HIV when compared with those who got a placebo! Stop kidding! How can that happen to 'the most advanced vaccine ever developed', the only 'vaccine of vaccines'? Dear author, have you gone round the bend? Well, read on and find out if the author is kidding or crazy.

Introduction

True to its name, the human immunodeficiency virus HIV has man as its only natural host. It does not have other animal hosts even though there are other retroviruses that infect other animals. In the lab, chimpanzees pick up HIV infection but, unlike man, they do not progress to AIDS. The SIV, simian immunodeficiency virus, for instance, infects monkeys. Even though the chimeric SHIV infects monkeys, experience has shown that its features are significantly different from HIV in man. In a nutshell, there are no ideal animal models for HIV experimentation. Besides, the chimpanzee is a costly and rare animal; keeping them for experimentation is also very costly. Similar limitations apply to monkeys though they are cheaper than chimpanzees. The author does not know of any centre that keeps monkeys or chimpanzees for HIV research in his country. So, whatever candidate HIV preventive vaccines one conceives must eventually come to human trials for efficacy and safety.

The author thinks that a brief review of the natural course of HIV infection will provide the necessary background for appreciating the peculiar problems that have militated against safe and effective HIV vaccine development worldwide.

The Natural History of HIV Infection

The human immunodeficiency viruses (HIV-1 and HIV-2) are retroviruses belonging to the lentivirus subfamily. Like all retroviruses, the HIV genome consists of two identical but linked RNA molecules. The HIV is an enveloped virus. It causes a progressive and relentless loss of immune function that ultimately leads to the opportunistic infections and malignancies that characterize the acquired immunodeficiency syndrome, AIDS. Although there is marked variation in the rate of disease progression, the average time from initial infection with the HIV to the development of AIDS is 10 years (range: 18 months–18 years). Therefore, HIV infection in man is verily and generally a very chronic infection.

HIV-1 is responsible for the global pandemic. HIV-2, first isolated in West Africa, is said to be related to the Simian Immunodeficiency retrovirus (SIV). HIV-1 and HIV-2 genomes exhibit 60% homology in genes that code for core and polymerase proteins and 30–40% homology in genes that code for other viral proteins [1].

The HIV mutates continuously and extensively — it is estimated that any infected person has 1–100 million mutants of the virus at any point in time. Infection by one HIV strain does not protect against infection by another strain.

The HIV targets cells with a cluster of differentiation class 4 (CD4) receptors on their cell membrane: the CD4+ T-lymphocytes (T-helper cells), monocytes, macrophages, microglia, dendritic cells and Langerhan's cells.

When it infects a cell, the HIV viral core (RNA, reverse transcriptase RT, integrase, protease and other viral enzymes) enters the cytoplasm of the infected cell as a consequence of a complex and permanent fusion of the viral envelope glycoproteins gp120 and gp41 (the numbers refer to the molecular weight in kilodaltons) and the cell membrane after the virus locks onto the CD4+ receptors. Even though reverse transcription actually begins during virus assembly and maturation, it is self limiting within viral particles and is dependent on nucleotide pools and other factors required for DNA synthesis.

When the viral genome core enters the cytoplasm in a suitable form, reverse transcription is completed, resulting in a haploid, double-stranded DNA provirus which, with the help of viral integrase, becomes covalently integrated into the host cell's DNA in the cell's nucleus [2, 3]. When a cell infected with the HIV undergoes mitosis, the daughter cells inherit the provirus incorporated in the DNA of the mother cell. This is the basis for sayings among clinicians, retrovirologists, and HIV/AIDS vaccine experts /researchers like "Once you are infected with the HIV, you are infected for life" or "HIV infection is incurable"

The integrated provirus may remain latent for a long time in resting infected cells. When the infected cell is activated, however, the provirus initiates the transcription of viral RNA and other viral enzymes, leading to the synthesis, again in the cytoplasm of the infected cell, of new virions that bud off the infected cell. Such infected cells are eventually destroyed by the synthesis, assembly and budding off of new HIV virions.

Initial primary HIV infection is usually asymptomatic but quite a number of people experience acute symptoms similar to those of mononucleosis within 2–6 weeks of infection. During this initial phase, the person remains anti-HIV antibody negative ('diagnostic window period') but seropositive for viral protein/peptide p24 antigen with high plasma viral load (the person is therefore highly infective).

As one would expect, the first antibody response (primary response) consists of IgM that is usually undetectable in the first 3 months after infection [4]. The IgG response (secondary response) occurs after the appearance of detectable IgM antibodies. Anti-gp160 and anti-p24 IgG antibodies appear first, followed by anti-gp120 and anti-gp41 IgG antibodies. Antibodies to the viral envelope proteins such as gp120 and gp41 persist for life, but anti-p24 antibodies may diminish to nondetectable levels in the late stages of the disease [5].

In early HIV infection when there are no neutralizing antibodies, the virus infects and destroys about 200 million CD4+ lymphocytes per day. Eventually, there is a gradual decline of circulating CD4+ lymphocytes as the disease progresses. Generally and without treatment, the CD4+ lymphocyte count in blood decreases by 40-80 cells/μL of blood per year in HIV infection. In AIDS, the virus destroys about 20 billion CD4+ lymphocytes per day. A CD4+ lymphocyte count of fewer than 200 cells/μL of blood in those with HIV infection is associated with a high risk of developing opportunistic infections and cancers associated with AIDS [6]. The author uses the CDC classification of A1-A3, B1-B3 and C1-C3 [7, 8] for his HIV-infected patients. By this classification, A1, A2, B1 and B2 are non-AIDS HIV infection whereas any C or 3 is categorized as AIDS.

Anti-HIV Antibodies in HIV Infection

The HIV has genes for gag, pol, env, regulatory (early and late) and virion-associated accessory proteins. These proteins are very immunogenic (antigenic). As clearly demonstrated by the universally used ELISA HIV screening test and the Western Blot used for confirmation of anti-HIV antibodies, a person infected with the HIV produces effective antigen-binding antibodies against, among others, viral p17, p24, p9 and p6 gag proteins, p10, p66/51 and p32 pol proteins, gp120 and gp41 env proteins, p14 tat proteins, p19 rev proteins, p27 nef proteins, p23 vif proteins, p15 vpu proteins, p15 vpr proteins and p16 vpx proteins.

Assessment of Humoral and Cell-Mediated Immune Responses

Antibody detection, assay and characterization are far easier to carry out than tests for CMI. Routine and easily performed tests abound for anti-HIV antibody screening and confirmation, but there are no such cheap, easy and simple tests to assess CMI. Tests to assess CMI are costly, take time and require not only special expertise, training and equipment but the use of appropriate animal models with which to assess it. Furthermore, frozen serum, plasma or other body fluids and even tissue samples can be stored for long periods and readily transported across the world for qualitative and quantitative antibody assays. Cells and tissues for CMI assessment are much more difficult to handle. Blood samples for CD4+ lymphocyte counts, for instance, must not be refrigerated and the test must be carried out within a few hours (< 6 hours) of sampling, otherwise the results would be very unreliable.

HIV infection usually elicits strong CMI responses involving CD8+ cytotoxic T-cells. Effector T-cell activity can be detected a few days after viral replication starts in many infections. In vivo, this disappears within a few days of the cessation of viral replication, indicating that individual effector cells have a short half-life [9]. Some memory cytotoxic T-lymphocytes (CTLs) however, may persist for a long time, just like the memory antibody secreting cells.

Evidence indicates that cell-mediated immunity may be the predominant mechanism for control of HIV in primary infection and in long-term non-progressors [10-12]. In spite of these immune responses to HIV infection however, the body is unable to clear the virus completely and the infection progresses relentlessly to AIDS and death.

Some Thoughts about the Immunogen Concept for HIV Vaccine Development

Undoubtedly then, the HIV is very immunogenic. HIV infection is associated with humoral and cell-mediated immune responses but these are unable to clear the infection. As mentioned earlier, the outpouring of anti-HIV antibodies after HIV infection is massive and extensive. The relentless progression of HIV infection to AIDS and death after, on the average, 10 years after initial HIV infection occurs in spite of these immune responses to the virus. In the author's view, any candidate HIV vaccines that aim to stimulate anti-HIV antibody production would likely be ineffective just as happens in natural HIV infection.

Besides, the author still cannot see how such a vaccine would ever cure HIV infection as he earlier explained when dealing with the meaning of cure of HIV infection. Even if such a vaccine were efficacious, how would one confirm such efficacy? How would one differentiate between vaccinated persons and those infected with the HIV when the universal method of screening for HIV infection is by the detection of anti-HIV antibodies in the blood? Recipients of such vaccines would also be as stigmatized as those with HIV infection. In a nutshell, the author thinks it is unscientific and naïve to consider developing any candidate HIV therapeutic vaccines that involve the production of anti-HIV antibodies.

In the light of our present knowledge of the immunopathology of HIV infection, the author is better off discarding the possibility of such vaccines. Until we realize that anti-HIV antibodies do not, and cannot provide cure of, or effective protection against HIV infection, we are likely to continue to harvest failure in our attempt to successfully develop safe and effective HIV vaccines. After all, a person already infected with one type or strain of HIV is not protected against infection by another HIV type or strain even though that person already has massive quantities of binding anti-HIV antibodies against various HIV proteins/peptides. The new HIV strain proceeds and successfully establishes itself in the person already infected with the HIV. In other words, the adage, 'He who is down needs not fear a fall' does not apply to HIV infection; any HIV-infected person is at risk of picking other strains of HIV infection.

It is trite immunology that any successful vaccine must contain the appropriate immunogen delivered appropriately. An appropriate immunogen is one that stimulates the necessary appropriate specific immune responses when administered. How was the author going to get an immunogen that would tackle all the millions of mutants of the HIV when in any infected person, there are millions of such mutants?

Besides that problem, how does the author get hold of an immunogen that would eliminate the HIV provirus covalently incorporated in the infected cell's DNA? This, at first sight, looked really formidable because immune responses take place extracellularly, not intracellularly. Is it possible to think of an immunogen that would eliminate the provirus from its sequestrated and protected position in the nucleus of the infected cell, a position that very effectively shields it from the host's immune responses? Unless and until one conceives and develops a vaccine that eliminates the provirus, one would just be wasting his time thinking of getting an effective HIV therapeutic vaccine.

It is generally believed and accepted that safe and effective HIV vaccines have been difficult to achieve not only because of the extensive genetic variability of the virus but also because of the problem of conceiving the appropriate immunogen(s) delivered appropriately. Accordingly, most candidate HIV vaccine concepts and strategies involve the use of immunogen(s) specific for the predominant subtypes found within a country or geographic region. HIV-1 subtype A, for instance, was reported in 1994 to be predominant in 21 African countries [13], but a more recent survey in the author's country Nigeria showed a clear dominance and widespread distribution of gp41 subtypes A and G, even though a subtype C and a subtype J were also identified [14].

Available evidence indicates that cell-mediated immunity may be the predominant mechanism for the control of HIV in primary infection and in long-term non-progressors [15-20]. HIV envelope subcomponent vaccines have limited ability to induce neutralizing antibody production against clinical HIV-1 isolates [21].

Immune Complexes in HIV Infection

The formation of immune complexes between specific antibodies and the various HIV gp and p fragments takes place continuously during HIV infection. The deposition of similar circulating immune complexes containing HBsAg appears to be a key factor in the pathogenesis of most extra-hepatic manifestations (arthritis, polyarteritis nodosa, erythema nodosum, glomerulonephritis, uveitis, Gullain-Barre syndrome) of acute and chronic hepatitis B infections [22]. We have not yet seen similar manifestations that may be related to the deposition of similar complexes in HIV infection or those taking our HIV therapeutic vaccine.

HIV/AIDS and Other Concurrent Infections

Opportunistic infections and cancers characterize the development of AIDS. Other concomitant viral or even non-viral infections in those infected with the HIV accelerate the downhill progression of HIV infection. Globally, hundreds of millions of people are infected with the Hepatitis C virus, HCV. More still are infected with the Hepatitis B virus, HBV. Both are lethal viruses.

The latest developments in treating HCV and HBV infections involve the use of antiretrovirals or their distant cousins. A 6-12 month combination of Interferon (an immune booster) and the antiviral Ribavirin is used to manage HCV infection. The 2 drugs combined clear the HCV in just 50 to 55 per cent of patients after 6-12 months treatment. They are very costly and may cause such severe side effects (hair loss and heart failure) that one patient in seven abandons the combination regimen in the United States. Similarly, the antiretroviral AZT is being used for the treatment of HBV infection. AZT too is costly and has severe side effects. Co-infection with HCV leads to a more rapid progression from HIV to full-blown AIDS. Conversely, co-infection with the HIV accelerates the deterioration from HCV infection [23].

Later, we will see the effects of the author's HIV therapeutic vaccine on concomitant HBV and HCV infections.

Modify HIV Vaccine Concepts to Meet the Extraordinary HIV Challenges

In the author's view, the position of HIV vaccine developers worldwide at the beginning of this millennium has not changed significantly eight years on. Then and now, the key obstacle to the development of an HIV vaccine is said to be the continuous lack of basic scientific knowledge about the specific immune responses that must be elicited in order either to prevent HIV from infecting cells (a sterilizing vaccine) or to stop disease from developing after infection has occurred. Vaccines that successfully protect against most common diseases work in the latter manner, that is, they keep a person from becoming ill but do not actually prevent infection.

Unlike most other viruses, the singular properties of HIV make it a uniquely difficult target for vaccine design and development. First, the HIV virus particles coat their surface proteins with sugar-like molecules, so that antibodies have difficulty binding to appropriate protein sites on them. At the same time, HIV constantly alters its outer coat through genetic mutations, thus staying one step ahead of the immune response to any given vaccine preparation. The HIV mutates every time it replicates, and its replication cycle is 6 to 8 hours!

As Nobel laureate, Dr. David Baltimore remarked in an article in *The Chronicle of Higher Education* (May 28, 1999):

> "Antibodies are the first line of defence against most viruses, and [HIV] has breached that line."

Indeed, it is doubtful whether antibodies alone can protect against HIV. Virtually all HIV-infected individuals produce measurable amounts of antibodies to HIV, but studies have shown that high levels of HIV-neutralizing antibodies – levels at least 200 times greater then those found in HIV infection – would be required to probably protect against HIV infection. But the author asks: 'At that level of immunoglobulins, would the normal physiological functions of plasma not be adversely affected?'

Also, one of the defining characteristics of HIV is that it can be transmitted not only through free-floating virus particles in blood and other body fluids, but directly through cell-to-cell contact in the mucosal linings of the vaginal and gastrointestinal (including oral and anal) tracts. *Most traditional vaccine preparations are said to elicit only the production of antibodies in blood and body fluids and do not stimulate a cellular immune response.* But because HIV can be transmitted sexually – and possibly directly from cell to cell without entering the blood – a successful HIV vaccine might need to elicit cell-mediated immunity in order to prevent infection. Additional studies suggest that other, as yet undefined, immune responses might also be needed for an HIV vaccine to be successful.

HIV poses other obstacles to the designing of an effective vaccine. In addition to the two major types of HIV (HIV-1 and HIV-2), there are already at least nine known strains or clades, of HIV-1 circulating worldwide and many genetic variants within each clade. It is considered unlikely that a single vaccine preparation will protect against all of them. Furthermore, HIV often remains hidden inside some body cells and tissues for long periods of time, thus evading antibodies. And, of course, HIV attacks and destroys the very immune cells that are supposed to learn how to recognize and respond to both an HIV vaccine preparation and a real HIV infection. *It is claimed that to date, there is no evidence that the immune system of any HIV-infected person has been able to destroy or eliminate the human immunodeficiency virus on its own.*

Lack of an Ideal Animal Model

Another clinical challenge in the development of an HIV vaccine is the lack of an ideal animal model for testing candidate vaccines. Chimpanzees, man's closest genetic relative, are the only animals that can be infected with HIV-1, but they do not usually develop clinical

AIDS from the virus. Monkeys develop an AIDS-like syndrome from an HIV-related monkey retrovirus, the simian immunodeficiency virus (SIV), but the virus differs from HIV-1 in important ways. Researchers have created hybrid (chimeric) viruses called SHIV viruses that combine SIV with HIV's outer coat, and will make it easier to test HIV candidate vaccines in monkeys. But such experiments cannot fully predict the safety or efficacy of a vaccine designed for use against HIV in humans.

Successful HIV Vaccines Development Requires Non-Conventional Approaches

Confronted with a virus unlike any, for which a vaccine currently exists, many pharmaceutical and biotechnology companies have not invested heavily in HIV vaccine research. Indeed, a 1996 AmfAR-funded report prepared by the AIDS Vaccine Advocacy Coalition (AVAC), *Industry Investment in HIV Vaccine Development* surveyed more than 25 industry scientists. It concluded that scientific uncertainty about the type of immune response necessary for protection against HIV infection was the primary reason for limited private sector investment in HIV vaccine research. Concern that sales to the developing world might not offset enormous research and development costs has also dampened corporate interest in developing an HIV vaccine, as have the considerable logistic and ethical challenges involved in conducting clinical trials of HIV candidate vaccines in humans.

Nevertheless, over the past several years, scientists claim they have gained a greater understanding of HIV and how it infects human cells. Generated by research worldwide, costing billions of dollars, it was hoped that these advances would provide new hope that a successful HIV vaccine can be designed.

The new hope was placed on DNA-based, Fusion-Competent, and/or Recombinant Vector Vaccines that are completely genetically engineered. To highlight the importance of human trials of HIV candidate vaccines and provide the information to potential trial participants, the *HIV/AIDS Vaccine Trial Directory* was launched in 1997. This Directory is said to be the world's only regularly published guide to HIV vaccine trials. Funding and technical assistance to help launch the AIDS Vaccine Advocacy Coalition AVAC) were, and are still being provided to support many of that group's activities, including its 1999 report *Eight Years and Counting: What Will Speed Development of an AIDS Vaccine?*

The ultimate goal of HIV vaccine research is a sterilizing vaccine that can protect against HIV infection and prevent disease. But it is still being said that such a product is unlikely to become available within the next decade.

The late Dr. Mary Lou Clements-Mann observed in *The Journal of Infectious Disease* (177:1230-1246):

> "To prevent chronic [HIV] infection, it is thought that a vaccine will need to induce neutralizing antibodies to eliminate virus from body fluids and [cytotoxic] T lymphocyte (CTL) activity to destroy infected cells."

However, it is said that a vaccine that could reduce levels of HIV in the blood and thus slow disease progression to clinical AIDS and hopefully decrease HIV transmission should be attainable within the next ten years. Such a preventive, or "therapeutic," HIV vaccine might not need to induce both antibody- and cell-mediated immune responses.

In addition to proving capable of stimulating the desired immune responses and being safe to use, it is said that a successful HIV vaccine will also need to be:

- Inexpensive and easy to administer;
- Easy to transport and store;
- Capable of inducing long-lasting immunity with a single or few injections;
- Compatible with other vaccines; and
- Protective against diverse strains of HIV.

Were such a vaccine available today, it is estimated that more than 300 million people would require immediate vaccination.

More than 40 potential or candidate HIV vaccines have been tested worldwide over the past decade, involving some 10,000 volunteers. To date, only a few candidate vaccines have entered large-scale Phase III clinical trials in humans.

Inevitably, according to HIV vaccine developers and experts, there will be scientists who will discover the crucial components of a successful HIV vaccine. How long it takes to make those essential discoveries – and to control the assault of HIV/AIDS on humankind – will depend not only on the number and quality of scientists committed to the goal of finding an HIV vaccine, but also on the level of resources committed to the goal of finding an HIV vaccine as well as on the level of resources provided in support of their work.

As Emilio Emini, M.D., Vice President, Antiviral and Vaccine Research, Merck and Co., Inc. put it:

> An AIDS vaccine will not be successfully developed unless we are willing to think innovatively and support basic research efforts that "push the envelope" of our understanding.

THE TIME International Magazine of March 29, 1999 says:

> The only sure way to stop the [HIV] epidemic is to prevent infection in the first place, and only a vaccine can do that. ... Until scientists find a vaccine, however, they may control but never cure the century's final scourge [AIDS]

A website [24] says,

HIV vaccine

An *HIV vaccine* is a hypothetical vaccine against HIV, the etiological agent of AIDS. As there is no known cure for AIDS, the search for a vaccine has become part of the struggle against the disease.

The urgency of the search for a vaccine against HIV stems from the AIDS-related death toll of over 25 million people since 1981. Indeed, in 2002, AIDS became the primary cause of mortality due to an infectious agent in Africa (UNAIDS, 2004).

Alternative medical treatments to a vaccine do exist. Highly active antiretroviral therapy (HAART) has been highly beneficial to many HIV-infected individuals since its introduction in 1996 when the protease inhibitor-based HAART initially became available. HAART allows the stabilization of the patient's symptoms and viraemia, but they do not cure the patient of HIV, nor of the symptoms of AIDS (Martinez-Picardo et al., 2000). And, importantly, HAART does nothing to prevent the spread of HIV through people with undiagnosed HIV infections. Safer sex measures have also proven insufficient to halt the spread of AIDS in the worst affected countries, despite some success in reducing infection rates.

Therefore, an HIV vaccine is generally considered as the most likely, and perhaps the only way by which the AIDS pandemic can be halted. However, after over 20 years of research, HIV-1 remains a difficult target for a vaccine.

Difficulties in Developing an HIV Vaccine

In 1984, after the confirmation of the aetiological agent of AIDS by scientists at the U.S. National Institutes of Health and the Pasteur Institute, the United States Health and Human Services Secretary Margaret Heckler declared that a vaccine would be available within two years (Associated Press, 1984).

However, the classical vaccination approaches that have been successful in the control of various viral diseases by priming the adaptive immunity to recognize the viral envelope proteins have failed in the case of HIV-1, as the epitopes of the viral envelope are too variable. Furthermore, the functionally important epitopes of the gp120 protein are masked by glycosylation, trimerisation and receptor-induced conformational changes making it difficult to block with neutralizing antibodies. In February 2003, Vaxgen announced that their AIDSVAX vaccine was a failure in North America as there was not a statistically significant reduction of HIV infection within the study population (Francis et al., 2003). In November 2003, it also failed clinical trials in Thailand for the same reason. These vaccines both targeted gp120 and were specific for the geographical regions (Billich et al., 2001).

The ineffectiveness of previously developed vaccines primarily stems from two related factors. First, HIV is highly mutable. Because of the virus' ability to rapidly respond to selective pressures imposed by the immune system, the population of virus in an infected individual typically evolves so that it can evade the two major arms of the adaptive immune system; humoral (antibody-mediated) and cellular (mediated by T cells) immunity. Second, HIV isolates are themselves highly variable. HIV can be categorized into multiple clades and subtypes with a high degree of genetic divergence.

Therefore, the immune responses raised by any vaccine need to be broad enough to account for this variability. Any vaccine that lacks this breadth is unlikely to be effective.

The typical animal model for vaccine research is the monkey, often the macaque. The monkeys can be infected with SIV or the chimeric SHIV for research purposes. However, the well-proven route of trying to induce neutralizing antibodies by vaccination has stalled because of the great difficulty in stimulating antibodies that neutralize heterologous primary HIV isolates (Poignard et al., 1999). Some vaccines based on the virus envelope have protected chimpanzees or macaques from homologous virus challenge (Berman et al., 1990), but in clinical trials, individuals who were immunised with similar constructs became infected after later exposure to HIV-1 (Connor et al., 1998).

The human body can defend itself against HIV, as work with monoclonal antibodies (MAb) has proven. That certain individuals can be asymptomatic for decades after infection is encouraging.

17 vaccine candidates are in phase I trials and four in phase I/II. There is only one in phase III (the NIH/Department of Defense's ALVAC vCP 1521 canary pox vector/AIDSVAX prime-boost vaccine trial now under way in Thailand).

Up to May 2000 over 60 phase I/II trials of candidate vaccines had been conducted worldwide. Most initial approaches focused on the HIV envelope protein. At least thirteen different gp120 and gp160 envelope candidates have been evaluated, in the US predominantly through the AIDS Vaccine Evaluation Group. Most research focused on gp120 rather than gp41/gp160, as the latter are generally more difficult to produce and did not initially offer any clear advantage over gp120 forms.

Overall, they have been safe and immunogenic in diverse populations, have induced neutralizing antibody in nearly 100% recipients, but rarely induced CD8+ cytotoxic T lymphocytes (CTL). Mammalian derived envelope preparations have been better inducers of neutralizing antibody than candidates produced in yeast and bacteria. Although the vaccination process involved many repeated "booster" injections, it was very difficult to induce and maintain the high anti-gp120 antibody titers necessary to have any hope of neutralizing an HIV exposure.

The availability of several recombinant canarypox vectors has provided interesting results that may prove to be generalizable to other viral vectors. Increasing the complexity of the canarypox vectors by inclusion of more genes/epitopes has increased the percent of volunteers that have detectable CTL to a greater extent than did increasing the dose of the viral vector. Importantly, CTLs from volunteers were able to kill peripheral blood mononuclear cells infected with primary isolates of HIV, suggesting that induced CTLs could have biological significance. In addition, cells from at least some volunteers were able to kill cells infected with HIV from other clades, though the pattern of recognition was not uniform among volunteers. As canarypox is the first candidate HIV vaccine that has induced cross-clade functional CTL responses, the first phase I trial of a candidate vaccine in Africa was launched early in 1999 in Ugandan volunteers, and determine the extent to which Ugandan volunteers have CTL that are active against the subtypes of HIV prevalent in Uganda, A and D.

Other strategies that have progressed to phase I trials in uninfected persons include peptides, lipopeptides, DNA, an attenuated Salmonella vector, p24, etc. Specifically, candidate vaccines that induce one or more of the following are being sought:

- broadly neutralizing *antibody* against HIV primary isolates;
- cytotoxic T cell responses in a vast majority of recipients;
- strong mucosal immune responses.

On December 13, 2004, a large phase II clinical trial of a novel HIV vaccine began enrolling volunteers at sites in North America, South America, the Caribbean and Australia. The organizers were seeking 3,000 participants. The trial was co-funded by the National Institute of Allergy and Infectious Diseases (NIAID), part of the National Institutes of Health

(NIH), and the pharmaceutical company Merck and Co. Inc. Merck developed the experimental vaccine called V520 to stimulate HIV-specific cellular immunity, which prompts the body to produce T cells that kill HIV-infected cells. In previous smaller trials, this vaccine was found to be safe and to induce cellular immune responses against HIV in more than half of volunteers.

V520 contains a weakened adenovirus that serves as a carrier for three subtype B HIV genes. Subtype B is the most prevalent HIV subtype in the regions of the study sites. Adenoviruses are among the main causes of upper respiratory tract ailments such as the common cold. Because the vaccine contains only three HIV genes housed in a weakened adenovirus, study participants cannot become infected with HIV or get a respiratory infection from the vaccine. *It was announced in September 2007 that the trial for V520 would be discontinued after it determined that the vaccination was ineffective. Additionally, it appears that V520 may have made recipients more receptive to infection by HIV-1.*

Organizers expected results in 2009, but declared the vaccine a failure in September 2007.

Novel approaches, including modified vaccinia Ankara (MVA), adeno-associated virus, Venezuelan Equine Encephalitis (VEE) replicons, and codon-optimized DNA have proven to be strong inducers of CTL in macaque models, and have provided at least partial protection in some models. Most of these approaches are in, or will soon enter, clinical studies.

Economics of HIV Vaccine Development

A June 2005 study estimates that $682 million is spent on AIDS vaccine research annually.

Economic issues with developing an AIDS vaccine include the need for advance purchase commitment (or advance market commitments) because after an AIDS vaccine has been developed, governments and NGOs may be able to bid the price down to marginal cost.

Controversy

Some conservatives, such as Reginald Finger, M.D., M.P.H., a member of the Advisory Committee on Immunization Practices (ACIP) in the U.S., have stated that the Committee would have to carefully consider an HIV vaccine's effects on sexual activity. ACIP is a government committee linked to the Centers for Disease Control. ACIP is charged with advising the President on prevention of vaccine-related diseases. Dr. Finger's term expired in June, 2006.

Similar controversy has arisen in response to the recent introduction of the HPV vaccine, which prevents infection with certain strains of human papillomavirus, another sexually transmitted disease [24].

The author noticed that the Home page of HIV Vaccine Trials Network HVTN is aesthetically pleasing. The first impression it gave to the author on his first visit was, 'Look!

May be, this is a network of serious scientists.' The caption there seems to underscore that impression; it reads:

> Our excitement is in the SCIENCE
> We are an international network working together to find a safe and effective HIV vaccine. >our Scientific Mission [25]

(Unfortunately, that first impression ends at the Home Page! Not all that glitters is gold! Their scientific mission is definitely different from their claim that they are working together to find a safe and effective HIV vaccine. HIV vaccines were developed since 1998 by the author and there have been several publications in reputable international Journals (References 2–8 in Chapter 11) about it. Do they not read such Journals? The author presumes that they do. It is therefore deliberate falsehood they are propagating by their misleading home page.

The author developed safe and effective HIV vaccines, not just a vaccine but vaccines, in the twilight years of the last century. With these facts, how can they honestly claim that their excitement is in the science and that they are working together to find a safe and effective HIV vaccine? The only good point in their beautiful home page is their use of the phraseology, 'safe and effective' to describe the vaccine they claim they are looking for. Verily indeed, once any medical remedy, vaccines included, is safe and effective, nothing else is needed before its use on those that need it, and are willing to take it.)

The website [26] carried the following editorial. The author has put his comments in parenthesis and italics:

Editorial - AIDS and the Next 25 Years

Researchers had been scheduled to gather at the Institut Pasteur in Paris to mark the quarter century since the human immunodeficiency virus (HIV) was discovered as the cause of acquired immunodeficiency syndrome (AIDS). Since then, over 60 million people have been infected with the virus and over 25 million people have died. These numbers make the results of two "proof of concept" vaccine efficacy trials—the STEP and Phambili trials—extremely disappointing. Indeed, these results have raised questions about whether investments in HIV vaccine research are misplaced and whether a vaccine is even achievable. Those views are misguided. *(They are misguided indeed because safe and effective vaccines have already been developed since 1998/99. The so-called search for safe and effective HIV vaccines is analogous to crying when one's head is off).*

The failure of candidate vaccines or drugs is to be expected. More than ever, investigations in humans are essential to explore concepts, test hypotheses, and delineate the human immune response to HIV immunogens. *(Humanity is not looking for concepts, hypothesis or the delineation of anything. With the scourge, humanity is in dire need of safe and effective HIV vaccines irrespective of who produced them, irrespective of how they are produced, irrespective of anything else.).* The STEP and Phambili trials, cosponsored by the pharmaceutical company Merck and Co. and the U.S. National Institutes of Health were designed to test the efficacy of a recombinant adenovirus vector cocktail expressing three HIV genes.

The vaccine candidate failed to limit viral replication in people who became infected with HIV and failed to prevent the acquisition of HIV. Most disconcertingly, a subset of volunteers appeared to show an increased probability of acquiring HIV (see the Perspective by Moore et al., p. 753). These results reflect our still-limited knowledge of HIV, its interactions with the human immune system, and the formidable, unprecedented challenges that it poses. *(The author thinks the results are telling you very loudly that the immunogen concept, design and delivery are not correct.)*

Why Has Developing an HIV Vaccine Been so Difficult?

One reason is that HIV has evolved highly sophisticated ways to evade the immune system. Its extraordinarily high degree of sequence diversity, caused by mutation and recombination, makes it especially challenging to design neutralizing antibodies that recognize the broad range of epitopes needed for effective immune protection. *(The author maintains that researchers have put the cart before the horse by outlining recipes for the vaccine before the vaccine is developed. A recipe is a methodology. It should follow discovery, not precede it.)*

Moreover, HIV wipes out some of the very cells needed to mount an effective immune response. Despite progress in characterizing cellular and humoral immune responses to the virus, we still don't know enough about the magnitude, breadth, or types of immune responses necessary for effective vaccine protection, in part because of the lack of a robust animal model that recapitulates critical features of both HIV and the human immune system.

Indeed, these are major challenges, but evidence of immunological protection in certain experimental models of HIV in nonhuman primates, and the intriguing observation that a small proportion of HIV-infected individuals ("elite controllers") can completely suppress the virus for years, suggest that a vaccine may be achievable (see the Review by Walker and Burton, p. 760). *(Safe and effective HIV vaccines were developed since 1998/99)*

Furthermore, new technologies in structural and computational biology are providing novel approaches for designing immunogens that might elicit broadly reactive neutralizing antibodies, and new insights into innate and mucosal immunity are expanding vaccine design strategies. *(There goes the wrong approach again, putting the cart before the horse. Get the safe and effective vaccine first before trying to find out how it works if you are keen on that. Instead of doing that, they are looking for immunogens that fit into their pre-suppositions.)*

At meetings over the past few months, including an international workshop convened last week by the Global HIV Vaccine Enterprise, there was broad agreement on many points, particularly that more, not less, basic and early-stage clinical research is needed. *(The broad agreement was irrelevant and unnecessary. The author developed these vaccines without any such agreement.)*

Understanding the human immune response to HIV remains a priority. *(The author disagrees. The priority should be getting safe and effective vaccines, not any understanding.)* We need to understand the role of both the innate and adaptive immune responses during HIV infection. Better assays are needed that reflect the functional biology of cellular immune responses and incorporate a systems biology approach - that is; encompass the integrative functioning of gene, protein, and biochemical networks - to monitor the immune system. We need to make it much more attractive for young researchers, including those from other fields, to enter the HIV vaccine field. And the continued engagement of industry is essential if we are ever to have a vaccine. *(There goes the cart before the horse again! How do they know it is essential? Since 1984, they have engaged industry and not succeeded. The author did not engage any industry and he succeeded.)*

Laboratory research has led to effective drugs against HIV that have prolonged the lives of infected individuals, and epidemiological studies have shown that interventions such as circumcision (see the Policy Forum by Potts et al., page 749) can reduce viral acquisition. However, we know from experience with other pathogens that a vaccine is the best way to stop a virus.

The only end for a journey that began 25 years ago should be the development of a safe and effective HIV vaccine. *(If the development of a safe and effective HIV vaccine is the only end for the journey that began 25 years ago, it means of course that the journey ended in 1998/99, the time the author developed his safe and effective HIV vaccines!)*

– Alan Bernstein

10.1126/science.1159797

Alan Bernstein is executive director of the Global HIV Vaccine Enterprise, New York.

Published by AAAS [26]

"The Vaccine of Vaccines", Merck's V520 HIV Preventive Vaccine

HIV vaccine researchers, developers, experts and interested parties worldwide have been frustrated and disillusioned since September 2007. Before then, they had started counting their chicken even before the eggs were hatched. They were all waiting for the 2009 results of Merck's V520 HIV preventive vaccine that they had described as the most promising HIV candidate vaccine ever developed. Many dubbed it 'the vaccine of vaccines'; it had taken over 10 years of modern genetic engineering techniques and the best brains in the world to develop it at a cost of several billion US dollars (not the September 2007 Zimbabwean dollar!). We were all told it had proved its worth in animal experiments. The FDA had given its nod for accelerated trials in order to bring it to the market in the shortest possible time. The author was literally the only lone voice in the world that would not be sucked in; he had been telling those who have hearing ears that the 'vaccine of vaccines' would likely fail because the immunogen(s) concept, design and delivery were wrong *ab initio,* like their other candidate HIV vaccines before and after it

There was no need to wait till 2009 for their long-awaited celebrations to begin for 'the vaccine of vaccines'. The CNN, on 22-23 September 2007, carried this on its NEWSBAR,

'Merck drops trials of HIV vaccine after test fails'

The author later found out that the CNN did not tell its viewers the whole story. Merck's HIV vaccine did not just fail; those who took the vaccine were worse off when they became infected with the HIV than those that got a placebo, those that did not get the vaccine! In addition, more recipients of the vaccine were infected with the HIV than the placebo group! Why did CNN omit these aspects of the Merck's vaccine failure? The reader's guess may be better than the author's! It may be more than just mellowing down the gravity of the failure.

Turning to the internet, the author discovered that it was a pandemonium of unbelief, surprise, mourning, weeping and gnashing of teeth from all quarters for the 'vaccine of vaccines'. The author would like to reproduce just the following randomly selected articles from the internet as examples. One says:

Disappointment for HIV Vaccine Developers, Merck

Posted: Sat, 22 Sep 2007 10:16:11 GMT
Author: Emma Price
Category: Health
Health News

And another one bites the dust. It was supposed to be the vaccine of vaccines, the one that would be the answer to stopping the AIDS epidemic. But it is not to be.

After 10 years of research and testing, Merck, the pharmaceutical giant that was developing the experimental HIV vaccine, announced on Friday September 21, that it was cutting short its test called STEP since it did not prove to be successful in preventing infection or in reducing the degree of infection in volunteers who instead were infected during the trial.

Merck reported that "the vaccine did not reduce the amount of virus in the bloodstream of those who became infected."

Experts believed that this vaccine, known as V520, would be the answer to all their hopes and prayers and therefore closely observed the trial.

The V520 was the first of a new group of H.I.V. vaccines to go as far as it did in the clinical trials. Now its failure has caused investigators to have second thoughts about this new approach.

"This was viewed as the most promising strategy," said Dr. Mark B. Feinberg, a vice-president of Merck, "so I think it is a disappointment for us and a disappointment for everyone in the AIDS vaccine area."

The doctors involved with the trial believe that failure of the vaccine highlighted the fact that H.I.V. is unlike any infection for which scientists have successfully developed a vaccine

Dr. Anthony S. Fauci, the director of the National Institute of Allergy and Infectious Diseases, which conducted the trial with Merck, said in an interview that "the results are obviously disappointing."

However he also pointed out that even if it was too early to make predictions about the capability of the new group of vaccines, the company has promised to reveal all the information it has collected with scientists.

Health officials consider the development of an HIV vaccine to be the most effective instrument in the control of the AIDS epidemic, but so far only one HIV vaccine has been through full-scale testing. It had been based on the traditional approach of stimulating the immune system to produce antibodies against an infectious agent.

It, however, like several other vaccines, was not successful. Scientists now reasoned that young people who are infected with HIV respond well to CD8 T-cells, which can be manipulated to recognize and kill HIV infected cells. They wondered if AIDS could be harnessed by rousing this different component of the immune system.

They therefore hoped that a vaccine capable of strong T-cell response against H.I.V could be administered before people were infected.

Merck had initially conducted experiments on animals and people which were promising enough to make them consider the development and the carrying out of the tests known as cell-mediated immunity.

They developed the V520 vaccine from a diluted adaptation of the common cold virus. The virus was capable of delivering three synthetically produced genes from the AIDS virus, called gag, pol and nef.

The subjects received three doses of the vaccine over a period of six months.

Beginning in the latter half of 2004 the trial involved 3000 volunteers who had not yet been infected. They were mainly from the Latin America and the United States, Australia and the Caribbean. This particular trial was the second of the three stage system that the Food and Drug Administration typically requires before the licensing of any vaccine or drug.

The scientists expected the initial results of the trial only by the end of 2008. However, in their very first analysis of 1500 of the volunteers they discovered that the vaccine was obviously ineffective in that of the 741 people receiving at least one dose of the vaccine, 24 had been infected thirteen months later. They compared the statistics with those who had received the placebo. Of those 762 people 21 had been infected.

On reviewing the data collected so far, the Data Safety Monitoring Board for STEP advised the discontinuation of the vaccine since it very obviously did not work. The vaccinated volunteers would however continue to be monitored.

"The results were very clear," said Dr. Feinberg of Merck.

In the meantime, Merck has also decided to stop its vaccination trials called Phambili that had been started in South Africa in 2006. Two additional phase I trials have also been suspended.

The AIDS Vaccine Advocacy Coalition assured the public however that the latest failure was definitely not the end of the search for an AIDS vaccine [27].

Under the caption *HIV Vaccines in the News*, another website [28] says,

Date: September 11, 2007
Title: South Africa: Vaccine trial volunteers contributing to AIDS fight
Source: Reuters
Summary: Several volunteers in HVTN's Phambili trial speak about their participation in helping to fight AIDS.

Date: September 21, 2007
Title: AVAC voices disappointment in trial result
Source: AVAC
Summary: Executive Director Mitchell Warren of the AIDS Vaccine Advocacy Coalition comments on the discontinuation of the Step Study.

Date: September 22, 2007
Title: Failure of Vaccine Test Is Setback in AIDS Fight
Source: New York Times
Summary: The Step Study was closely watched because experts considered the vaccine one of most promising to be tested on people so far. This was also the first of a new class of H.I.V. vaccine to get this far in clinical trials. The failure of the vaccine raises questions about whether the new approach will work.

Date: September 28, 2007
Title: Failed HIV vaccine study disappoints local participants
Source: Southern Voice
Summary: Interview with a vaccine trial volunteer in Atlanta. Scott Smith, 39, a volunteer for the vaccine research for just over two years said, "I was bummed. But I knew what the chances were." Smith will continue going to his scheduled appointments for however long researchers want to follow participants to find other useful information in the failed trial. "Every test helps us get closer to a vaccine," he said.

Date: October 6, 2007
Title: Try, try again
Source: The Philadelphia Inquirer

Summary: Lessons learned from the discontinued Step and Phambili trials.

Date: October 25, 2007
Title: Warning Is Sent to AIDS Vaccine Volunteers
Source: The Washington Post
Summary: HIV/AIDS researchers in South Africa began warning 801 volunteers who participated in an HIV vaccine trial about a possible increased risk of HIV.

Date: October 25, 2007
Title: AIDS Vaccine May Raise Infection Risk: Researchers
Source: Reuters
Summary: More than 3,000 people who volunteered to receive an experimental Merck and Co. AIDS vaccine are being told to come back and get extra tests because the jab may itself raise the risk of infection. Researchers stress that they do not yet have enough information to say whether those who got the shot indeed are more susceptible to infection with HIV.

Date: November 12, 2007
Title: Fallout from failed AIDS vaccine could dampen research
Source: Forbes
Summary: Experts are concerned that the news of the Step Study will keep would-be trial participants away from future AIDS vaccine studies.

Date: November 12, 2007
Title: Finding the way again after failed AIDS vaccine
Source: MSNBC
Summary: The vaccine development world is now in a state of stunned shock since the trial that many believed had the greatest chance of success was halted. So what should be done next? Clearly many scientists must carry out as many experiments as possible to understand the STEP results. Dr. Seth Berkley, head of the International AIDS Vaccine Initiative, emphasizes the race to find a vaccine is a "marathon not a sprint" and we should not lose sight of the goal.

Date: December 18, 2007
Title: A Shot at Stopping AIDS
Source: Washington Post
Summary: Editorial by Seth Berkley, chief executive and president of the International AIDS Vaccine Initiative. Despite some setbacks, there are good reasons to think we can win against AIDS. The failure of one vaccine product does not rule out success on that front.

Date: December 27, 2007
Title: One Step Forward, Two Steps Back — Will There Ever Be an AIDS Vaccine?
Source: New England Journal of Medicine
Summary: About a quarter-century after the discovery of HIV, there is neither a marketable vaccine nor a credible expectation about when there will be one [28].

Another website [29] has this article:

Fallout and Frustration: Merck's Failed HIV Vaccine Trials

World AIDS Day
Article Date: *11/26/2007*
By Duane Wells

Just a few short months ago, a spirit of cautious optimism surrounded the prospects for a viable HIV vaccine. As Merck began testing its highly anticipated V520 vaccine, which it had reportedly been developing over a ten year period, there was an undercurrent of excitement among researchers in the HIV community about the radical new approach, which was expected to attack, seek out, and destroy infected cells. There was a sense of promise: For the first time in years, the study might yield a significant breakthrough in the ongoing fight to contain the global HIV/AIDS epidemic.

Two months into the study, those hopes were dashed and the HIV community sent reeling as the international Merck trials were shut down after preliminary results demonstrated the vaccine appeared to be doing more harm than good.

With researchers collectively scratching their heads in confusion, the Merck failure has created some serious impediments for future HIV vaccine trials, forcing the HIV research community to rethink its science, priorities and goals.

The Merck HIV vaccine trials included 3,000 participants, mostly male, in North and South America, the Caribbean and Australia, all of whom were considered to be at high risk of exposure to the virus because of their sexual activity or drug use. A sister trial in Africa was also shut down.

Unlike previous experimental HIV vaccines that attempted to stimulate the body to produce antibodies that would ward off infection, Merck's V520 focused on T-cells that attack and kill cells that HIV had already infected.

But rather than stimulate an immune response to ward off HIV invasion, the vaccine, which employs a few synthetic fragments of HIV loaded onto a genetically modified cold virus (called an adenovirus) may well have altered the immune system to facilitate infection of study participants. Moreover, the vaccine did not reduce viral loads in volunteers who became infected with HIV during the trial.

Despite this disappointing initial data, there are those in the HIV research community who insist that all hope is not lost.

The first piece of good news: Though the V520 vaccine may have increased the chance of infection, Merck, along with the majority of HIV experts agree that the vaccine itself did not and cannot cause HIV infection.

The other piece of good news to come out of the Merck HIV Vaccine trials is that there are valuable lessons to be learned from its failure. According to Dr. Stephen J. Brown, Medical Director for AIDS Research Alliance, which was the only Los Angeles site conducting clinical trials for the Merck Vaccine, "The closing of the Merck vaccine study may have an important impact as to the future of most HIV vaccines candidates currently in clinical trials because, like the Merck vaccine, many are designed to similarly stimulate strong cell-mediated immune responses."

Further, in a published statement, AIDS Research Alliance was quick to not discount the outcome of the Merck experiment.

"The results of this study may also provide valuable information as to the future direction of HIV vaccine research. Since all vaccine candidates in the pipeline are designed to stimulate only one arm of the immune system, maybe an efficient vaccine against HIV will need to stimulate both arms (including neutralizing antibodies, or other cells such as natural killer cells) of the immune system in humans," the statement said.

Despite these arguably positive, if unanticipated, results, there remains substantial concern about the long-term perception that the high profile failure of the Merck trial might have on future studies.

According to the *Philadelphia Inquirer*, Hildegund C.J. Ertl, an immunologist at the Wistar Institute in Philadelphia, who is preparing to test another HIV vaccine based on a chimpanzee cold virus next year, has said that the Merck effort will likely alter her study.

Gary J. Nabel, director of the Vaccine Research Center of the National Institutes of Health, has postponed until at least mid-2008 his group's PAVE 100 HIV-vaccine trial. That trial uses three shots of DNA followed by a cold-virus booster, albeit one with different components from the Merck product.

Meanwhile, according to various news reports, The National Institutes of Health, which helped sponsor Merck's aborted clinical trial, recently halted recruitment for vaccine trials involving several diseases, including Ebola, because those vaccines, like the failed Merck one, are made with an adenovirus.

Perhaps the greatest problem that lies ahead for future HIV vaccine studies may not be the science or the trials themselves but the recruitment of now skittish volunteers to take part in them.

"I can tell you that as a volunteer in the study, and as someone who worked on the last phase III clinical trial of an AIDS vaccine, I'm less disappointed than I am scared by the early results of this trial," says Jim Key, Chief Public Affairs Officer for the Los Angeles Gay and Lesbian Center. "What scares me, of course, is the indication that study volunteers who received the product, and not the placebo, may be at greater risk of HIV-infection than those who didn't receive it. This is a scary concern not just for volunteers in the study, but for the success of future studies. It's already difficult to recruit volunteers for vaccine studies. The results of this trial are likely to make recruitment for future studies considerably more difficult. "I don't believe hopes were high for the Merck vaccine, so I'm not overly surprised it didn't prove efficacious," Key added. "What's important to remember, however, is that every clinical trial of a vaccine helps advance the science and if we don't continue to develop and test promising vaccines we'll never stop AIDS."

Still others like Michael Weinstein, President of AIDS Healthcare Foundation, seem to believe that the implosion of the Merck trial is only more indicative of the need to balance the quest for a vaccine with developing long-term treatment options and the availability thereof.

"Development of a safe and effective AIDS vaccine is clearly a noble and worthy goal; however, the sad truth remains that more than 33 million people worldwide are living with HIV/AIDS today, yet barely two million of them have access to lifesaving antiretroviral AIDS treatments, Weinstein said in a statement.

"Treatments that actually do work and help keep those fortunate enough to have access to them alive and well, and which also have also been around, and continually improved, for over a decade. These recent failures in vaccine development underscore just how tenuous the quest for an AIDS vaccine remains, and reminds us of what effective, but underused tools, including antiretroviral treatment, we already have available to us today. While we long for the day when there is an effective preventive AIDS vaccine, we also call for a re-evaluation of the distribution of limited government resources in the battle against AIDS, and renew our call for a greatly stepped-up commitment to bringing antiretroviral treatment to many, many more of those people still in need worldwide."

The final effects of the collapse of the Merck HIV vaccine trials may not be seen for quite some time to come. Whether the results of the study will ultimately help or hinder HIV research is debatable, but one thing is for certain. Though hope for a vaccine may spring eternal, its prospects have, for the moment, most certainly been dealt a short-term setback at minimum.

On November 5, 2008, the author encountered this on the Internet [30]:

Experimental HIV vaccine may have increased infection risk: study

Trials of a once-promising experimental HIV vaccine were cut short in 2007 because the drug may have increased the likelihood of HIV infection rather than preventing it, according to a new study.

The HIV-1 vaccine, which raised hopes in the fight against AIDS as it was being developed by US pharmaceutical giant Merck and Co., was undergoing second stage trials when the problem was discovered in September 2007, said researchers at the Montpellier Institute of Molecular Genetics in France.

The vaccine relied on a modified form of a common cold virus -- Adenovirus 5 (Ad5) -- to carry elements of HIV (Human immunodeficiency virus) into the body.

The smaller HIV parts, the Merck trials contended, would trigger the human immune system to start fighting off later infection with the virus.

One of main worries about the approach was that widespread immunity to the vaccine might cause the drug to be rejected by the body before an effective anti-HIV response could develop.

But three years after the first trial, researchers discovered that more of the vaccine recipients who had prior immunity to the Ad5 virus had been infected with HIV than those not exposed to the vaccine, according to the study, published online in the Journal of Experimental Medicine.

The presence of long-lasting antibodies specifically catering to the Ad5 virus, generated during natural infections with the common cold, could have altered the response to the HIV vaccine, the study said.

HIV infection spread through cell cultures three times faster in the presence of antibodies from individuals immune to the Ad5 virus, because the HIV virus came in contact with more of its preferred "T" cells -- prompted to grow by the vaccine -- to infect.

The study said the vaccine reached the second phase of its trials because primates, used in the first phase, do not naturally come into contact with the human common cold, so the problem went unrecognized.

The vaccine prototype was tested on 700 HIV-negative persons in five hospitals in South Africa between February and September 2007, in the first clinical HIV trial of its magnitude ever conducted in Africa.

Meanwhile, tests had been conducted since 2004 in the United States, Australia, Peru, Brazil and Puerto Rico.

HIV can lead to acquired immunodeficiency syndrome (AIDS).

According to the World Health Organization, 33 million people around the world are infected with the AIDS virus, mostly in the sub-Sahara Africa.

Some two million people died worldwide of AIDS in 2007.

Well-Deserved Harvest of Disappointment and Anguish

In the author's opinion, they are all still reaping their deserved reward for pretence and deliberate falsehood, and if they do not return to the path of sanity, honesty, truthfulness and correct scientific approach by acknowledging the fact that all human beings irrespective of race, nationality, religious belief or place of domicile possess the inalienable ability to reason and conceive possible candidate HIV vaccines and building on any successful foundation of HIV recipes conceived by others for the development of their own safe and effective HIV vaccines, many more harvests of similar bitter grief, frustration and financial loss are likely waiting in store for them.

The author developed safe and effective HIV therapeutic and preventive vaccines since 1999. The CNN, BBC, CBS, VOA, AFP, and the other international media institutions are all aware either because the author wrote and informed them, or they visited and interviewed the author about his HIV vaccines, or they attended Press or Scientific Conferences where the author's HIV vaccines were discussed, or they should have read the publications in reputable scientific journals about the author's HIV vaccines but they all connived and decided to give the news a black-out that they believed would be the kiss of death when they deliberating refused to let the world know about the development. Their science correspondents must have come across the publications (References 2 – 8 in Chapter 11) on the author's work.

Similarly, the United Nations and its Agencies like the WHO, UNAIDS and UNICEF, the Governments of virtually all the countries of the world especially the arch-leader Nigeria, the US, Britain, and France, the US Congress, the multi national Pharmaceutical companies especially Pfizer, GlaxoSmithKline and Roche, and the world's medical community all know about the author's HIV vaccines either because they read the publications about the author's work, or the author wrote and informed them, or the author sent them copies of his report and the preceding editorial published in the *Vaccine* Journal in 2004, or, in the case of the US Congress, the Chairman of the US Congressional Task Force on HIV/AIDS Congressman Jim McDermott and his team visited the author at his small Hospital in Gwagwalada in Nigeria's Federal Capital Territory of Abuja at about 1500 hours on Tuesday, August 1, 2000 and discussed the development of the author's HIV vaccines with the author for about an hour, or, in the case of the world's medical/scientific community, they must have read about the author's work on HIV vaccines that has been published in a number of international medical scientific Journals (References 2-8 in Chapter 11).

For reasons best known to them, they have all teamed up to bury the author's efforts by fraudulently pretending that nothing like that exists even though they know that by their action, they have deliberately killed, are still killing, and will kill millions of people. The author is convinced that the present generations, posterity and history will not forgive them, particularly Nigeria's Governments from February 1999 to date for this deliberate and atrocious genocide.

Conclusion

Experts have calculated that a vaccine that is 50% effective, given to just 30% of the population could reduce the number of HIV infections in the developing world by more than half over 15 years. More effective vaccines could cut the infection rate by more than 80%. Everyone seems to agree that "Developing a safe and effective vaccine against HIV is critical to our efforts to control the devastating pandemic of HIV and AIDS" - *Dr Anthony S. Fauci, Director of NIAID*

Unfortunately, the same experts have kept on drumming it into our heads that developing HIV vaccines has been a very difficult challenge because of many reasons that include the following:

- Nobody has ever recovered from HIV infection, so there is no natural mechanism to imitate.
- HIV destroys the immune system cells that are meant to fight against it.
- Soon after infection, HIV inserts its genetic material into human cells, where it remains hidden from the immune system.
- HIV occurs in several *subtypes,* each of which is very different from the others.
- Even within each subtype, HIV is highly variable and constantly changing.
- There are no good animal models to use in experiments [27].

To some, 'an HIV vaccine is a hypothetical_*vaccine* against *HIV,* the *etiological* agent of *AIDS.* As there is no known cure for AIDS, the search for a vaccine has become part of the struggle against the disease' [24].

The author joins others to acknowledge that these difficulties still confront virtually all HIV experts, scientists and researchers worldwide because they are extremely dishonest.

If they had been reading scientific medical publications in international journals, they would have known since 2004 that these statements are all obsolete. The likelihood is that they must have been reading such journals, and must have come across one or more publications about the author's HIV vaccines. The only reasonable conclusion to reach is that they are deliberately telling lies with these statements and assertions for reasons best known to them. It would appear that the fear that has always been associated with HIV/AIDS has also frightened honesty out of the political leadership and out of the medical and scientific community worldwide! Anyway, it is still the fact that all these assertions and purported difficulties faded into history a decade ago when the author developed safe and effective HIV vaccines. The author has a pool of human beings who have recovered from HIV infection with the author's HIV therapeutic vaccine.

References

[1] Mascola JR, Snyder SW, Weislow OS, et al. Immunization with envelope subunit vaccine products elicits neutralizing antibodies against laboratory-adapted but not primary isolates of human immunodeficiency virus type 1. *J. Infect. Dis.* 1996; 173: 340-48.

[2] Lori F, di Marzo Veronese, De Vico AL. et al (1992). Viral DNA carried by human immunodeficiency virus type I virions. *J. Virol.* 66:5067-5074.

[3] Tono D (1992). Partial reverse transcripts in virions from human immunodeficiency and murine leukaemia viruses. *J. Virol* .66:4893-4900.

[4] Lange JMA, Parry JV, De Wolf F, Mortimer PP, Gondsmit J (1988). Diagnostic value of specific IgM antibodies in primary HIV infection. *AID*S 2:31-35.

[5] Broder S, Merigan TC, Bolognesi D (2000). *Textbook of AIDS Medicine*. Baltimore: Williams and Wilkins 4:47.

[6] MacDonell KB, Chimiel JS, Poggensee L, Wu S, Phair JP (1990). Predicting progression to AIDS: combined usefulness of CD4 lymphocyte counts and p24 antigenemia. *Am. J. Med.* 89:706-712.

[7] Stein DS, Korvick JA, Vermund SH (1992). CD4+ lymphocyte cell enumeration for prediction of clinical course of human immunodeficiency virus disease: a review. *J. Infect. Dis.* 165:352-363.

[8] Centres for Disease Control and Prevention. 1993 Revised classification system for HIV infection and expanded surveillance of definition for AIDS among adolescents and adults. *MMWR* 1992; 41 (RR170).

[9] Ada GL, Jones PD (1986). The immune response to influenza infection. *Curr. Top Microbial Immunol*.128:1-54.

[10] Borrow P, Lewicki H, Hahn BH, et al. Virus-specific CD8+ cytotoxic T-lymphocyte activity associated with control of viraemia in primary human immunodeficiency virus type 1 infection. *J.Virol*.1994; 68: 6103-10.

[11] Rinaldo C, Huang XL, Fan ZF, et al. High levels of anti-human immunodeficiency virus type 1 (HIV-1) memory cytotoxic T-lymphocyte activity and low viral load are associated with lack of disease in HIV-1-infected long-term nonprogressors. *J. Virol.* .1995; 69: 5838-42.

[12] Cao Y, Qin L, Zhang L, et al. Virologic and immunologic characterization of long-term survivors of human immunodeficiency virus type 1 infection. *N. Eng. J. Med.* 1995; 332: 201-08.

[13] HIV type 1 variation in World Health Organization-sponsored vaccine evaluation sites: genetic screening, sequence analysis, and preliminary biological characterization of selected viral strains. WHO network for HIV isolation and characterization. AIDS Res Hum Retroviruses 1994; 10:1327-43.

[14] Agwale SM, Zeh C, Robbins KE, et al (2002). Molecular surveillance of HIV-1 field strains in Nigeria in preparation for vaccine trials. *Vaccine* 20, 2131-2139.

[15] Koup RA, Safrit JT, Cao Y, et al (1994). Temporal association of cellular immune responses with the initial control of viraemia in primary human immunodeficiency virus type 1 syndrome. *J. Virol.* 68: 4650-55.

[16] Cao Y, Qin L, Zhang L, et al (1995). Virologic and immunologic characterization of long-term survivors of human immunodeficiency virus type 1 infection. *N. Eng. J. Med.* 332: 201-08.

[17] Wolinsky S, Korber B, Neumann A, et al (1996). Adaptive evolution of human immunodeficiency virus-type 1 during the natural course of infection. *Science* 272: 537-42.

[18] Barker E, Mackewicz CE, Levy JA (1995). Effects of TH1 and TH2 cytokines on CD8+ cell response against human immunodeficiency virus: implications for long-term survival. *Proc. Natl. Acad. Sci. USA* 92: 11135-39.

[19] Rinaldo C, Huang XL, Fan ZF, et al (1995). High levels of anti-human immunodeficiency virus type 1 (HIV-1) memory cytotoxic T-lymphocyte activity and

low viral load are associated with lack of disease in HIV-1-infected long-term nonprogressors. *J. Virol.* 69: 5838-42.

[20] Borrow P, Lewicki H, Hahn BH, et al (1994). Virus-specific CD8+ cytotoxic T-lymphocyte activity associated with control of viraemia in primary human immunodeficiency virus type 1 infection. *J. Virol.* 68: 6103-10.

[21] Mascola JR, Snyder SW, Weislow OS, et al (1996). Immunization with envelope subunit vaccine products elicits neutralizing antibodies against laboratory-adapted but not primary isolates of human immunodeficiency virus type 1. *J. Infect. Dis.* 173: 340-48.

[22] Borrow P, Lewicki H, Hahn BH, et al (1994). Virus-specific CD8+ cytotoxic T-lymphocyte activity associated with control of viraemia in primary human immunodeficiency virus type 1 infection. *J. Virol* .68: 6103-10.

[23] Ismail G, Macgregor K, Margolis M, et al. Hepatitis C - The insidious spread of a killer virus. Newsweek International Magazine, May 20, 2002, 42-45.

[24] http://www.earthtimes.org/articles/show/112056.html

[25] http://en.wikipedia.org/wiki/HIV_vaccine

[26] http://www.hvtn.org/index.html

[27] http://www.hvtn.org/media/Bernstein_editorial

[28] http://en.wikipedia.org

[29] http://www.247gay.com/article.cfm?section=70andid=17324

[30] http://uk.news.yahoo.com/18/20081104/tts-experimental-hiv-vaccine-may-have-in-3c8ed92.html

Chapter XV

About Time, Too, for the 1984 Mirage

Abstract

The whole world has been blindly following Gallo's recipe for HIV vaccine development since 1984, even though Gallo himself had no previous experience of vaccine production against anything at the time he detailed his recipe. In 2000, UNAIDS came out with its bizarre guidelines on HIV preventive vaccine research, a document that entrenched Gallo's recipe by insisting that only the developed countries can conceive how HIV vaccines may be developed. More than 24 years since Gallo literally forced his recipe down the world's throat, and over eight years since UNAIDS guidelines were formulated, the medical scientific world claims safe and effective HIV vaccines are yet to be developed. During these past 24 years, the HIV/AIDS scourge has taken millions of lives, created millions of orphans, and has left many societies economically and socially ruined. The author, in complete disregard for Gallo's recipe and the UNAIDS guidelines, gave himself an unencumbered free hand on HIV vaccines concept and development, and he succeeded in 1998. But the worldwide adherents of Gallo's recipe and the UNAIDS guidelines are so shocked by that development that they are not prepared to accept the fact that safe and effective HIV vaccines have been developed on this terrestrial ball since 1998. If the USA, for instance, were to be under the siege with which HIV/AIDS has held many countries in sub-Saharan Africa since the AIDS epidemic broke out in 1981, the author is convinced that the USA's response(s) would have been different all these years. Discoveries always precede methodology or recipe, and not vice versa. The author advocates that all interested HIV vaccine researchers in every country should be left to work out their own recipes for safe candidate HIV vaccine development; such safe candidate vaccines may then be assessed for efficacy by the developer. A comparison of polio and AIDS diseases sheds more light on the issues raised in this chapter.

Introduction

In Chapters 12–14, we saw that the initiator of the approach to be used to develop HIV vaccines is Robert Gallo (Figure 15-1) who laid the foundation at Margaret Heckler's 1984 Press Conference.

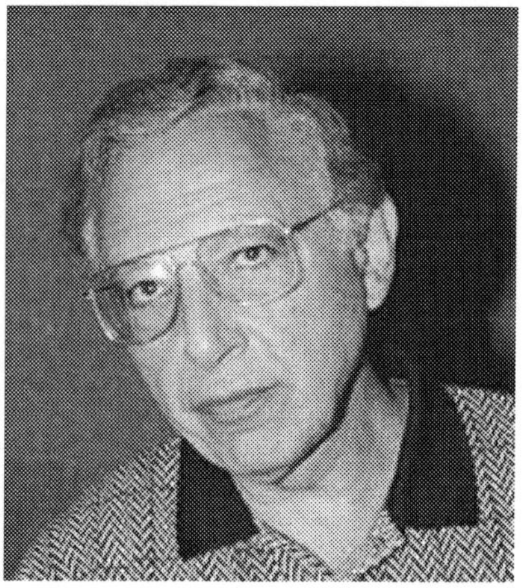

Figure 15-1. Robert Gallo of the US.

We have also discussed in some detail how he succeeded in not only rallying the entire medical scientific community worldwide to follow his approach without raising any question up till today but he himself has insisted that his infallible approach is the only way to develop HIV vaccines—remember his interview in Israel in 2005?

Gallo's worldwide flock consists not only of the scientific community of HIV vaccine researchers and developers worldwide, not only of the entire United Nations and all its agencies, not only of all the superpowers, all the upcoming powers, all the ordinary powers, all the developing powers and all the poorest powers in the world together with all their ministries, departments, agencies and institutions, not only of the multinational, national and local pharmaceutical companies, but also of 'lawyers, activists, social scientists, ethicists, vaccine scientists, epidemiologists, representatives of NGOs, people living with HIV/AIDS, and people working in health policy' worldwide.

How can the author find words to reflect his opinion on this matter? He can only say, 'Gallo, how great thou art!'

Gallo Earns His Greatness

Is it for His Work on the Causative Agent of AIDS?

What work did Gallo do to achieve this unbelievable feat? Was it because he was the first person to isolate the causative agent of AIDS? No, the author does not think it is because he was the first or only person to isolate, before others, the causative agent of AIDS. After all, it was agreed after the presidents of their countries intervened and settled a 3-year-old bitter dispute (over royalties for HIV blood tests) between the USA and France, two superpowers and long-term friends for centuries, that Robert Gallo and Luc Montagnier should be recognized as co-discoverers of the HIV. If it were because he co-discovered the HIV with Luc Montagnier of France, why has the latter not achieved any such comparable feat? Besides, many actually believe that the French were the first to isolate the AIDS virus in 1983 whereas the Americans isolated the same virus a year later.

Is It for His Numerous Scientific Publications?

Did Gallo achieve this fantastic feat because of his numerous scientific publications? No, it cannot be because in that, he is not alone. There are many researchers worldwide with equally formidable scientific publications.

How did Gallo achieve his feat then? The author cannot say with certainty that he knows the answer because Gallo has never revealed it, as far as the author knows. However, the author can give a reasonable guess based on the facts known to him.

Is It for Surfing with the Tide?

It is the author's opinion that Gallo was clever and smart enough to go beyond the issue of isolating the causative agent of AIDS during Margaret Heckler's 1984 Press Conference. Even though Gallo knew that Luc Montagnier's group was actually the first to isolate the virus, he was smart enough to appreciate the fact that for being the first to announce to the world that he had isolated the causative agent of AIDS, he had the world at his feet, to lead as he wishes. He did not need to do any further work before winning his star prize on a platter of gold. All he needed to do was go ahead and tell them how a vaccine against the virus should be made and how soon it would be available even though he knew he had never made any vaccine against anything before that 1984 press conference. Even though he knew that then, he did not know enough about the characteristics of the virus he had isolated, even though he knew from medical history then that his chance of being the first to develop HIV vaccines was less than 10 percent.

Is It for Being Like Joseph before Pharaoh?

Let the author please recall the story of a prisoner called Joseph and Pharaoh, the King of Egypt. Joseph had been thrown in prison for years for an offense he did not commit. While he was languishing in prison, Pharaoh had a very troubling dream of seven very fat cows followed by seven lean cows that joined the seven fat cows to graze beside the River Nile, but surprisingly, the seven lean cows ate up the seven fat cows. The King woke up frightened and sweating profusely because of the dream. He immediately summoned all the astrologers and magicians in his Kingdom, told them his dream and asked for the interpretation, but none of them could tell him the meaning. At that point, the King's selfish butler remembered Joseph as a dream interpreter and he told the King about him. Moving with lightening speed on his highway from grass to grace, Joseph was plucked willy-nilly out of prison and brought before Pharaoh. The author still wonders what thoughts went through Joseph's cerebral hemispheres during his short journey from prison to face the King in the Palace, a place he had never visited before in his life. Did he think he was being summoned for execution?

Anyway, Joseph interpreted the King's dream. After consultations with his advisers, the King decided that Joseph was best qualified to prepare his Kingdom for the seven years of famine that would come seven years from then. Joseph never went back to prison. From a prisoner, he immediately became the Vice-Pharaoh (the VP of Egypt indeed).

The author finds this story may be compared, in some ways for similarities and differences, with the situation in 1984. AIDS had been around since 1981 and no one knew the cause, like Pharaoh's dream that his astrologers and magicians could not decipher. At the behest of Barrister Margaret Heckler, then US Secretary of Health and Human Services, Gallo hurried back home from Italy. Unlike Joseph though, Gallo knew he was being summoned to fame, and so, he confirmed at the press conference that his lab had indeed isolated the virus that caused AIDS. He did not give any credit to the French team for the achievement; he did not even acknowledge the French contribution at all at that press conference. Even though no one asked him about how he thought an HIV preventive vaccine should be produced, Gallo went on a voyage of his own, detailing a recipe of how such a vaccine should be made, even though at that time he had no experience at all in vaccine preparation for any infectious agent, unlike Joseph that had extensive experience in dream interpretation.

Is It for Dropping the Bombshell Without Provocation?

Gallo told the world how the vaccine should be prepared, stating emphatically that he would take such a vaccine if he were a high risk person. Working in his lab then with the new virus whose characteristics had not yet been worked out, was Gallo not a high risk person for HIV infection? Anyway, he then buttered his bread by telling the world that such a vaccine should be ready for testing in two years. The deed was done!

He had literally paved his highway for rapid transfiguration from grass to grace, from being just the first person to announce the isolation of the virus—Gallo must have realized that Luc Montagnier and France would come fuming after him with fire and brimstone for double-crossing them by his press conference in complete disregard of the agreement he had reached with Montagnier earlier on—to the one that would dictate to the world how the vaccine should be made.

He would never share that crown with Montagnier! The author guesses that Gallo's reasoning went further—he knew that by outlining how the vaccine should be prepared, he had laid the foundation for worldwide recognition of his contribution irrespective of who developed the vaccine. He would always take the lion's share of the credit since he had become the first person to give the recipe for producing the vaccine.

There we are! The author doffs his hat for you, Gallo! Whether the author is right or wrong in his analysis of the situation in 1984 when Margaret Heckler and Gallo announced to the world that Gallo's lab had isolated the causative agent of AIDS, the undisputable fact on the ground is that Gallo has been crowned the great infallible shepherd of how to develop HIV vaccines.

The author is not jealous of Gallo for achieving that feat. Gallo has the author's sincere and unlimited congratulations for the feat. Gallo's worldwide followership since 1984 is enough justification for the author to offer him unreserved congratulations.

The author's offer of his unreserved congratulations to Gallo is without any prejudice to the fact that the author is diametrically opposed to Gallo's presence and utterances at that 1984 Press conference, utterances that have done incalculable harm to the cause of science, research, scientific approach to the HIV/AIDS pandemic and humanity, not to mention the loss of millions of lives and the creation of millions of orphans especially in sub-Saharan Africa as a result of the HIV/AIDS scourge since that cursed day in 1984 when Gallo made those utterances, not to mention the socio-economic calamity that has befallen many societies, communities and nations especially in sub-Saharan Africa because of the HIV/AIDS pandemic that would perhaps have been treated otherwise if Gallo had not made those damnable utterances at that 1984 press conference.

Remorselessly Admitting the Most Significant Failure

During his 2005 interview in Israel, Gallo agreed that since 1984, HIV preventive *'Vaccine has been the most significant failure of the scientific quest. In our institute there has been some important progress. I don't want to say breakthrough, I don't even want to say yet milestone, but the progress that has been made is proving that you can get a vaccine candidate that will make an immune response of the type we believe to be what's needed to block HIV from entering the cell. A type which raises neutralizing antibodies and can do it against the majority of strains of HIV. But we don't have other technical problems solved yet; we can't make that vaccine last a long time. We want to get it to the right levels; those are problems we are still working on with collaborators. While I'm here in Israel it's important for me to point out that intellectually the contributions for this vaccine came from one of my colleagues Dr. Devito, but also from an Israeli scientist, a young guy from the Weizmann institute then, he's now in Tel-Aviv, John Gershoni, who made important intellectual contributions to this pathway.'*

After over 20 years of failure with the approach Gallo gave to the world in 1984, Gallo has not reviewed the approach and he shows clearly that he harbours no such plan for the foreseeable future. He still maintained at his 2005 interview that his team is looking for the type of HIV candidate vaccine 'which raises neutralizing antibodies and can do it against the majority of strains of HIV'. He then went on to praise two people who had made intellectual contributions for that type of vaccine. Angling again to make sure he keeps his flock in Israel and elsewhere firmly behind him without raising any questions that might threaten his leadership since 1984, he heaped praises on 'an Israeli scientist, a young guy from the Weizmann institute then, he's now in Tel-Aviv, John Gershoni, who made important intellectual contributions to this pathway.' Hear the great infallible Gallo? To him, they are 'important intellectual contributions to this pathway' as long as the contributions are in tandem with his recipe! Any other contributions to any other pathway would attract his invectives, and Gallo's tongue is permanently sharpened to unleash such piercing invectives on any one that dares to suggest any other pathway.

At this point, the author would like to echo the words of Gordon Brown the British Prime Minister in October 2008 and say to Prof Gallo and others like him:

"The extraordinary HIV/AID pandemic has been calling for bold and far-reaching solutions that break new grounds; not the time for conventional thinking or outdated dogma but of fresh and innovative intervention that gets to the heart of the problem."

Tightening the Noose Indeed

Even though the author has never met Gallo and has never been in any form of communication with him, a colleague who attended an international scientific conference with Gallo a couple of years or so ago informed the author that Gallo publicly criticised the author and his HIV vaccines at the conference and dismissed them with a wave of his hand. Of course, the great shepherd had to do that because he considers the author a rebel for daring to abandon his 1984 approach to HIV vaccine development. Accordingly, he had to seek a forum of an international Conference to publicly rebuke and condemn the author's HIV vaccines work to let the others know that a similar fate awaits them from the great shepherd if they should ever think of abandoning his ship, the only ship for HIV vaccines development.

The Response of the USA to Polio Epidemics

The author wonders if Gallo is not a human being with flesh and blood and human feeling especially of sympathy for the millions of victims of HIV/AIDS since 1984. If the number of deaths and HIV infection in any country in sub-Saharan Africa were to be the lot of the USA today, the USA scientists, researchers and society may immediately abandon the great shepherd Gallo and start looking frantically and realistically for HIV vaccines. The very first step they might take, the author guesses, may be to abandon the approach that has failed for over 20 years. Let us remember that in 1916 when the USA had over 27,000 cases of polio with 7,179 deaths (negligible figures when compared to the carnage HIV/AIDS has been wrecking in sub-Saharan Africa), 'there was panic in New York where over 2,000 died. People fled Manhattan, only to meet armed robbers in the suburbs. Some hospitals refused to admit cases for fear of infecting others. Cities impounded cats and dogs because authorities mistakenly thought they could transmit the virus to humans. Parents sealed windows and doors and refused to let their children outside to play. Miracle cures like ox and frog blood, cedar shavings, and radium water abounded.'

Let us also remember that in 1954 when the USA had 38,476 cases of polio (again, very negligible figures compared to HIV/AIDS in sub-Saharan Africa), 'the National Foundation organized field trials in 44 States when 1,830,000 school children received the unregistered Salk vaccine. 20,000 doctors and public health officials, 40,000 registered nurses, 14,000 school principals, 50,000 teachers and 200,000 lay volunteers participated in the field trials'. The USA using an unregistered vaccine on almost 2 million children in 44 States?! Crazy talk! Go and say that to the Marines!

Suppose the USA were under Heavy HIV/AIDS Bombardment

Imagine the Following Hypothetical Situation

"More than one in every three adults who live in the USA is infected with HIV. Let that number sink in: 35.8% of the school teachers, doctors, scientists, politicians, bankers, engineers, parents, pilots, astronauts, university students, university lecturers, journalist, lawyers, judges, drivers, etc are infected with a lethal virus that, in most cases, will cut their lives short by decades. Canada and Mexico are only slightly better off, where the number is one in five adults. In five other countries in Central America, it is more than one in ten. All told, North and Central America now accounts for two-thirds of the estimated 40 million HIV-infected people in the world, and AIDS on that continent is the leading cause of death for adults. Hundreds of thousands of children are infected, and even more have been orphaned. Life expectancy, which had been around 75 during the past several decades, is rapidly declining: In California, for example, the World Health Organization (WHO) says the average child born today will live to be about 40; the same child could have expected to live to 75 in the absence of HIV."

What are the Possible Responses of the US to the Attack?

The reader, at this point, may wish to stop reading, carefully work out his/her own possible US responses to the attack, and then resume further reading so that the reader may compare notes with the author's own.

Shock and Awe

In the scenario we are considering, the author imagines some rascally and thoughtless elements in the US society may firebomb the house of Robert Gallo for misleading the world since 1984, arguing perhaps that if he had not done so, there might not have been any HIV to devastate God's own country. In case the reader thinks the author is being unrealistic, let us recall with trepidation that

> Prejudice against people with HIV continued in America. The Ray family lived in Arcadia, Florida, and they had three sons, each of whom was a haemophiliac and was HIV positive. During 1986 the family was told their sons could not attend school. In 1987 the family moved to Alabama, and once again they were refused entry to school. Threats against the family grew louder and more frequent, and on August 28th the Rays' small single-storey house was doused with gasoline and torched [1].

There we are! After several months of open discrimination and ostracization, some Yankees eventually firebombed three young HIV-positive haemophiliacs and their parents out of their Florida home in 1987. Yet, it was even possible that some of those in the mob that carried out the arson were themselves HIV positive and had donated their blood for these chaps who became infected through tainted blood products.

More Eerie Episodes

Let us also bear in mind with that eerie, scary feeling that still creeps all over the author's body that the USA has, for the past 20 years, been operating a policy that bars any HIV-positive but non-US citizen from visiting the US even for one day. In June 1987, the U.S. Public Health Service added AIDS to its list of diseases for which people on public health grounds could be excluded from the USA [2]. Subsequently in July, the "Helms amendment" created by Senator Jesse Helms added HIV infection to the exclusion list [3]. Few foresaw the implications of the addition and it went virtually unnoticed [4]. In March 1993, the House of Representatives in the USA voted overwhelmingly to retain the ban on the entry into the country of HIV positive people [5]. Meanwhile, on April 2, 1989, Hans Verhoef, a Dutch man with AIDS, was jailed in Minnesota under the federal law banning travellers with HIV from entering the USA [6].

No Room for Logic

How one wishes that man was a creature of logic! And that the American Government and people were just a wee bit more logical and humane! Dale Carnegie, an American warned us several decades ago when he wrote,

> 'When dealing with people, let us remember we are not dealing with creatures of logic. We are dealing with creatures of emotion, creatures bristling with prejudices and motivated by pride and vanity' [7].

Talk of double standard and man's inhumanity to man? Talk of a senseless and illogical display of sheer emotion bristling in a potpourri of prejudice, pride and/or vanity? Otherwise, why has the same USA still not passed any resolution banning HIV-positive US citizens from visiting any other country even for one day? The fact is that what the US considers is good food for the US and its citizens may never be considered good food for other countries and their citizens, even if that other country is France (or have you forgotten how the Americans Gallo, the then US Secretary for HHS Mrs. Margaret Heckler and her top officials at the HHS betrayed and back-stabbed the French on April 23, 1984?), or Holland (or have you forgotten that, in April 1989, the US jailed a Dutchman with AIDS for having the effrontery to enter the US?), or any other country.

Rattlesnake Blood and Human Urine May Perhaps be Called upon for Rescue

Under the scenario we are considering, the author imagines the US society would turn to all sorts of things to treat, cure or prevent HIV/AIDS, things that will presently be beyond our wildest imagination. Instead of frog and ox blood that some New Yorkers used for polio, may be, some would use condoms soaked in rattlesnake blood to make sure the HIV is rattled away from them and from God's own country. US doctors and other health professionals may stop working for fear of picking the HIV from patients. Husbands may stop having anything to do with their HIV-positive spouses. Parents may abandon their HIV-positive children. All sorts of remedies like the urine of those not infected with HIV, radium or deuterium water, moon soil brought by astronauts, 'soil' from the surface of Mars at very exorbitant prices may start flourishing (the FDA and other US law enforcement agents would just look the other way, and not raise the issue of licensing before use, etc! After all, 1 in 3 of them is also infected with the lethal virus!)

The Responses of the US Government

The author imagines that the US Government and the US society may then remember the author and would do everything within their power to get him to give them his formula for HIV vaccines. With the active connivance of the author's own Government – a few million dollars would break down any unexpected resistance from his country's Government, anyway - the US may even arrange to use their modern laser, infrared and other technologies, etc to locate the author wherever he may be in his country, pluck him up and forcefully take him to the US to give them his recipe after which the author would be silenced for ever. After all, Nigeria has no mountainous hideouts similar to the one along the Pakistani-Afghanistan border where the US believes Osama Bin Laden has been hiding since 2001!

It Won't be Another Iranian Rescue Mission, Osama Bin Laden or Nigeria's Alhaji Umaru Dikko

After all, the author is not Osama bin Laden who has been able to evade US capture, dead or alive, since 2001! Besides, the ancestors of the Yankees were able to take millions of the author's ancestors as slaves to America. It is just an easy matter to take one more nondescript fellow from the place that provided the US with millions of slaves and whisk him off from Nigeria to the US. There would be no possibility of a failure in such a mission that cannot be compared in any way with the failed rescue commando mission for the US Embassy staff in Iran on April 28, 1980 when the mission ended in fiasco with US helicopters crashing in the Iranian desert and the loss of 8 lives for the US. The Nigerian mission would not fail! It cannot end like the failed attempt by Nigeria's Military Government led by Major General Muhammed Buhari around 1984 that crated their country's former powerful Minister Alhaji Umaru Dikko in England en-route his forceful return to Nigeria in a civilian aircraft.

An Iraqi-Type Invasion

Does the author not know that when the US decided to topple Saddam Hussein of Iraq, the then US Secretary of State Colin Powell showed to the UN and the world satellite photograph evidence of the weapons of mass destruction that Saddam had? On that basis, the US and Britain along with other coalition partners invaded Iraq and have occupied there since. Now the world knows that the satellite photograph evidence they were shown were 'American wonder' indeed, a visual hallucination and a mirage that emanated from US technological wonder, not a reality at all. It brings back to the author's memory the beautiful childhood songs that primary school children used to sing. One of them was all about 'Come and see American wonder'!

The world by now should know that the US carries out its wish anywhere in the world even if there is no logical basis for her actions. After all, the Yankees know very well that human beings are not creatures of logic!

Of course, the chief architects of the March 20, 2003 invasion of Iraq, President Bush of the US and Prime Minister Tony Blair of Britain have insisted up till today that they have no regrets for the invasion even though the invasion has cost both countries the loss of over 5,000 troops and has resulted in the loss of Iraqi lives far greater than those lost under Saddam Hussein's rule. According to the unrepentant duo, the important thing is that Saddam is dead, and the world is better off without him. The animalistic side of humanity on display, eh! Do the families of the fallen US and UK troops as well as the families of the fallen Iraqis agree that the world has become a better place because of the Iraqi invasion?

Interim Measures for Ordinary US Citizens

In the interim, the author also imagines that thousands of US citizens who are unaware of their Government's top secret plan for the author would start trooping to the author in Nigeria for HIV treatment and prevention.

He also imagines the US would probably operate several flights to Nigeria at highly reduced fares to enable their citizens come to the author for HIV treatment or prevention, all part of a grand decoy to cover up the small military operation to capture the author and land him on US soil.

In the interest of US citizens, the US Government, the author imagines, under the scenario we are discussing, might immediately direct its Ambassador in Nigeria to immediately get in touch with the author and prepare the ground to make it smoother and faster for their citizens to get the author's HIV vaccines.

The author further imagines the US Government might get across to Nigeria's 'co-operative' Government with huge incentives to ensure Nigeria's Government gets across to the author and does everything in its power to obtain and pass on to the US the author's formula for HIV vaccines in the interest of the lives and health of US citizens wreaking under the HIV/AIDS scourge.

Lastly but not least, the author imagines urgent arrangements might be made for the US President to visit a few African countries with Nigeria being one of them not for the official reasons that would be given to the world but for the real purpose of getting the Nigerian Government to secretly bring the author to meet the US President over the HIV/AIDS scourge in God's own country.

As in 1945, the US May Have to Drop Another Big Boy

All these decoys would not deter the mighty US from dealing a final blow to the stupid author whose remaining days on this floating ball will be spent in the US with suggestions from some hawks in the US Government that the author, on landing in the US, should be sent to Gitmo Bay for some time on charges of acting against US citizens and US interests by failing to disclose, on his own, to the US his recipe for HIV vaccines, stressing that Gitmo interrogation and experience will teach him some lessons about what the US can, and will do to those not willing to bow to US interests and supremacy in everything including the search for HIV vaccines. Stupid author! He has been deceiving himself since 1999 that keeping off 'American soil by all means' will protect him from being grabbed by the long and sure arm of the US!

Is it All Just Imagination?

The author may be wrong but he does not think so. Meanwhile, because the scenario does not exist, and the author hopes it never comes to pass, the author has been treated as a pariah not only by his own country's Governments from February 1999 to date, but by others including the US, Britain, the UN and its Agencies, the multinational pharmaceutical companies, the CNN, BBC, VOA, CBS, and AFP, the international medical scientific community, etc while Gallo, the great infallible shepherd, continues to wax from strength to strength, firmly holding on to his worldwide flock of sheep that continues to follow him even though sheep and shepherd alike have remained completely lost in the wilderness in their over 20 years wayward search for HIV vaccines.

But Change is Possible under the New American Leadership

Please hold on, Jeremiah! The US held elections on 4 November 2008 that ushered in the new leadership of President Barack Obama and his Vice President Joe Biden. In their campaign, they promised the Americans change: change that they need, change that they can believe in, change that they want, and change that the whole world needs, believes in and desperately wants. They were sworn into office on 20 January 2009. Jeremiah, do not be surprised about any change that may occur under the new US leadership! The author wholeheartedly congratulates the American people on the historic election. He similarly congratulates President Barack Obama and his Vice President Joe Biden and wishes them well as they 'steeply tackle' the problems facing the US and the world.

A Comparison of the Diseases Polio and Aids

The author thinks it is interesting to compare some aspects of the struggles against polio (infantile paralysis) with those against AIDS. Here it is.

A COMPARISON OF THE DISEASES POLIO AND AIDS	
THE DISEASE POLIO	THE DISEASE AIDS
Was known to man since c. 1500 B.C.	Was known to man since 1981 A.D.
The causative agent, a virus, was first isolated by Landsteiner in 1908	At a Press Conference on April 23, 1984, the US Secretary of Health and Human Services Mrs. Margaret Heckler was the first to announce at a press conference that Robert Gallo's lab in the National Cancer Institutes had isolated the virus that caused AIDS. Actually, the French team led by Luc Montagnier of the Pasteur Institute in France was the first to isolate the virus in 1983, but they had given a sample of the putative AIDS virus to the Gallo's team to study. Both teams agreed to give a joint press conference later. Gallo undercut them! Robert Gallo had published 2 articles in 1983 and argued then that the HTLV-1 and HTLV-2 that his lab had identified were the possible cause of AIDS. At the 1984 Press Conference he attended without letting the French know, Gallo refined his stand, and argued that AIDS was caused by HTLV-3, another member of this viral family. As it later turned out, however, Gallo's HTLV-3 was not as similar to HTLV-1 and HTLV-2 as he had presumed.
After working on the polio virus for 18 months, an American, Flexner predicted in 1911 that within 6 months, a remedy for polio would be announced. His prediction was not correct.	At the 1984 Press Conference, Margaret Heckler, at Gallo's prompting, announced that an AIDS vaccine would be available for human testing in 2 years. The Americans also announced at that Press Conference that an AIDS vaccine should be in the market in 3 years. *Spontaneously and with bubbling enthusiasm, Gallo who had no previous experience at all in any vaccine development against any infectious agent, announced at that Press Conference his recipe for producing an AIDS vaccine despite the fact that some journalists at the Conference cautioned him several times against such optimism.* That 1984 dramatic Press Conference concluded with "yet another terrible disease is about to yield to patience, persistence and outright genius".
Franklin Delano Roosevelt (1882-1945), the 32nd President of the US (1933-1945), was crippled by polio in 1921 at the age of 39. 1934 marked the beginning of the personal involvement of President Roosevelt in raising funds for polio victims. He organised charity balls on his birthday "to dance so others may walk". He established the President's Birthday Ball Commission for Infantile Paralysis (polio) that was renamed The Commission for Infantile Paralysis in 1935. In 1937, he replaced it with The National Foundation for Infantile Paralysis, colloquially called the March of Dimes.	Ronald Wilson Reagan (1911-2004), the 40th President of the US (1981-1989) never suffered from AIDS. For many years, Ronald Reagan refused even to say the word "AIDS" in public, and of course, his top aides had as difficult a time with AIDS as their boss. By October 1982, over a year after the first cases of AIDS were reported by the CDC, Reagan's spokesman Larry Speakes did not know the disease existed even though it had appeared on the network news and on the front pages of major daily newspapers in the US. By June1983, the same Larry Speakes, Reagan's Press Secretary was publicly joking about 'gay cruising'. Reagan's Secretary of Health and Human Services for 3 months, Mrs Heckler, on her part, did notunderstand, in June 1983, that homosexuals engaged in anal intercourse!
A COMPARISON OF THE DISEASES POLIO AND AIDS	
THE DISEASE POLIO	THE DISEASE AIDS

From 1938 to 1940, the American Jonas Salk (1914-1995) acquired experience in inactivated influenza vaccine development (1938-1940). In 1942, Salk started working on polio vaccine. In 1949, another American John Enders in Boston developed the technique of growing the polio virus in monkey testicles or kidneys instead of nervous tissue cultures in use before then. Salk used Enders' technique to develop his own polio virus tissue-culturing system. In 1952, Salk successfully tested his polio vaccine in monkeys, on himself and a few willing participants, keeping it all secret from the public; his vaccine had boosted anti-polio virus antibodies that were known to protect against the disease. Salk announced at a Press Conference in February 1953, 11 years after he started his work on polio vaccine, that he had developed the polio vaccine. The unregistered Salk vaccine was used in a large field trial on school children in 1954. The results of the field trials were announced in April 1955 - the vaccine was safe and efficacious. Two hours after the announcement of the results of the field trial, the vaccine was licensed in the US.	On March 31, 1987, three years after Heckler's Press Conference and still no AIDS vaccine, it was announced at a ceremony at the White House attended by President Reagan that an agreement had been reached regarding ownership of the HIV antibody test patent - the Pasteur Institute would end its legal challenge and share the profits from the test with the US Department of Health and Human Services. The question of who first discovered the HIV and identified it as the cause of AIDS was left hanging. It was generally agreed that "historians can decide who found the AIDS virus first". But to many people it appears clear that the HIV was isolated in Paris a year before it was isolated in the USA. More than 24 years on, in 2008, the Americans and the rest of the world maintain that there is still no vaccine anywhere in the world against the virus that causes AIDS. Instead, they now say that if such a vaccine will ever be developed at all, humanity is at least a decade away from the dawn of such vaccines, *meaning indeed that yet another terrible disease is not about to yield to patience, persistence and outright genius even after more than 24 years.*
The Salk polio vaccine was developed in 1953, 45 years after the causative agent of the disease was isolated, and 11 years after Salk, who had some experience in influenza vaccine development took up the challenge of trying to develop a polio vaccine. After searching extensively in the internet, the author failed to find any account of intrigues, betrayals, back stabbing, dishonesty, credit grabbing, political manoeuvring, recipes before development, etc for polio vaccines development.	(1) Gallo's greatest regret is that the 1984 press conference was held at all, as it violated an agreement he had made with Montagnier and the other Pasteur researchers earlier that month – and seriously incensed them. "I was terribly, terribly nervous," remembered Gallo. "I had massive conflicting emotions. I felt this shouldn't have been done. I didn't act strong enough that we should have waited until we compared the virus with the French and made a joint announcement." Gush! Gallo betrayed the French, back-stabbed them and broke his agreement with them for absolutely no just cause. (2) In the summer of 1983, the French gave the Americans the virus, which they called LAV, a sample of the putative AIDS virus, to study it. At the 1984 Press Conference, Gallo failed to acknowledge this. Put mildly, the author says it was most unbecoming of Gallo to fail to admit this fact at the Press Conference even when journalists present reminded him many times about the French, with one of them mentioning Luc Montagnier by name. (3) At the Press Conference, no one asked Gallo about an AIDS vaccine recipe before he announced that such a vaccine would be ready for testing in two years. Gallo knew he had no experience in any vaccine development prior to the Press Conference. (4) Gallo must have known much about Salk's polio vaccine that had been developed in his own country, but decided to ignore all the lessons from it. (5) The plan was for Heckler to make the announcement about Gallo's discovery on May 4, 1984 to coincide with the publication of Gallo's articles in the *Science* Journal. For political reasons and misplaced patriotic zeal, Heckler brought the announcement forward because the *New York Times* had revealed on April 22 that the French had isolated the virus that caused AIDS. Therefore, Heckler felt compelled to ask

	Gallo to hurry back home from Italy where he was attending a scientific meeting. The author would like to believe that Heckler explained all this to Gallo. If she did not, Gallo should have enquired. Italy, by the way, is next door to France. Gallo could have alerted the French before he left Italy, but he did not. It was even possible that some members of the French team were at the Italian conference with Gallo when Gallo got Heckler's urgent summons. (6) At the pre-conference discussions with HHS big guns and with Heckler herself, Gallo had all the opportunity to explain his agreement with the French to Margaret Heckler and the other HHS officials, but he failed to do so. (7) All the other officials from the CDC, NCI and NIH all shied away from giving a time frame for an AIDS vaccine but Gallo went on his own voyage of self-confidence and told Heckler before the press conference that a vaccine would be ready for testing in 2 years. In the author's view, all these facts show clearly that Gallo's presence and utterances at that Press Conference were unjustified, impetuous, unreasonable and despicable. Gallo just went all out for unmerited credit grabbing at Margaret Heckler's 1984 Press Conference.

Conclusion

Arise, then, ye noble men of the world.
Are ye all blind and dumb?
Can ye not open thy eyes?
And the envelope of thy understanding?
Leave not any rookie to lead you by the nose.

Refrain: Thy salvation from the HIV/AIDS scourge
Lies not in irrational recipes or methodology,
Or any extant ethical guidelines and protocols
Because discovery must always precede them.
Adieu, adieu, adieu and fare thee well

Victory over the scourge lies not in
Impetuous recipes by any rookie;
For rookies we all are
When it comes to HIV vaccines.
Therefore, back to the basics, everyone.

Let every able researcher
Toil hard, night and day
To develop for humanity
Safe and effective HIV vaccines
From his or her own concept.

Just two universal encumbrances;
First and foremost,
Thy candidate HIV vaccine
Safe indeed it must be.
Then thou should confirm its efficacy.

Accept ye not, and
Listen ye not to
Any other encumbrance
From anywhere or anyone.
Depart thee with confidence.

If ye abandon any and every recipe,
And discard extant guidelines and protocols,
And from basics, work hard on thy own concepts,
Before many years pass, safe and effective
HIV vaccines shall be thy bountiful harvest.

Are ye then keen on developing
Safe and effective HIV vaccines
In the shortest possible time
For the happiness of all mankind?
Then depart thee not from this admonition.

References

[1] Department of Health and Social Security (1987) 'Don't die of ignorance', leaflet

[2] Jambs J.S. (1991), 'HIV travel/immigration ban: background, documentation' in www.aids.org

[3] Senate Record Vote Analysis (1987) 'Supplemental appropriations/AIDS testing for immigrants', 100th Congress, 1st session, June 2, Vote No. 142 in www.senate.gov

[4] Wachter R.M. (1991) *The Fragile Coalition*, St. Martin's Press, New York, p.29

[5] Cooper K.J. (1993) 'House backs HIV immigration ban nonbinding resolution at odds with Clinton's campaign pledge', *The Washington Post*, March 12

[6] Olszewski L. (1989) 'S.F. Protest planned over INS detaining of Dutch man with AIDS', *San Francisco Chronicle*, April 6

[7] Carnegie D (1956). *How to Win Friends and Influence People*. Published by Pocket Books, New York, p.14.

Chapter XVI

Surgical Op on UNAIDS Ethical Considerations in HIV Preventive Vaccine Research

Abstract

Ask the average person on the street in any country today, "What do you think are the most important issues that an orthodox western-trained medical doctor should consider when treating any patient?" The answer would likely spill out immediately, "Ethical considerations and following the UN and other protocols!" Of course, that answer to the question is very wrong. It shows the extent to which the West and its awful machinery of mass communication have gone to twist and falsify issues.

All modern orthodox doctors are bound by the Physician's Oath to which they pledge at the beginning of their medical careers. In that document, there is no mention of the words or terms "ethics", "ethical consideration", or "protocol" at all. But the Oath spells out in very clear language what the first consideration of every doctor should be. The author believes the reader will enjoy this chapter that thrashes out these issues.

Introduction

The following account is part of the proceedings during Margaret Heckler's 1984 Press Conference:

> Another sharp reporter asked whether they intended to test a live- or a killed-virus vaccine. These are the traditional methods of making a viral vaccine: either killing the virus or weakening a live version of it. These modified versions of the virus then safely can teach the immune system how to defend itself should the real thing ever invade. "Can you comment on the difficulty of human clinical trials of such a vaccine?"
>
> Brandt, an earnest and well-meaning man, did not seem to understand this question either. "Well, we're going to develop the vaccine first," he said. "Then we'll be able—it depends entirely on what kind of vaccine comes out of it. So we certainly are not going to test in humans any vaccine that would put those people at risk of the disease."
>
> The reporter, obviously baffled, kept pressing Brandt, who accused the journalist of "presupposing the kind of vaccine" they intended to develop. "I'm not presupposing anything," the journalist snapped back.

> "We don't have a vaccine at the moment," said Brandt. "And we would certainly take all . . ."
> "You're talking about having one in a couple of years," the journalist interrupted, raising the question again about how they planned to stage tests of the vaccine in healthy volunteers.
> "Well, as soon as we see the vaccine, then I'll be able to answer that question."

Had Brandt understood vaccine development better, this testy exchange need not have happened. Long before AIDS came around, scientists well recognized that the testing of a vaccine against a lethal disease raises difficult ethical questions. Inevitably, the issue comes down to weighing risks against benefits—and carefully describing the two sides of the scale to anyone who volunteers for the trial. What is more, Brandt's charge that the journalist was "presupposing" the type of AIDS vaccine that would be developed was particularly off-base because if anyone was presupposing anything about the formula for an AIDS vaccine, it was Gallo, as he revealed in a subsequent answer [1].

The Physician's Oath and Ethics

All doctors practising orthodox medicine worldwide are bound by the Physician's Oath to which they pledged. That Oath says:

> "I SOLEMNLY PLEDGE to consecrate my life to the service of humanity;
> I WILL GIVE to my teachers the respect and gratitude which are their due;
> I WILL PRACTISE my profession with conscience and dignity;
> THE HEALTH OF MY PATIENT WILL BE my first consideration;
> I WILL RESPECT the secrets, which are confided in me, even after the patient has died;
> I WILL MAINTAIN by all means in my power, the honour and the noble traditions of the medical profession;
> MY COLLEAGUES will be my Brothers;
> I WILL NOT PERMIT consideration of religion, nationality, race, party politics or social standing to intervene between my duty and my patient;
> I WILL MAINTAIN the utmost respect for human life from the time of conception;
> Even under threat, I WILL NOT USE my medical knowledge contrary to the laws of humanity;
> I MAKE THESE PROMISES solemnly, freely and upon my honour."

The author, an orthodox medical practitioner. took the Physician's Oath in 1972 and has been bound by it since then. The health of the patient has always been the author's first consideration, and will continue to be his first consideration as long as he lives. The author would like the reader to note that the words "ethical consideration" and "protocol" do not appear at all anywhere in the Physician's Oath. In the case of any conflict between any ethics or protocol and the Physician's Oath, the latter must prevail.

The author's understanding is that ethics refer to principles of behaviour based on the moral sense of right and wrong. The author firmly believes that whatever one does as a normal human being should be guided and influenced by ethical considerations, medical practice or any vaccine development inclusive.

When prescribing any drug or remedy for any patient, all doctors are trained to compare the benefits of the prescription with the risks and side-effects of the prescription on an imaginary scale. If the risks and side effects clearly outweigh the benefits, then the doctor should not prescribe the drug or remedy. If, on the other hand, the benefits clearly outweigh the risks and side effects, then the doctor should give the prescription. Clearly, this is purely a professional decision so far; it is not a matter of ethics. However, there are borderline cases where the doctor is not sure which one outweighs the other. In such borderline or indeterminate circumstances, the doctor must consider other factors before deciding one way or the other.

THE World Medical Association (WMA)'s Declaration of Helsinki (DoH)

The *Declaration of Helsinki (DoH)* is the WMA's best-known policy statement. The first version was adopted in 1964 and has been amended six times since, most recently at the General Assembly in October 2008. The current (2008) version is the only official one; all previous versions have been replaced and should not be used or cited except for historical purposes. The WMA thanks all those who submitted comments and suggestions for the most recent (2007-2008) revision of the DoH [2]

WORLD MEDICAL ASSOCIATION DECLARATION OF HELSINKI
Ethical Principles for Medical Research Involving Human Subjects

Adopted by the 18th WMA General Assembly, Helsinki, Finland, June 1964, and amended by the:

29th WMA General Assembly, Tokyo, Japan, October 1975
35th WMA General Assembly, Venice, Italy, October 1983
41st WMA General Assembly, Hong Kong, September 1989
48th WMA General Assembly, Somerset West, Republic of South Africa, October 1996
52nd WMA General Assembly, Edinburgh, Scotland, October 2000
53th WMA General Assembly, Washington 2002 (Note of Clarification on paragraph 29 added)
55th WMA General Assembly, Tokyo 2004 (Note of Clarification on Paragraph 30 added)
59th WMA General Assembly, Seoul, October 2008

A. INTRODUCTION

1. The World Medical Association (WMA) has developed the Declaration of Helsinki as a statement of ethical principles for medical research involving human subjects, including research on identifiable human material and data.

   The Declaration is intended to be read as a whole and each of its constituent paragraphs should not be applied without consideration of all other relevant paragraphs.

2. Although the Declaration is addressed primarily to physicians, the WMA encourages other participants in medical research involving human subjects to adopt these principles.

3. It is the duty of the physician to promote and safeguard the health of patients, including those who are involved in medical research. The physician's knowledge and conscience are dedicated to the fulfilment of this duty.

4. The Declaration of Geneva of the WMA binds the physician with the words, "The health of my patient will be my first consideration," and the International Code of Medical Ethics declares that, "A physician shall act in the patient's best interest when providing medical care."

5. Medical progress is based on research that ultimately must include studies involving human subjects. Populations that are underrepresented in medical research should be provided appropriate access to participation in research.

6. In medical research involving human subjects, the well-being of the individual research subject must take precedence over all other interests.

7. The primary purpose of medical research involving human subjects is to understand the causes, development and effects of diseases and improve preventive, diagnostic and therapeutic interventions (methods, procedures and treatments). Even the best current interventions must be evaluated continually through research for their safety, effectiveness, efficiency, accessibility and quality.

8. In medical practice and in medical research, most interventions involve risks and burdens.

9. Medical research is subject to ethical standards that promote respect for all human subjects and protect their health and rights. Some research populations are particularly vulnerable and need special protection. These include those who cannot give or refuse consent for themselves and those who may be vulnerable to coercion or undue influence.

10. Physicians should consider the ethical, legal and regulatory norms and standards for research involving human subjects in their own countries as well as applicable international norms and standards. No national or international ethical, legal or regulatory requirement should reduce or eliminate any of the protections for research subjects set forth in this Declaration.

B. BASIC PRINCIPLES FOR ALL MEDICAL RESEARCH

11. It is the duty of physicians who participate in medical research to protect the life, health, dignity, integrity, right to self-determination, privacy, and confidentiality of personal information of research subjects.

12. Medical research involving human subjects must conform to generally accepted scientific principles, be based on a thorough knowledge of the scientific literature, other relevant sources of information, and adequate laboratory and, as appropriate, animal experimentation. The welfare of animals used for research must be respected.

13. Appropriate caution must be exercised in the conduct of medical research that may harm the environment.

14. The design and performance of each research study involving human subjects must be clearly described in a research protocol. The protocol should contain a statement of the ethical considerations involved and should indicate how the principles in this Declaration have been addressed. The protocol should include information regarding funding, sponsors, institutional affiliations, other potential conflicts of interest, incentives for subjects and provisions for treating and/or compensating subjects who are harmed as a consequence of participation in the research study. The protocol should describe arrangements for post-study access by study subjects to interventions identified as beneficial in the study or access to other appropriate care or benefits.

15. The research protocol must be submitted for consideration, comment, guidance and approval to a research ethics committee before the study begins. This committee must be independent of the researcher, the sponsor and any other undue influence. It must take into consideration the laws and regulations of the country or countries in which the research is to be performed as well as applicable international norms and standards but these must not be allowed to reduce or eliminate any of the protections for research subjects set forth in this Declaration. The committee must have the right to monitor ongoing studies. The researcher must provide monitoring information to the committee, especially information about any serious adverse events. No change to the protocol may be made without consideration and approval by the committee.

16. Medical research involving human subjects must be conducted only by individuals with the appropriate scientific training and qualifications. Research on patients or healthy volunteers requires the supervision of a competent and appropriately qualified physician or other health care professional. The responsibility for the protection of research subjects must always rest with the physician or other health care professional and never the research subjects, even though they have given consent.

17. Medical research involving a disadvantaged or vulnerable population or community is only justified if the research is responsive to the health needs and priorities of this population or community and if there is a reasonable likelihood that this population or community stands to benefit from the results of the research.

18. Every medical research study involving human subjects must be preceded by careful assessment of predictable risks and burdens to the individuals and communities involved in the research in comparison with foreseeable benefits to them and to other individuals or communities affected by the condition under investigation.

19. Every clinical trial must be registered in a publicly accessible database before recruitment of the first subject.

20. Physicians may not participate in a research study involving human subjects unless they are confident that the risks involved have been adequately assessed and can be satisfactorily managed. Physicians must immediately stop a study when the risks are found to outweigh the potential benefits or when there is conclusive proof of positive and beneficial results.

21. Medical research involving human subjects may only be conducted if the importance of the objective outweighs the inherent risks and burdens to the research subjects.

22. Participation by competent individuals as subjects in medical research must be voluntary. Although it may be appropriate to consult family members or community leaders, no competent individual may be enrolled in a research study unless he or she freely agrees.

23. Every precaution must be taken to protect the privacy of research subjects and the confidentiality of their personal information and to minimize the impact of the study on their physical, mental and social integrity.

24. In medical research involving competent human subjects, each potential subject must be adequately informed of the aims, methods, sources of funding, any possible conflicts of interest, institutional affiliations of the researcher, the anticipated benefits and potential risks of the study and the discomfort it may entail, and any other relevant aspects of the study. The potential subject must be informed of the right to refuse to participate in the study or to withdraw consent to participate at any time without reprisal. Special attention should be given to the specific information needs of individual potential subjects as well as to the methods used to deliver the information. After ensuring that the potential subject has understood the information, the physician or another appropriately qualified individual must then seek the potential subject's freely-given informed consent, preferably in

writing. If the consent cannot be expressed in writing, the non-written consent must be formally documented and witnessed.

25. For medical research using identifiable human material or data, physicians must normally seek consent for the collection, analysis, storage and/or reuse. There may be situations where consent would be impossible or impractical to obtain for such research or would pose a threat to the validity of the research. In such situations the research may be done only after consideration and approval of a research ethics committee.

26. When seeking informed consent for participation in a research study the physician should be particularly cautious if the potential subject is in a dependent relationship with the physician or may consent under duress. In such situations the informed consent should be sought by an appropriately qualified individual who is completely independent of this relationship.

27. For a potential research subject who is incompetent, the physician must seek informed consent from the legally authorized representative. These individuals must not be included in a research study that has no likelihood of benefit for them unless it is intended to promote the health of the population represented by the potential subject, the research cannot instead be performed with competent persons, and the research entails only minimal risk and minimal burden.

28. When a potential research subject who is deemed incompetent is able to give assent to decisions about participation in research, the physician must seek that assent in addition to the consent of the legally authorized representative. The potential subject's dissent should be respected.

29. Research involving subjects who are physically or mentally incapable of giving consent, for example, unconscious patients, may be done only if the physical or mental condition that prevents giving informed consent is a necessary characteristic of the research population. In such circumstances the physician should seek informed consent from the legally authorized representative. If no such representative is available and if the research cannot be delayed, the study may proceed without informed consent provided that the specific reasons for involving subjects with a condition that renders them unable to give informed consent have been stated in the research protocol and the study has been approved by a research ethics committee. Consent to remain in the research should be obtained as soon as possible from the subject or a legally authorized representative.

30. Authors, editors and publishers all have ethical obligations with regard to the publication of the results of research. Authors have a duty to make publicly available the results of their research on human subjects and are accountable for the completeness and accuracy of their reports. They should adhere to

accepted guidelines for ethical reporting. Negative and inconclusive as well as positive results should be published or otherwise made publicly available. Sources of funding, institutional affiliations and conflicts of interest should be declared in the publication. Reports of research not in accordance with the principles of this Declaration should not be accepted for publication.

C. ADDITIONAL PRINCIPLES FOR MEDICAL RESEARCH COMBINED WITH MEDICAL CARE

31. The physician may combine medical research with medical care only to the extent that the research is justified by its potential preventive, diagnostic or therapeutic value and if the physician has good reason to believe that participation in the research study will not adversely affect the health of the patients who serve as research subjects.

32. The benefits, risks, burdens and effectiveness of a new intervention must be tested against those of the best current proven intervention, except in the following circumstances:

    - The use of placebo, or no treatment, is acceptable in studies where no current proven intervention exists; or

    - Where for compelling and scientifically sound methodological reasons the use of placebo is necessary to determine the efficacy or safety of an intervention and the patients who receive placebo or no treatment will not be subject to any risk of serious or irreversible harm. Extreme care must be taken to avoid abuse of this option.

33. At the conclusion of the study, patients entered into the study are entitled to be informed about the outcome of the study and to share any benefits that result from it, for example, access to interventions identified as beneficial in the study or to other appropriate care or benefits.

34. The physician must fully inform the patient which aspects of the care are related to the research. The refusal of a patient to participate in a study or the patient's decision to withdraw from the study must never interfere with the patient-physician relationship.

35. In the treatment of a patient, where proven interventions do not exist or have been ineffective, the physician, after seeking expert advice, with informed consent from the patient or a legally authorized representative, may use an unproven intervention if in the physician's judgement it offers hope of saving life, re-establishing health or alleviating suffering. Where possible, this intervention should be made the object of research, designed to evaluate its safety and efficacy. In all cases, new information should be recorded and, where appropriate, made publicly available.

Pre-Operative Preparation

Just consider the following hypothetical scenario about a safe and effective death-preventing vaccine. The world that has for long been looking for the vaccine admits it has not yet been developed. As a result, some lawyers, activists, social scientists, ethicists, vaccine scientists, epidemiologists, representatives of NGOs, people who have lost loved ones and people working in health policy from 33 countries and others met between 1997 and 1999 in several countries at the instance of the UN to look into the failure to develop effective death-preventing vaccines in spite of the huge funds that had been spent globally for the research.

Meanwhile, death of course continues to kill millions of human beings every year. The goals of the meetings were to: (1) identify and discuss ethical elements specific to development of death-preventing vaccines; (2) reach consensus when possible, and elucidate different positions, when not; (3) progress in ability to address these matters during pending or proposed death-preventing vaccine research. At the end, the UN produces a Guidance Document that seeks to offer guidance emanating from these meetings. The document does not purport to capture the extensive discussion, consensus, and disagreement which occurred at these meetings. Rather it highlights, from UN perspective, some of the critical elements that must be considered in death-preventing vaccine development activities.

Incidentally, an individual researcher who had been working quietly on the vaccine in one of the developing countries claimed in 1999 that he had developed such a vaccine but his country and the rest of the world have continued to say they would not consider, investigate or recognize the claim because the purported discovery had not followed the guidelines in the UN's Guidance document. Meanwhile, all those who have been following the UN guidelines have still not developed any safe and effective death-preventing vaccine. The author wonders what the readers think about this scenario though hypothetical!

The author would like to let readers know that in accordance with his entire life's principles, his accounts in this book are the truth, the whole truth and nothing but the truth.

As will be detailed later in this book, the author is a practising surgeon who decided to involve himself in the hobby of HIV vaccine research at the beginning of 1992. He knew very little about HIV then (and even now) and had no previous experience whatsoever in any vaccine preparation.

The author graduated from Medical School in June 1972. The first cases of AIDS were reported in the US in 1981, 9 years after the author left medical school. The first announcement that the causative agent of AIDS had been identified was at Margaret Heckler's Press Conference in April 1984, almost twelve years after the author graduated from Medical School, but the author did not even hear about that Press Conference until around 2000.

The author comes from a developing country Nigeria, received his medical training in his country and has been practising the profession in his country. Nigeria was not part of the global village in those days at all! The author did not know anything about the Heckler Press Conference until the availability of Internet in his country around 2000! The author, like all doctors (including Luc Montagnier of France, Robert Gallo of the US, and Peter Piot of UNAIDS) worldwide who finished Medical School before 1984, was not lucky to be taught anything about HIV/AIDS within the walls of Medical School.

Communication Blues

When the author was on Clinical attachment in Surgery in Liverpool in the UK in 1977/78, he had to book for at least 72 hours before he could get a phone call across to his family in Zaria in Nigeria, and he could only take the call at the telephone exchange building in the Centre of Liverpool. The GSM was available in Nigeria to commoners like the author around 2000, and the cost then was very prohibitive. Even at the time the author was writing this manuscript in 2008, fax facilities are extremely difficult to get in Nigeria because land telephone lines went "dead" since around 2005.

The author has a Fax machine but it is of no use. In May 2009, the author travelled about 80 kilometres to his country's capital city of Abuja for the sole purpose of faxing a document but failed after several hours in the City centre—he just could not find a place from which to fax the document. In the University satellite town of Gwagwalada where the author resides and practises his profession, there are times when there would be Internet problems for 24 to 48 hours such that one cannot access Yahoo! Mail even at the Cyber Cafes.

The upshot of the foregoing is that in the field of HIV/AIDS, most doctors including the author are beginners indeed, just like children in kindergarten. The HIV/AIDS scourge took mankind by surprise. There was no record in history of such a disease before 1981, unlike other diseases such as polio, smallpox, measles, syphilis, rabies and tuberculosis that were known to humanity long before our era.

The author must admit that he did not know about the existence of any United Nations ethical guidelines on HIV preventive vaccine research until 2000 when he received a copy of the prepublication version of it.

The National Agency for Food and Drug Administration and Control (NAFDAC) is Nigeria's regulatory authority equivalent to the Food and Drug Administration (FDA) in the US. The author had initiated correspondence with NAFDAC about his HIV vaccines. Details of the correspondences will be found in Chapter 39 in this book. On May 5, 2000, the then Chief Executive Officer of NAFDAC wrote a letter to the author about the author's HIV vaccines. Here are excerpts from that letter:-

> "I herewith enclose the following documents for your guidance:-
> NAFDAC Guidelines on Drug Registration
> NAFDAC Guidelines on Vaccine Registration; and
> Ethical Consideration in HIV Preventive Vaccine Research (UNAIDS, guidance document - March, 2000)"

The 19-page document 'c' attached to his letter is captioned ***"Ethical Considerations in HIV preventive vaccine research. UNAIDS guidance document. Prepublication version. March 2000"***, and has 18 'Guidance points'. The complete document is available in Chapter 39.

Operation Notes

With lightening speed, the author studied the document by reading it over several times. Before receiving the document, the author had been operating with the Physician's Oath and his own ethical standards as his guide, so the author was naturally and avidly hungry to know what the UNAIDS guidelines stipulated. In the following excerpts from that UNAIDS Guidance Document, the author has inserted his comments in *italics* and in parentheses:

"As we enter the third decade of the AIDS pandemic, there still remains no effective HIV preventive vaccine *(As elaborated later, this is not true!)*. As the number of those infected by HIV and dying from AIDS increase dramatically, the need for such a vaccine becomes ever more urgent *(The more urgent the vaccine need, the quicker the procedure should be to identify safe and effective vaccines against the pandemic)*. Several HIV candidate vaccines are at various stages of development. However, the successful development of effective HIV preventive vaccines is likely to require that many different candidate vaccines be studied simultaneously in different populations around the world *(How did UNAIDS know this likelihood?)*. This in turn will require a large international cooperative effort drawing on partners from various health sectors, inter-governmental organisations, government, research institutions, industry, and affected populations. It will also require that these partners be able and willing to address the difficult ethical concerns that arise during the development of HIV vaccines.

In an effort to elucidate these ethical concerns, and to create fora where they could be discussed in full by those presently involved in, or considering, HIV vaccine development activities, the UNAIDS Secretariat convened meetings in Geneva (twice), Brazil, Thailand, Uganda and Washington during 1997/1999. These meetings included lawyers, activists, social scientists, ethicists, vaccine scientists, epidemiologists, Representatives of NGOs, people living with HIV/AIDS, and people working in health policy *(Too many cooks spoil the broth indeed! The author is unaware of any precedent like this one in the history of vaccine development against any human viral disease. This again shows that human beings hardly learn anything from the lessons of history! What formed the basis for the guidelines when no one had yet succeeded in developing effective HIV preventive vaccines? How can you produce guidelines on how to achieve any target when no one has yet achieved that target?)*.

In the regional meetings, efforts were made to include people from a number of countries from that particular region. The entire process involved people from a total of 33 countries. The goals were to: (1) identify and discuss ethical elements specific to development of HIV preventive vaccines; (2) reach consensus when possible, and elucidate different positions, when not; (3) progress in ability to address these matters during pending or proposed HIV vaccine research.

In the present document, UNAIDS seeks to offer guidance emanating from this process. This document does not purport to capture the extensive discussion, consensus, and disagreement which occurred at these meetings. Rather it highlights, from UNAIDS perspective, some of the critical elements that must be considered in HIV vaccine development activities. ... *(How scientific or rational is it for anybody to offer guidance under the extant circumstance, accepted by UNAIDS, that no one has yet developed effective HIV preventive vaccine? In any case, there are only 2 crucial or critical elements to be considered in any remedy for any disease, safety and efficacy)*

It is hoped that this document will be of use to potential research participants, investigators, community members, government representatives, pharmaceutical companies, and ethical and scientific review committees involved in HIV preventive vaccine development. It suggests standards, as well as processes for arriving at standards, and can be used as a frame of reference from which to conduct further discussion at the international, national, and local levels. *(Charity begins at home! Why has UNAIDS not used its own Guidelines to produce a safe and effective HIV preventive vaccine up till now? Is that failure not a clear pointer to the worthlessness of the UNAIDS Guidelines?)*

The global burden of disease and death related to HIV is increasing at a rate unmatched by any other pathogen. For many countries, it is already the leading cause of death. Currently available treatments are inadequate because they do not lead to cure *(UNAIDS did not tell us its definition of 'cure' of HIV infection)*, but at best slow the progression of disease *(This is not true because the HIV therapeutic vaccine developed by the author has cured some people infected with the HIV. And by 'cure' of HIV infection, the author means sustained serodeconversion to HIV antibody negative status as a result of the administration of his HIV therapeutic vaccine)*. The most effective treatment for slowing HIV-related disease progression, antiretroviral medication is complicated to administer, requires close medical monitoring, is extremely costly, and can cause significant adverse effects *(Very untrue! The author's HIV therapeutic vaccine is not complicated to administer, does not require close medical monitoring, is not costly, does not cause any significant adverse effects, and results in cure of HIV infection)*. Because of this, antiretroviral medication is not readily available to the vast majority of people affected by HIV/AIDS. These are people living in developing countries and in marginalized communities in developed countries. There is therefore an ethical imperative to seek, as urgently as possible, a globally effective and accessible vaccine, to complement other prevention strategies.

Genetically distinct subtypes of HIV have been described, and different HIV subtypes are predominant in different regions and countries. Yet the relevance of these sub-types to potential vaccine-induced protection is not clearly understood. ... *(What the world needs are safe and effective HIV vaccines, not the understanding or relevance of any other thing)*

Some candidate vaccines may be conceived and manufactured in laboratories of one country (sponsor country or countries), usually in the developed world, and tested in human populations in another country (host country or countries), often from the developing world. ... *(What is the scientific basis for asserting that only laboratories in the developed world can conceive and manufacture HIV candidate vaccines? None. The UNAIDS document seems to be founded on Robert Gallo's assertions in 1984 when Margaret Heckler, at a Press Conference, announced his lab's isolation of the virus that caused AIDS. The document deals only with HIV preventive vaccine, and as such, it upheld Gallo's view that only modern genetic engineering techniques would result in an HIV preventive vaccine. This is sheer human and scientific pride emanating from nothing other than the sheer belief that only modern genetic engineering techniques and recombinant technology can be used to conceive and develop candidate HIV vaccines, something the developed countries have been doing for over 20 years now, without success. During this period of over 20 years, well over 20 million have died from the pandemic.)*

HIV/AIDS is a condition that is both highly feared and stigmatised. This is in large part because it is associated with blood, death, sex, and activities which are often not legally sanctioned, such as commercial sex, men having sex with men, and substance abuse. ...

Given the global nature of the epidemic, the devastation being wreaked in some countries by it, the fact that vaccine(s) may be the best long term solution by which to control the epidemic, especially in developing countries, and the potentially universal benefits of effective HIV vaccines, there is an ethical imperative for global support to the effort to develop these vaccines. This effort will require intense international collaboration and co-ordination over time, including among countries with scientific expertise and resources, and among countries where candidate vaccines could be tested but whose infrastructure, resource base, and scientific and ethical capacities could be insufficient at present *(How did UNAIDS know that global support or intense international collaboration and co-ordination over time is required in the effort to develop these vaccines when UNAIDS admitted that the vaccines have never been produced? The author does not know of any vaccine developed in the past for human viral infections that had such requirements)*. ...

... HIV vaccine development activities take time, are complex, and require infrastructure, resources and international collaboration ... *(UNAIDS claims they seek effective HIV vaccines as urgently as possible. Yet, in another breath, it says HIV vaccine development activities take time etc. And there is no scintilla of scientific data to support their assertions that HIV vaccine development activities take time, are complex, and require infrastructure, etc. Very strange, the author would say.)*

As health and research communities build HIV preventive vaccine research programmes, attention needs to be given immediately to how a successful vaccine, and other benefits resulting from the research, will be made readily and affordably available to the communities and countries where such a vaccine is tested, as well as to other communities and countries at high risk for HIV infection. This process of discussion and negotiation should start as soon as possible and should be carried on through the course of the research.

At a minimum, the parties directly concerned should begin this discussion before the trials commence. This discussion should include representatives from relevant stakeholders in the host country, such as representatives from the executive branch, health ministry, local health authorities, and relevant scientific and ethical groups. It should also include representatives from the communities which participants are drawn, people living with HIV/AIDS, and NGOs representing affected communities. The discussions should include decisions regarding payments, royalties, subsidies, technology and intellectual property, as well as distribution costs, channels and modalities, including vaccination strategies, target populations, and number of doses.

> Furthermore, the discussion concerning availability and distribution of an effective HIV vaccine should engage international organisations, donor governments and bilateral agencies, representatives from wider affected communities, international and regional NGOs and the private sector. These should not only consider financial assistance regarding making vaccines available, but should also help to build the capacity of host governments and communities to negotiate for and implement distribution plans. ...

In order to be ethical, clinical trials of vaccines should be based on scientifically valid research protocols, and the scientific questions posed should be vigorously formulated in a research protocol that is capable of providing reliable responses. Valid scientific questions relevant to HIV vaccine development are those that seek:

- to gain scientific information on the safety, immunogenicity (ability to induce immune responses against HIV) and efficacy (degree of protection) of candidate vaccines
- to determine that immunological correlates or surrogates in order to identify the protective mechanisms and how they can be elicited
- to compare different candidate vaccines; and
- to test whether vaccines effective in one population are effective in any other populations.

Furthermore, the selection of the research population should be based on the fact that its characteristics are relevant to the scientific issues raised; and the results of the research will potentially benefit the selected population. In this sense, the research protocol should:

- justify the selection of the research population from a scientific point of view
- outline how the risks undertaken by the participants of that population are balanced by the potential benefits to that population
- address particular needs of the proposed research population
- demonstrate how the candidate vaccine being tested is expected to be beneficial to the population in which testing occurs, and
- establish safeguards for the protection of research participants from potential harm arising from the research.

> .... Participation in HIV preventive vaccine research may involve physiological, psychological and social risks. ...

Participation, if it becomes publicly known, may also cause stigma and discrimination against the participant if s/he is perceived to be HIV-infected *(only if one follows their so-called modern approach, the only approach they can conceive. Because the author's HIV vaccines do not cause the production of any anti-HIV antibodies, they do not stigmatise those who receive them and they do not interfere with the way we normally diagnose HIV infection through the detection of anti-HIV antibodies in the blood).*

Finally, some people may develop a positive HIV test (because the only vaccines they can conceive stimulate anti-HIV antibody production) after receiving a candidate HIV vaccine (conceived and manufactured using the HIV viral protein/s), even though they are not truly infected with HIV, i.e. a 'false positive' HIV test. This may result in the same negative social consequences that exist for those actually HIV-infected (Is this serious side effect of the HIV vaccines they have been conceiving not enough to make them make a U-turn and start thinking of other approaches that may not have this stigmatizing consequence?)...

A vaccine with proven efficacy in preventing infection or disease from HIV does not currently exist (This is deliberate falsehood being propagated by UNAIDS. As shown in Chapters 26 and 27 in this book, the author wrote to inform the WHO of the availability of these vaccines in early 1999 but they bluntly refused to even investigate his claim just because the development was not a product of their stereotyped concept of developing these vaccines). Therefore, the use of a placebo control arm is ethically acceptable in appropriately designed protocols. ... HIV preventive vaccine trials require informed consent at a number of stages (This applies only to their chosen concept of HIV vaccine development, a choice that very unscientifically does not recognize the possibility that other approaches to HIV vaccine development exist!) ...

Reducing the risk of HIV infection throughout the trial among participants is an essential ethical component of HIV preventive vaccine trials. All trial participants should receive comprehensive counselling concerning methods of decreasing the risk of transmission of HIV. This should include the basic principles of safe sexual practice and safe use of injection equipment, as well as education concerning general health and treatment of sexually transmitted infections (STIs). Investigators should provide trial participants appropriate access to condoms, sterile injecting equipment (where legal) and treatment for other STIs. All trial participants should also be counselled prior to enrolling in a clinical trial regarding the potential benefits and risks of post-exposure prophylaxis with antiretroviral medication, and how it can be accessed in the community. ...

The provision of counselling to reduce risk should be monitored to ensure quality and to minimise the potential conflict of interest between the risk-reduction goals and the vaccine trial's scientific goals. As new methods of prevention are discovered and validated, these must be added to the preventive methods being offered to trial participants. ...

Women, including pregnant women, potentially pregnant women and breastfeeding women, should be eligible for enrolment in HIV preventive vaccine trials, both as a matter of equity and as a function of the fact that in many communities throughout the world women are at high risk of HIV infection. Therefore, the safety, immunogenicity, and efficacy of candidate vaccines should be established for women, and for their fetus and breastfed child, where applicable. In these situations, the clinical trials should be designed with the interest of establishing the effects of the candidate vaccine on the health of the woman and the fetus and/or breastfed infant, where applicable. ..."

Post-Operative Management

The Health of the Patient Should Always Be the Physician's First Consideration

It seems to the author that those who met and came out with the UNAIDS's Guidance document on HIV preventive vaccine research and development made ethical consideration and protocol their most important priority. The author doubts if any of them is a committed Physician. What position does the HIV-infected patient occupy in their consideration, the patient that is highly stigmatized and knows he has a fatal infection? That patient's health is always the author's first consideration, not all these distracting and worthless sermons about guidelines, protocols, etc.

Is This not a Case of Being Penny Wise and Pound Foolish?

How many lives have been lost to HIV/AIDS these past years that these sermons on ethical considerations have held humanity captive? How many orphans have been created by HIV/AIDS during the period that UNAIDS has been preaching its sermons on guidelines and protocols without ceasing? The author does not agree with this strange approach that leaves the issues and attends to the irrelevant and extremely worthless matter of protocols and guidelines.

An adage says one does not abandon his burning house in order to chase a rat escaping from the fire! With the greatest respect, the author is convinced that UNAIDS and its adherents have abandoned humanity's house that is on fire from HIV/AIDS and have, instead, been senselessly chasing protocols and guidelines since the pandemic came. As they themselves have admitted even while claiming to adhere to their bizarre ethical considerations, recipients of their candidate HIV vaccines develop stigmatizing anti-HIV antibodies. So, where lies the usefulness of their ethical considerations?

During these past years of promoting adherence to their ethical guidelines, HIV/AIDS has claimed tens of millions of lives and produced tens of millions of orphans across the world. To rub salt on the injury, so to say, neither UNAIDS nor any of its disciples of guidelines and protocols have produced any safe and effective HIV vaccines, and they are still telling us that if ever such vaccines will ever be produced, we are at least a decade away from the dawn of such vaccines.

Man's Inalienable Rights to Life, Liberty, and the Pursuit of Happiness

The author agrees with those that signed, on July 4, 1776, '*The Declaration of Independence*' of the United States of America where they declared, inter alia:

> 'We hold these Truths to be self-evident, that all Men are created equal, that they are endowed by their Creator with certain inalienable Rights, that among these are Life, Liberty, and the Pursuit of Happiness'

In practice however, the very Americans who made that declaration found nothing wrong with depriving others, for centuries, of their inalienable rights to life, liberty, and the pursuit of happiness for, at the end of it all, that was what the trans-Atlantic Slave Trade amounted to – deprivation of the slaves to their rights to life, liberty and the pursuit of happiness. It was a terrible anomaly and travesty that made great mockery of their own convictions in their Declaration of Independence.

The author does not consider it proper for UNAIDS or anyone else to deprive HIV-infected persons, the author or anyone else of their inalienable rights to Life, Liberty, and the Pursuit of Happiness. It is the alienable right of every capable human being to conceive and develop HIV vaccines in pursuit of his inalienable rights to Life, Liberty, and the Pursuit of Happiness. The author reiterates that every able-bodied and interested human being should be left to conceive and develop HIV vaccines to try and combat the serious HIV/AIDS pandemic that has been ravaging humanity since 1981, provided the concepts are safe. (S)he may then proceed and test such safe candidate HIV vaccines for efficacy.

The developed nations do not have the monopoly of thinking and/or conceiving HIV vaccines development. All normal human beings have the endowment of thinking. The author does not know of any precedence in history where the right of conceiving possible solutions to any ravaging epidemic is given to just a particular section of humanity.

It was in an impetuous show of arrogance, falsehood and completely unscientific approach in April 1984 that Robert Gallo limited the recipe for HIV vaccines development to those with genetic engineering techniques, that is to say, to the developed nations. For making that declaration alone, he deserves severe condemnation. The developed world, the UN and others have blindly followed Gallo's recipe for over 24 years now. They all deserve the same condemnation for ascribing to themselves alone the capability to conceive and develop candidate HIV vaccines. They have carried out their wish for over 24 years and persistently failed to develop safe and effective HIV vaccines. In those 24 years, see the havoc the HIV/AIDS has wrecked on humanity!

Stop the Muzzling of HIV Vaccine Research and Development

UNAIDS guidelines and protocols have imprisoned the development of HIV vaccines worldwide. The world should have been left with an open field in every country with everyone trying hard to develop HIV vaccines since 1984 with just the two necessary guidelines that researchers must ensure safety first followed by efficacy of their candidate HIV vaccines. If that had been the case these past years, the author thinks that it is likely that by now, several countries would have come up with their HIV vaccines just as the author has single-handedly produced safe and effective HIV vaccines since 1998. The author gave himself an open, unencumbered field that did not presuppose anything..

The author would be the happiest person the day he learns that India has produced its safe and effective HIV vaccines using its own recipe, that Brazil has done the same using a completely different approach, that the developed countries have done the same using yet another completely different approach (of course, they are at complete liberty to continue to use modern genetic engineering techniques as Gallo declared in 1984, if they so wish), that Kenya or Malawi or South Africa has done the same using their own recipe, etc. Every person would then have a choice of which HIV vaccines to take. That would be great for medicine, great for science, great for humanity and above all, great for HIV-infected persons or those who would wish to take an HIV preventive vaccine. It is the availability of such open unencumbered fields that has resulted in the various safe and effective vaccines that are in use today. It is the presence of such open unencumbered fields that have produced all the new inventions and discoveries that litter not only our terrestrial ball, but our outer space today.

'By their fruit, ye shall know them'. Similarly, the author says emphatically that by the barrenness of the UNAIDS guidelines and protocols that have been in place for many years, ye shall know indeed that the guidelines and protocols are verily worthless.

Also, 'the taste of the pudding is in the eating'. Those who have tasted the guidelines all over the world should by now know its barren taste of fruitlessness. Those who, like the author, wish to ignore the UNAIDS guidelines should be left to discard them without any further delay, my brethren. The author knows from basic scientific principles and the lack of any dividends over the years that the UNAIDS guidelines for HIV preventive vaccine research are verily barren guidelines produced by the blind, for the blind and of the blind!

The author did not follow them before he developed safe and effective HIV vaccines, and he has just refused to allow anyone to compel him to follow the anonymous, useless and unscientific concoction being paraded as an UNAIDS document. The author is not a signatory to any document authorizing UNAIDS to prevent him from thinking! Let those who wish to continue to follow them do so, but let no one force the guidelines down the throat of others who do not wish to be bound by a document that has demonstrated its worthlessness over several years.

Conclusion

History tells us that no one has made any new discovery by complying with any laid down guidelines or protocols. Where, for example, is the guideline or recipe that Christopher Columbus, the Italian navigator in Spanish service, followed before he discovered the New World in 1492? How could there have been such a guideline or recipe when no one in Europe knew of the existence of the New World before him? New discoveries, by definition, are the by-products of some minds somewhere that stray away and beyond the prevailing dogmas or recipes of their day, minds that think out their own recipes and ignore the ranting of those that claim either monopoly of concepts or recipes for the subject matter at hand or are opposed to ideas that are at variance with established knowledge and therefore incredible just as was done to Edward Jenner over 200 years ago.

Accordingly, the author says again:

Arise, then, ye noble men of the world.
Are ye all blind and dumb?
Can ye not open thy eyes?
And the envelope of thy understanding?
Leave not any rookie to lead you by the nose.

Refrain: Thy salvation from the HIV/AIDS scourge
Lies not in irrational recipes or methodology,
Or any extant ethical guidelines and protocols
Because discovery must always precede them.
Adieu, adieu, adieu and fare thee well

Victory over the scourge lies not in
Impetuous recipes by any rookie;
For rookies we all are
When it comes to HIV vaccines.
Therefore, back to the basics, everyone.

Let every able researcher
Toil hard, night and day
To develop for humanity
Safe and effective HIV vaccines
From his or her own concept.

Just two universal encumbrances;
First and foremost,
Thy candidate HIV vaccine
Safe indeed it must be.
Then thou should confirm its efficacy.

Accept ye not, and
Listen ye not to
Any other encumbrance
From anywhere or anyone.
Depart thee with confidence.

If ye abandon any and every recipe,
And discard extant guidelines and protocols,
And from basics, work hard on thy own concepts,
Before many years pass, safe and effective
HIV vaccines shall be thy bountiful harvest.

Are ye then keen on developing
Safe and effective HIV vaccines
In the shortest possible time
For the happiness of all mankind?
Then depart thee not from this admonition.

References

[1] Cohen J (2001). Chapter 2 "The Next Breakthrough", In: *Shots in the Dark: the wayward search for an AIDS vaccine*. W.W. Norton and Company, New York. The quotations are from the author's copy that he kindly emailed to me in 2004 after *Vaccine* published my report.

[2] http://www.wma.net/e/ethicsunit/helsinki.htm

[3] http://www.wma.net/e/policy/b3.htm

Chapter XVII

The Third Decade of Holocaust and Shipwreck

Abstract

AIDS was first diagnosed by US doctors in 1981 among US gay citizens living in the US. The causative agent of the disease, the HIV, was first isolated by Luc Montagnier's team in France in 1983, but they did not announce it. In April 1984, the US Secretary of Health and Human Services announced at a press conference attended by Gallo himself that Gallo's lab in the National Cancer Institutes had isolated the virus that caused AIDS. At that press conference, an ebullient swinging Gallo prescribed for the world the recipe for the development of an AIDS vaccine, adding confidently that a vaccine would be ready for testing in two years and for the market another year later. The following month, the journal *Science* published Gallo's work on the virus that caused AIDS. We are now several years into the third decade since the advent of HIV/AIDS that has been described as the worst pandemic in human history. In this short chapter, the author hopes to encapsulate the HIV holocaust and shipwreck that have been described in greater detail in the preceding chapters.

Introduction

Since 1981 when the Americans first reported a new disease AIDS among five young gay Americans living in the US, the world has had no peace. On the issue of isolating the causative agent of AIDS, there was a bitter dispute between the US and France; the presidents of both countries had to intervene before an out-of-court settlement was reached after three years in 1987. The Americans were responsible for causing that bitter 3-year dispute with the French, a dispute that arose from the Americans' ill-advised press conference in April 1984. The same Americans, by their premature and heady outbursts at that 1984 press conference have caused humanity much agony, morbidity, mortality, heavy investments in toxic but non-curative antiretrovirals, failure of their scientists to develop HIV vaccines, etc., by leading the world blindly along a recipe for HIV vaccine development that they had proudly enunciated at that press conference as if they alone have the monopoly of thinking.

HIV vaccines were developed since 1998/99 but the same Americans have been in the forefront of making sure that humanity is deprived of knowing about, and benefitting from them. Here then are the key features of the holocaust and shipwreck that have been humanity's lot since April 1984.

A Précis of the Holocaust and Shipwreck

We have been confronted, since the early 1980s with the worst pandemic in history HIV/AIDS, a pandemic that threatens to unravel societies around the world, just at the time that we have all become interdependent in a "global economy". Accordingly, the search for an effective HIV vaccine is perhaps the most important scientific challenge of our generation, if not the most crucial ever in the history of science

Alice Park, writing in *TIME* Magazine's March 29, 1999, edition on AIDS, said:

> "For the nearly 35 million people around the world now living with HIV, there may never be a cure. Once cells are infected with HIV, it's excruciatingly difficult - perhaps impossible - to rid them of the virus. The only sure way to stop the epidemic is to prevent infection in the first place and only a vaccine can do that. ... As scientists learn more about how HIV co-opts the human body to survive, they are realizing that drugs alone may not be enough. To contain the virus effectively, it may take a balance between drug therapy that keeps HIV levels low and a bolstered immune system that can then target and destroy the remaining virus. Until scientists find a vaccine, however, they may control but never cure the century's final scourge."

All told, the Joint United Nations Programme on HIV/AIDS (UNAIDS) estimated in June 2000 that sub-Saharan Africa had 15 million deaths from AIDS, 12 million AIDS orphans, and 24.5 million people living with the virus—a whopping 70 percent of the global AIDS total, even though this region has a mere 10 percent of the world's population. "Despite millennia of epidemics, war and famine," stated UNAIDS, "never before in history have death rates of this magnitude been seen among young adults of both sexes and from all walks of life." A vaccine, the report concluded, represented "our best hope" of stemming the epidemic.

> "More than one in every three adults who live in Botswana or Zimbabwe is infected with HIV. Let that number sink in: 35.8% of the schoolteachers, doctors, cement mixers, mothers, engineers, truck drivers, seamstresses, and politicians are infected with a lethal virus that, in most cases, will cut their lives short by decades. Lesotho, Namibia, South Africa, Swaziland, Zambia, and Zimbabwe are only slightly better off, where the number is one in five adults. In five other countries in sub-Saharan Africa, it is more than one in ten. All told, sub-Saharan Africa now accounts for two-thirds of the estimated 40 million HIV-infected people in the world, and AIDS on that continent is the leading cause of death for adults. Hundreds of thousands of children are infected, and even more have been orphaned. Life expectancy, which steadily had been climbing during the past several decades, is rapidly declining: In Botswana, for example, the World Health Organization (WHO) says the average child born today will live to be about 40; the same child could have expected to live to 70 in the absence of HIV.
>
> While HIV crumbles sub-Saharan Africa, shaking it like an earthquake that will not stop, Americans largely have lost interest in AIDS. With the advent of powerful cocktails of anti-HIV drugs in the late 1990s, journalists began trumpeting the idea that AIDS was history, which the American public readily accepted. Death rates from AIDS plummeted for a time, furthering the notion that the epidemic has abated and will soon disappear altogether. AIDS activists, politically savvy and effective rabble-rousers who for a decade drew attention to the disease and sped development of treatments, have become as anachronistic as hippies.

Most of the world cannot afford the wonder drugs that have staved off disease and death for infected people in wealthier countries. And even in the United States, the advances celebrated a few short years ago are slipping, in no small part because the virus eventually develops resistance to every drug thrown at it. Look at AIDS deaths alone. In 1997, the year after the advent of the powerful drug cocktails, the U.S. death rate from AIDS plunged by 42%. The next year, the drop was only 20%, and the number of new AIDS cases had also nearly doubled from 1997. This is, in short, no time for any country to let down its guard against HIV, especially the United States, which spends more money on AIDS research than all other countries combined.

There are many ways to slow the spread of HIV. Using condoms and clean needles, abstaining from sex, treating other sexually transmitted diseases, male circumcision, and screening blood products all have proved effective—to a point. But the best hope the world has to thwart this virus is the same weapon effectively used against smallpox, polio, hepatitis B, rabies, and other devastating viruses: a vaccine.

Much effort indeed has gone into finding an AIDS vaccine, and the scientific problems are staggering. Yet there are problems that supersede science. This book describes in detail how scientists came to the impasse they are facing, explaining plainly the complicated mixture of scientific, business, political, and ethical forces that haphazardly steer the enterprise. I also offer a solution to the non-scientific problems that, I believe, ultimately would speed the search for a vaccine, possibly shaving years off the time it takes to slow HIV. My proposal is neither revolutionary nor unique: I argue that scientists should approach the problem in a logical, stepwise fashion, testing vaccines in meaningful animal experiments and following up on all promising leads. This book documents how, amazingly, this has not happened to date, and shows the strong forces in the U.S. scientific culture that resist such an approach. And I am convinced that similar problems dog the search for vaccines against malaria, tuberculosis, and hepatitis C—and will hamper vaccine research for new diseases that in the future will suddenly assault populations the way AIDS did in the 1980s.

I doubt that my book, which I began researching in 1989 and completed with help from a Sloan Foundation grant, will single-handedly change the U.S. scientific culture. But maybe, when the public and scientists alike take a careful look at the shortcomings of the AIDS vaccine research effort, a momentum will build to attack the problem with all of the might the world can muster. If one in four adults in the United States were infected by HIV, I am confident that such a critical rethinking of the scientific community's battle plan already would have happened."

Today let us look within and step up to the challenge of our time, a challenge with consequences far more immediate for the life and death of millions around the world. AIDS will soon overtake tuberculosis and malaria as the leading infectious killer in the world. More than 29 million people have been infected, 3 million in the last year alone, 95 percent of them in the poorest parts of our globe.

"Nigeria's HIV/AIDS prevalence rate of 5.8% may seem small in comparison to some Southern African nations with seropositivity rates of over 30% of the adult population.

However, the West African nation composes nearly one-tenth of the world's HIV/AIDS-infected persons with 3.5 million infected people (UNAIDS 2001 estimate), the largest HIV-positive population in Africa after South Africa. Nigeria's population is expected to double by the year 2025, which will multiply the spread of the HIV virus astronomically. In addition to the devastation HIV/AIDS has caused and continues to cause among Nigeria's adult population, half of the current population is under the age of 15. With only 55% of primary school-aged children in school and the high HIV/AIDS prevalence rates among adults, Nigeria faces serious challenges and significant obstacles in the education and health care sectors (USAID Congressional Budget Justification, 2004). In late July 2001, the government of Nigeria announced a major AIDS treatment program. President Obasanjo declared that his government would provide cheap generic drugs to AIDS patients beginning September 2001. Patients are expected to pay about $7 a month for the treatment. The government of Nigeria plans to distribute anti-retroviral drugs to an estimated 10,000 patients, but numerous obstacles have inhibited the implementation of this program."

Researchers are scheduled to gather at the Institut Pasteur in Paris to mark the quarter century since human immunodeficiency virus (HIV) was discovered as the cause of acquired immunodeficiency syndrome (AIDS). Since then, over 60 million people have been infected with the virus and over 25 million people have died.

The urgency of the search for a vaccine against HIV stems from the AIDS-related death toll of over 25 million people since 1981. Indeed, in 2002, AIDS became the primary cause of mortality due to an infectious agent in Africa (UNAIDS, 2004).

Economics of Vaccine Development

A June 2005 study estimates that $682 million is spent on AIDS vaccine research annually.

The world is not better off today than in 2001 as far as the HIV scourge is concerned. In fact, the world is worse off. *NEWSWEEK*, The International Newsmagazine, June 11, 2001 carried a SPECIAL REPORT on pages 38–48 on "*AIDS AT 20*". Excerpts:

> 'The plague that's killed 22 million isn't done with us yet. While we hunt for a vaccine, people continue to die – from AIDS or the drugs intended to treat it. BY SHARON BEGLEY.
>
> "With the current resources," says Dr. Peter Piot of UNAIDS, "it is not going to be possible to contain this epidemic." Drugs won't do it. ---
>
> The worst plague in modern history is far from done with us. ---
>
> In announcing the isolation of HIV (in 1984), (U.S.A) federal health officials famously predicted that a vaccine would enter clinical trials within two years and reach the market within three. Seventeen years later experts still agree that a vaccine is our best hope of ending the pandemic. They also agree that we'll be lucky to have even a crude one on the market by 2007.
>
> Why is a vaccine so critical? – But even at discounted prices, these medications (antiretroviral drugs for HIV) are far beyond reach for most of the world's 40 million HIV-infected people. The cost would exceed what some countries spend on all health services combined. ---
>
> "Prevention campaigns haven't fully worked on a global scale, and I'm not sure they ever will," Berkley says. "That's why you come back to the need for a vaccine." ---
>
> As far as we know, no one has ever recovered from the infection and gained protective immunity. The result is that vaccine developers don't know quite what they're looking for. They can only hope that immunity is possible and guess at the best ways to achieve it. ---
>
> Even a successful vaccine is less profitable than a drug that people take every day. ---
>
> "From the standpoint of maximizing return on investment," Berkley concedes, "you'd stay far away from a vaccine."

Eight Routes to a Vaccine

Because no one recovers from HIV infection, scientists aren't sure what it will take to make people immune. Here are some of the approaches now under investigation.

Live attenuated HIV: Weakened version of the virus triggers a robust immune response, but the vaccine itself could cause AIDS. Human tests unlikely.

Whole killed HIV: Safer than live virus but less effective because virus doesn't generate proteins. Vaccines based on pieces of HIV are easier to prepare.

Recombinant HIV proteins: Molecules mimicking HIV's outer surface trigger the production of antibodies, but the antibodies may not block infection.

Peptide epitopes: Tiny fragments of HIV proteins are easy to make and safe to use, but may not elicit a broad-enough response to handcuff the virus.

Live bacterial vectors: Genetically altered bacteria generate HIV proteins, which the immune system learns to recognize and destroy. Safe, simple.

Live viral vectors: Harmless viruses are engineered to generate HIV proteins, which elicit an immune response. More stable than bacterial vectors.

Naked DNA: HIV genes are introduced into the recipient's cells, which then produce the viral proteins needed to activate the immune system.

Combinations: Researchers hope that cocktails incorporating more than one element will elicit the broad immune response needed to ward off infection.

An insert, a graph shows NIH, U.S.A's National Institute of Health, funding for HIV vaccines rose from $100 million in 1993 to $400 million in 2002. ---

No one expects the first generation of AIDS vaccines to work perfectly. But with 15,000 people contracting HIV every day, even a partially effective immunization could work wonders. ---

The Oxford researchers had never fancied themselves vaccine developers. ---

No one is close to having a vaccine ready for universal use, and no one is suggesting that we abandon care or treatment to speed the search for one. But as the AIDS pandemic expands, the need for a vaccine grows ever clearer.

Conclusion

For the twenty years from 1984 to 2008, the amount spent on AIDS vaccine research is thousands of millions of US dollars, and there is nothing to show for it. What a shipwreck of a financial catastrophe to rub salt brutally into the wounds of the worldwide loss of tens of millions of lives and the creation of tens of millions of orphans with attendant socio-economic disruptions! But irrespective of whatever name anyone would like to call them, the fact and the truth are that the author's safe and effective HIV therapeutic and prophylactic vaccines have been available since 1998/99!

Section IV:
Gestational Period of Safe, Effective HIV Vaccines (1992-98)

Chapter XVIII

Desperate Measures for Desperate Situations

Abstract

With the dawn of the deadly and incurable HIV in his country, the author had to decide on what to do to face the serious risk he faced as a surgeon. The author eventually opted to include trying his hand on HIV preventive vaccine development as one of his strategies; if he succeeded, he would be able to protect himself against the rampaging HIV. This chapter recounts the circumstances that led the author to making that decision and the implications for him in a country that lacks the basic scientific culture of research/development. The author will tell readers more about himself in this Section of the book. Accordingly, readers will read about the early years of the life of the author in this chapter.

Introduction

It was announced by the Americans in 1984 that the virus that causes AIDS had been identified. In Nigeria then, most people did not even know about that announcement until many months later. When its transmission routes were also made public, many African countries, including the author's country, claimed they were not affected. As a practicing surgeon in Nigeria, the author kept his ears to the ground to try to learn more about this new infectious disease AIDS that started as a gay issue. In 1986 a paediatrician, Prof. Ransome-Kuti, Nigeria's then Health Minister, announced that HIV/AIDS indeed existed in Nigeria. Public campaigns were mounted to enlighten the unbelieving public.

As a practising general surgeon involved in emergency and elective surgical operations, the author had reason to worry. HIV screening tests were not available in those days where he practised, so he had no idea whether any of his patients was infected with the "dreaded and incurable" virus. And yet, he continuously faced the hazard of needle pricks during operations, like any other surgeon anywhere in the world. How was he to handle this desperate problem that threatened him and his career?

Assessing the Options

By 1991 when it had become clear that HIV/AIDS was common in the author's country, it became even more urgent for him to be protected against HIV if he was to continue surgical practice and keep his dignity—the disease was, and still is, highly stigmatized everywhere, including in the author's country Nigeria. But there was no vaccine against the deadly and incurable HIV infection.

The other option was to leave surgical practice and do something else for a living. That option had serious problems. How would he fulfil his social obligations while training for another career? And who would be responsible financially for his training in whatever new career he decided to choose?

In the author's country, polygamy is very rampant. It is commonplace to have a man married to 10 or more wives at the same time, especially among those who live traditionally including the traditional chiefs and chieftaincy title holders, very privileged people in Nigeria. In some parts of the author's country, a man with one wife does not qualify to be awarded a traditional title because it is indicative of either poverty or inability to manage or keep many wives. Marriage contracted under the traditional system in Nigeria may be terminated especially by the husband at any time without much ado. An aggrieved party may go to the Customary Courts, but in the end, the dissolution of the marriage is always upheld.

Among Moslems—and they form the biggest religious group in Nigeria—a man is entitled to a maximum of four wives at any point in time, but he could without much ado, get rid of any or all of them at anytime and replace them with new wives as soon as he gets rid of any of the current wives, provided that he does not exceed four at any point in time.

All it takes for a Moslem in Nigeria to end his marriage to any of his wives is to tell her repeatedly that the marriage is over. Once he does that, there is no room for anyone to try to save that marriage; the wife leaves. There is no remedy in law for her either because the Sha'aria Courts that exist for Moslems will dismiss her protest in a few seconds.

For those who marry in Churches in Nigeria, there is no law that forbids them taking additional wives, but usually the additional wives would not have the Church's blessing. Christians who take additional wives normally do so using a customary wedding for subsequent wives.

There is the Court marriage for the relatively very few who opt for it. That is the only marriage that is similar to the type of heterosexual marriages known to the Western world. The marriage can only be terminated by the order of the High Court.

Of course, there is no limit to the number of concubines a married man may keep in Nigeria. The more concubines a married man keeps, the more respect he gets from his own peers, the family into which he was born, and the society at large. Not too long ago, a gentleman gleefully and proudly told an audience that included the author that he had 49 children but that he could not say off hand the number of ladies that gave him that number of children! That gentleman was one of the Honourable Members of Nigeria's House of Representatives when he made that disclosure. Nigeria's House of Representatives is the Lower House of the country's National Assembly, the Upper House of which is called The Senate. The National Assembly in Nigeria is the equivalent of the US Congress. Instances abound in Nigeria where a wife goes all out to get another wife for her husband.

In the author's country, it is the culture that the senior children, as soon as they are old enough to live independent of their parents, look after their younger siblings. In addition, all children especially the oldest males are by culture the ones to look after their aging parents. They are also responsible, in part at least, for looking after other relations of their father and mother.

Nigeria has over 250 tribes. Each tribe has its own distinct culture. Generally, however, the extended family system applies with very minor differences to all Nigerian tribes. In the author's tribe called *Igala* in Central Nigeria, there is no word for aunt on one's mother's side just as there is no word for uncle on one's father's side. There is no word in Igala for cousin also. All one's cousins are one's brothers and sisters. All the maternal aunts and female cousins of one's mother are that person's mother, and all the paternal uncles and male cousins of one's father are that person's father. The same thing applies to sisters and brothers. The author therefore has uncountable numbers of fathers, mothers, sisters, brothers, grandparents, etc. Readers may therefore appreciate the author's difficulty in 1991 when he had all these responsibilities to bear in the family into which he was born.

The author had also to cater to the family in which he was the husband (of one wife) and the biological father of 3 children. As a result of his membership in this family, he had to take some responsibility, too, for his wife's extended family that is just like his own extended family.

In December 1991, the author was 43 years old. Like most people at that age, he was a member of two families. He was husband and father combined in one family where he had to look after his wife and children. He still continued to be a member of his first family where he is the second of seven living children born to the same couple, his father and mother. The author was lucky that his parents were monogamous. Was it realistic for him to leave his career and job and start training for a new career at the age of 43? How would he get the resources to meet his numerous social obligations? And who would be responsible for training him in any new career that he decided on? Oh HIV/AIDS! Thou has indeed brought too many problems for mankind!

As a compromise, the author took the decision to apply and, if admitted, start a part-time University program for a degree in Law at the University of Abuja's Distance Learning Programme. In that way, he would be able to struggle and train himself while continuing to practise as a Surgeon. That decision did not solve the fears and danger he faced of picking up HIV under the circumstances in which he worked, and carried out both elective and emergency surgical operations on patients whose HIV status he could not even determine. He would have to just keep his fingers crossed that his luck would carry him safely through the seven years it would take before he could qualify to be a legal practitioner in his country.

At the same time, the author decided at the beginning of 1992 to face the challenge by falling back on his knowledge of, and training in Immunology to try to develop a preventive HIV vaccine for himself. After all, he reasoned, it could indeed turn out to be a good hobby in the open field of HIV infection that the world had declared 'incurable'. In his reasoning then, all the leading vaccine developers in the world were 'rookies' as far as HIV vaccines are concerned. He might as well join them as another 'rookie'. What would he lose if he tried and failed? He would lose nothing other than the fact that he had tried and failed, and in that, instead of being alone, he would be one in a large company of many others that had been failing worldwide.

Besides, his father had inculcated in him from a very early age that in matters like this, it is far more honourable and rewarding to try one's hands and fail than to just sit, do nothing and possibly end up a victim of the problem. 'Come on then, are all men not born equal?' he told himself. 'Join the others elsewhere in the world that are trying to find HIV vaccines. They are humans like you. With regards to this problem of HIV vaccines, they do not have any monopoly of knowledge and more importantly, they are rookies like you.' That's how he joined the club of rookies looking for HIV vaccines.

Lonely Adventurer in His Country

The author did not know then (1991), and still does not know now of anyone or institution in his country that was, or is involved in HIV vaccines research or development. Everyone in his country was, and is still waiting for an announcement of the successful development of HIV vaccines from the developed world. After all, all other human technological developments including modern medical remedies came to Nigerians and other sub-Saharan African countries from there. The author would be regarded as insane in his country if it became known that he was trying his hands at HIV vaccine development within the shores of his country. Only a mad indigenous Nigerian living in Nigeria would try such a thing when the 'white man' had been trying without success. The author's plan was not just taboo, but beyond the normal range of human behaviour in his society.

In any case, he was not going to have any financial support from anywhere. In the author's country, any funds voted for 'scientific research/development' are in practice, funds earmarked for the pockets of some individuals. The author knew, and still knows that there is no culture of scientific research and development in his country. He remained adamant. He was facing a desperate situation and he just had to take desperate measures to tackle it. The author would be a lonely adventurer! At this point the author would like to tell readers about his early life on this planet.

The Author's Early Years

Place of His Birth

The author' country Nigeria, like all other countries in sub-Saharan Africa had no culture of writing in their history. Nigeria's first contact with writing occurred when the trans-Saharan Arab Slave Traders came in from the North and introduced Arabic literature. Later, the southern parts of the country, the coastal areas got their baptism of writing when the Europeans landed with Slave Trading in tow. Accordingly, all the Nigerian languages were not in any written form before the arrival of the Arabs and the Europeans who were joined later by the Americans in the lucrative but inhuman Slave Trade. The Central parts of Nigeria were the last groups to have contact with either the Arabs or the Europeans, and as such, they lagged behind the far North in Arabic knowledge, culture and writing, and also lagged behind the Coastal areas of the country in Western culture, education and writing. Generally however, the Central parts of Nigeria are ahead of the South in Arabic knowledge, civilization, writing and culture and ahead of the far North in Western culture, education, writing and civilization.

The author's recollection of his existence on this terrestrial ball was a toddler in a little rural Igala settlement called Ajiolo Aj'edim'oche located in a thick tropical forest in Central Nigeria, east of the confluence of Rivers Niger and Benue, Nigeria's two biggest rivers. The settlement was separated by thick forest from another settlement just about 200 metres away to the east, called Ajiolo Aj'onuch'aboko. These two settlements were said to be founded by 2 brothers (first cousins actually). Almost all the buildings in both communities were thatched mud huts. These mud huts were built or rebuilt haphazardly all over the settlement with no regard for any sort of planning and they needed to be rebuilt yearly at the longest. No lawns were kept because it was against the culture to leave any grass near one's hut. The best building in both settlements was the Church that had corrugated iron roofing sheets, popularly called zinc in Nigeria, for its roof but it had no ceiling; the Church was located in the eastern settlement but used by both communities.

There was no singleconvenience in any house in both settlements in which the author was born and brought up. Everyone eased himself or herself in the forest some reasonable distance away from the buildings. House flies and mosquitoes were all over the place. No one associated them with any illness. The community and tribe, like other tribes in Nigeria, had absolutely no knowledge of the existence of micro-organisms of any description. From time to time, children would pass round worms in their stools; no one bothered to ask how they got the worms. Some would prepare herbs for the worms while others would go for spiritual remedy. Others would hold witches and wizards responsible, and take appropriate actions like going to the oracles to deal with the witch or wizard responsible. House flies were considered harmless because they were said to be domesticated! Many, if not most Nigerians still believe that to this day.

The sick received free treatment from those with wisdom with plants and herbs. The author's father was one of such in the community, and he passed his knowledge to Tom and Jeremiah.

Infant and Maternal Mortality Was Very High in the Community

The only operation that the community practised routinely and commonly was male circumcision (female circumcision is not practised among the Igala people). There was no knowledge of sterilization. The same sharp knife used for shaving all the hair from the head of adults was used for these circumcisions for which a number of children may be lined up for the procedure that would be done quickly one after the other. The knife however would be wiped in the palms after every circumcision or shaving. Strong adults would hold the crying children for the procedure. The faster the surgeon is the better of course. Some had it as neonates while others had theirs any time up to age of about ten.. The author was circumcised by his dad at the age of 7 days.

There was no knowledge of anaesthesia. The ability to put someone to sleep and operate on them without their feeling any pain was one of the wonders that only the white man could perform. The author listened to various accounts of operations carried out at the Hospital at Idah by a white doctor, stories that set every body wondering whether they were really true or they were just fabricated stories. The story-tellers all swore they were recounting real life stories. The author therefore grew up with the idea that performing a surgical operation on someone under anaesthesia, cutting away the disease without the sleeping person feeling any pain during the cutting, and the person waking from the sleep back to life with the disease removed was the peak of human achievement in medicine that only the white man could perform.

All the medicines available to the community and the tribe were of two types; those to be taken orally and those to be rubbed on the skin. A sick person who could not eat or drink, or who was vomiting faced imminent death within a few days, particularly infants and children with gastroenteritis. It is therefore not surprising that less than 50 per cent of children saw their fifth birthday. Similarly, maternal mortality from childbirth was very high.

What about injections? Oh, they belonged only to the white man as part of what God had given to that race. The author grew up with the firm indoctrination that white people are not humans like the blacks. White people were believed to be somewhere between God and man; that God had given them all powers except the power to bring the dead back to life whereas blacks had no such gifts from God.

The Igala tribe into which the author was born has a traditional ruler called the Attah of Igala. He had, and still has his Palace at Idah (6 10N 6 40E), a town that lies on the eastern Bank of the River Niger south of Lokoja. At the time of the author's childhood, every Igala person held the Attah of Igala in the highest esteem the reader can imagine. He was the absolute leader to whom every Igala person owed unquestioning allegiance. It had been so from time immemorial, the author was told from his early days. He was also possessed of supernatural powers passed on to him by his forefathers, the author learnt in his infancy.

At the time the author was a kid, Idah was, to him and his community, the centre of life on this planet. A visit to Idah was taken as the fulfilment of life. To just see the Attah of Igala even from a distance was taken by the person and his community as a great favour from their forefathers.

Like all traditional positions in Nigeria and Europe, the position of the Attah of Igala was, and still is, hereditary; it was not an elective office open to every contestant. Only members of the Attah ruling houses are eligible for consideration and appointment to the Attahship when there is need to get another Attah. That need only arises when the incumbent Attah sleeps with his ancestors. And there are king makers whose job it is to appoint the successor. The holder of the Attah title occupies the office for life. It is an abomination hitherto unknown to the Igala to have two living Attahs at the same time.

Life in the Community of His Birth

It was completely an agricultural settlement with rudimentary farming techniques of shifting cultivation using hoes, cutlasses and machetes. The community had absolutely no knowledge of any sort of fertilizers. Sheep, goats, dogs, ducks and hens were the only domestic animals kept in the community. The community's source of water was a flowing and sparklingly clean stream called Ajiolo about a mile from the village. Dotted along the banks of the stream were many rural settlements all bearing the name Ajiolo and differentiated by adding the name of the first settler of the community. The source of the stream is close to the community where the author was born and raised, and as such our point of using the stream was the farthest up stream; there was no other point where humans used the stream that was further up stream than ours. We all bathed in the streams naked, children, ladies, and men, young and old. Dirty clothes and cooking utensils were also washed in the stream using very good local soap (made from palm oil and other ingredients) that the author still knows how to make.

The author would not be surprised if some readers are shocked by this community way of life especially group bathing in the nude in open space in a stream. The author would like the readers to know and note that what he went through no longer happens in the community of his birth. In any case, there are now popular television programmes showing nude adult ladies and men, some married and some single, bathing together and being telecast to the whole world. Such a 2008 programme has been running on South Africa's BBA (Big Brother Africa) 3. BBA 1 and BBA 2 were telecast in 2006 and 2007. The BBA programme lasts for 91 days! The current BBA 3 started on Sunday 24 August 2008 with 6 ladies and 6 men (one of the men is married with a daughter) from 12 different African countries, and since the programme will last for 91 days (13 weeks), it would last till Sunday 23 November 2008. In these programmes, whenever any housemates engaged in coitus, they are telecast live to the whole world! Britain has been running a similar programme too! What the author went through in his infancy and childhood in his community was not under cameras that boomed the pictures live to anybody, and it never involved copulating couples being seen or watched by others!

Besides, nude clubs are said to exist in some developed countries; in these clubs, adult members are sometimes shown nude on CNN and other stations. Such clubs do not exist in the author's country and society! In the author's society and country, marriage is heterosexual. It is crazy to contemplate a marriage contracted by two men or two ladies! But in the developed world of our days, it is taken as one of the hallmarks of modernity to engage in homosexual activities (lesbianism or gay relationships) to the extent that the association is legally recognized as union or marriage in some cases. And the author hears that some people in the developed world have started campaigning that they be allowed to marry their pets! One man's meat indeed may be another man's poison!

Many wild animals and birds inhabited the thick forests all around our settlement. The author still remembers encountering many when hunting with catapults in the forest with other kids or when answering the calls of nature. The community's source of meat came from group or individual hunting of the abundant wild game with traps of various types and bows and arrows and the newly introduced 'dane' gun owned by relatively few adults. In the community, it was a taboo to give eggs, meat and fish to children.

Domestic animals were kept mainly for economic reasons rather than for food. Chicken eggs were plentiful but children were not allowed to eat the eggs. The hatched chickens almost always ended as prey for hawks. Children were repeatedly warned that if caught eating eggs, the two hands would be clasped together and tied over a hot egg taken out of boiling water and left like that until the egg cooled down in the palms. Of course the child would wail and wail, but there would be no rescue. By the time the hands are untied when the egg would have cooled to body temperature, both palms peel off.

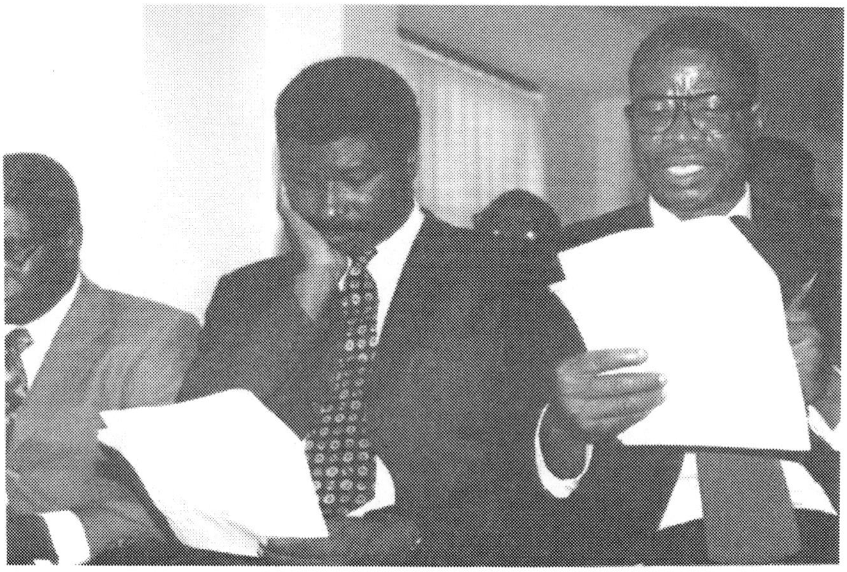

Figure 18-1. From left, the author's elder brother Tom, Barrister Isaac Okpanachi and the author at the HRPR, 30 Aug 2000.

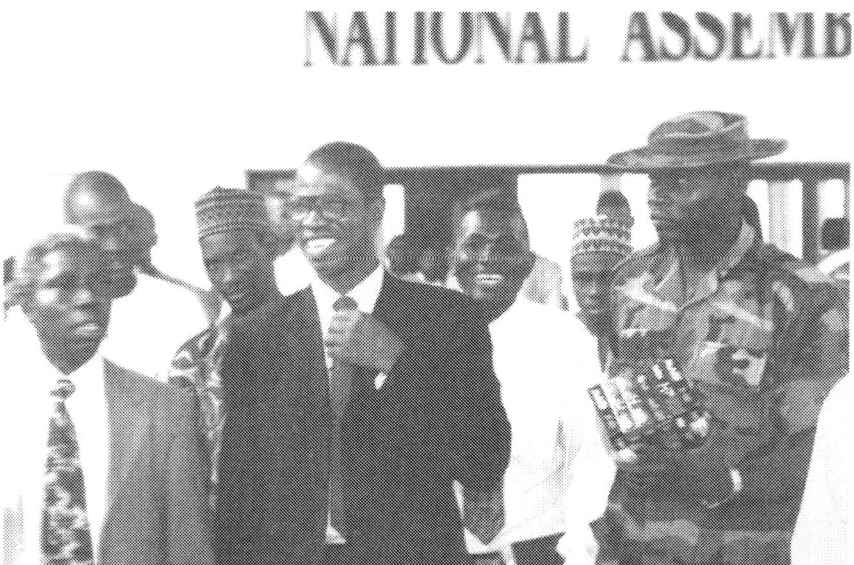

Figure 18-2. The author's elder brother Tom (first left) and the author leaving the National Assembly venue of the HRPR, 30 Aug 2000.

Jeremiah and his elder brother Tom (Figures 18-1 and 18-2) discussed the issue at length, and reached the conclusion that eggs must be very sweet. They could not risk stealing their mother's chicken eggs because of the punishment. In any case, it was not easy to steal the eggs and not be caught because one had to boil or roast it. They decided to ask their mother to give each of them one chick to rear as theirs. For a little job for their mother, they deservedly got a female chick each. They looked after them and luckily got them to maturity; they escaped the hawks. When they started laying eggs, they asked for their mother's permission to boil one of the eggs in her pot to eat. She refused. They then had no option but to roast them in the hot ash in big fires used for making palm oil. They were so eager to taste the sweet egg. They were so disappointed that the cooked egg was just tasteless. They found no sweetness in either the albumin or the yolk. They ended up wasting the egg because neither of them would eat it. Their mother laughed her head off at them, and told them to learn their lesson. What was the lesson? Always obey the elders because they know better!

The community had a lot of wild palm trees from which many things were obtained. The red palm oil was particularly widely used for cooking and eating almost every type of food. The source of light at night came from a by-product of extracting palm oil from the fruit. The palm kernel was also obtained from the trees. Palm wine, baskets and brooms for sweeping also come from the tree.

We had abundance of fresh fruit in the forests. All the kids were experts at climbing trees and shrubs for the fruits. So were Tom and the author. Tom and Jeremiah especially were expert in doing girls' jobs such as preparing palm oil, manually grinding cereals using stone, fetching water from the stream in clay pots, looking after babies and preparing the local foods and drinks because they were their mother's first 2 children. They had to help her with these chores until she had big-enough daughters to take over from them. The author recalls the episode when one of his father's friends from another community visited. The visitor asked the author's father about his 2 sons. The response of the author's father left both father and his visitor laughing for a long time. Alabi had told his visitor that in practice, he had only one son, Tom. Jeremiah, he said just had the appearance of a boy but in practice, he was a girl always doing the lady's chores and not helping him with the jobs that sons should do!

Once darkness fell, the children would gather round the elders for story telling, after supper. Jeremiah noticed that he was hard of hearing compared to other children. Two people would discuss with him sandwiched between them but he would not hear anything if they talked in whispers. That handicap has been with him throughout his life. Medical examination later in his life showed his cochlear had been damaged probably by quinine that his parents admitted they forced him to take in his infancy and early childhood. Out of ignorance, they probably overdosed him or he was overdosed because of concomitant dehydration at the time he took some doses of the alkaloid.

If there was moonlight, peers would play different games in the moonlight including hide and seek. With the warm tropical weather, clothes were more of a nuisance because of sweating. The author used to go about stark naked in the village up to the end of 1963 when he was 15 years old but had not reached puberty. Of course, there were no shoes or any form of foot wear for the children and most of the adults, too. Yaws was endemic then in Central Nigeria; Tom and the author suffered from it as kids. Jiggers, bedbugs and lice were common, too and we suffered from them also.

Almost all of us in the settlement were related by blood or marriage through one or both parents. Virtually everyone in the community was a traditionalist and pagan worshipper including the author's parents before the advent of missionaries. When an American Missionary called Mr. David Gross brought Christianity to our people around 1926, a few people embraced the new religion. The Mission he founded was called The Christian Missions in Many Lands, CMML. The author's parents were among these early converts before the author was born. Then and now in the author's country, converts to either Islam or Christianity take on Islamic or Biblical names at their conversion. The author's dad took on the Biblical name of Daniel at his conversion to Christianity, and his mum took on the name of Martha at her conversion. They gave all their children Biblical names at birth.

Community Beliefs

Belief in spirits was rampant. No one died naturally; someone somewhere must have used or evoked supernatural and evil forces to cause the death. From time to time, one would hear about the confessions of witches and wizards who would then receive severe punishment from those that had the power to handle such practitioners of wicked spiritualism.

Masquerades were rampant, and we were told from our early days that they were not human beings but the reincarnation of our ancestors. Of course, they were feared and revered, and one took in these words of the elders as gospel truth.

In Nigeria then and now, the best indigenous technological achievement in the country is the masquerade. Accordingly, Nigerian members of the Nigerian society would stop all other activity to watch masquerades. Foreign and local dignitaries are entertained by masquerades. What the masquerade is to the Nigerian is what the spacecraft is to the American today, assuming the spacecraft is America's highest technological achievement. The reader should bear this in mind as he reads this book.

From a very tender age, we were indoctrinated about corpses to which serious supernatural forces and capabilities were, and are still attributed. Dead bodies are feared and revered. Children were not allowed to see a dead body. White men, at death, became blacker in colour than black itself, we were taught from infancy – the author learnt later in his life that none of those who taught them this falsehood had ever seen the corpse of a white person! The corpse was, and still is more important to the Nigerian than the living person. Great honour and burial ceremonies await the dead. Up till now, in the author's country, very few relations will contribute money to treat an ill relation, but once the person is dead, funds would start pouring in for his/her funeral and burial, all because of the culture that makes the dead far more important than the living!

Nigeria has just two seasons in a year: the dry and rainy seasons. Lightening and thunder storms are common during the rainy season. Thunder is dreaded, but not the lightening! It was believed that some people have the power to control thunder; they could send thunder to kill someone. We have separate names in Igala for thunder and lightening, but out of ignorance, everybody believed it is the noisy thunder that does all the havoc while nothing is ascribed to lightening.

Fetishes, charms and belief in their supernatural forces were common place. Infant mortality rates were very high. These fetishes invariably have processed dead cow's skin (hide) as the fulcrum of the supposed powers that Nigerians still ascribe to them, powers that are ultra science and as such cannot be explained by science and its laws! Right from his infancy, the author could not come to terms with these beliefs. He would hide, open up these fetishes and find they contained nothing that could be any source of power. They all contained either ordinary sand or a piece of paper with some Arabic writing enclosed in the hide. They author therefore knew from his childhood that fetishes were just fake items being used to psychologically deceive the unwary.

These weird beliefs in the supernatural are not unique to the Igala tribe; they are commonplace not only in Nigeria but in other parts of sub-Saharan Africa. The author thinks the following recent Editorial on page 8 in the *Daily Sun* newspaper in Nigeria on Friday, July 25, 2008 will likely shed more light on the author's assertion:

> "Jungle justice in Kaduna
>
> The recent gruesome killing of Kingsley Mbagwu Onuoha by irate youths in Kaduna State over alleged missing genitals has brought to the fore the level the Nigerian society has degenerated to and the value it places on human life.
>
> According to Police report, the victim, a trader and an indigene of Imo State, was abducted from the Jagindi Police Station and lynched by people of the area for allegedly causing the disappearance of the sex organ of one Seth Israel, an indigene of Jagindi.
>
> The report also stated that Israel from Zambina, Damakasuwa District in Kauru Local government Area of Kaduna State, later mobilized his schoolmates from Government Secondary School, Jagindi and other youths from the same district to Jagindi police station. At the station, the late Onuoha was forcefully removed from police custody and set ablaze. The youths also burnt down the police station worth about N2 million, injured some policemen, set ablaze the house of one Jerome John, a cousin of the deceased, and destroyed property worth about N45 million.
>
> The incident generated a lot of heat and tension in Kaduna between the Igbo and their host community following threats to avenge the death of their kinsman over an issue that bordered on false alarm and accusation. The matter became more serious as medical examination has confirmed that the sexual organs of Israel are still normal and intact.
>
> Already Igbo leaders in the north have expressed their anger over the matter.
>
> In a petition to Kaduna State Governor Mohammed Namadi Sambo and copied to Ohanaeze-Ndi-Igbo, the Governor of Imo State and the Emir of Jema'a, the Igbo community said that the way the government reacts to this sordid action of the Jagindi people will determine their next line of action.
>
> The killing of Onuoha in a police station is barbaric and unimaginable in the Nigeria of the 21st Century. We condemn this heinous crime perpetrated in utter disregard of civilized ways of seeking redress through the legal process. There is indeed no need for resort to self-help in this situation. The law should have been allowed to take its normal course. What were the police doing when this sordid act took place? It is not enough for the police to tell us that the horrendous murder was contrary to sections 97, 240, 114, 106, 337 and 224 of the penal code. The police should tell us why they allowed the mob to take Onuoha away and lynch him so that the institution does not lend itself to accusations or suspicions that border on complicity.
>
> This jungle justice meted out to Onuoha rudely reminds us of the case of Gideon Akaluka whose head was cut off in Kano in 1991 by an irate mob operating under the guise of religion without recourse to due process. This type of killing has serious security implications for the country that is striving for nationhood.
>
> Now that the perpetrators of this wilful murder are in police net, they should be prosecuted and punished accordingly to deter others from taking the laws into their hands next time around. Treating them with kid gloves will embolden others to do similar things in the future.
>
> People should always act on verifiable evidence and not wallow in superstitious beliefs that have no bearing with truth or reality."

There was a single dusty motorable track through the community. Once in a while, a big lorry would ply it. As children we would rush to the roadside to cheer the passing vehicle and waive at it in ecstasy. We were told all sorts of funny stories about vehicles and aeroplanes and motor cycles. Every four days, many of these lorries would pass westwards in the morning to the market at Abocho (7 35N, 6 56E), the District headquarters 7 miles away to the west and return in the evening.

The white man, we were told from infancy, is next to God; that God gave the white man all powers except the power to bring the dead back to life. That was the explanation for the motor cycles, motor vehicles, and aeroplanes made by white people.

It was taboo for a husband and wife or wives to live under the same roof in the author's community and tribe. The man had his own separate house and each of the wives had hers.

Christian Upbringing

The author was born into a Christian family. He grew up and found himself taking part in Sunday services and Sunday school where they learnt Biblical stories and the ways of Christianity. Once in a while, the white missionaries (citizens of the USA, Canada or Britain) would visit their community. That would be special for the kids especially. They would show them moving cinema at nightfall before their departure. The children would have the opportunity to move close to their VW bus for a close-up look, and try to sneak and touch the vehicle! They would teach the village kids new Christian songs and choruses. Success at the Sunday school lesson would earn the child beautiful colour photographs of models from which they understood that white ladies have red lips. The village lads did not know about lipsticks then because it did not exist in their world. Sometimes, the missionaries would go with them to the stream and baptize those who qualified for it. Oh! These village kids enjoyed the visits by the missionaries especially Mr. Paul Gross who spoke Igala and knew more Igala culture and language than the Igala elders in their community. The author still recollects vividly Mr. Paul Gross, his wife and his 4 daughters. His parents, Mr. David Gross and his wife died at Anyigba and were buried there. Paul himself passed on in the US around 1982 from heart attack.

For about an hour every Sunday afternoon, the elders would bring out the 'gramophone' and play Christian songs for the children, something the kids adored. The lads would leave there and argue seriously about the source of the songs when no one was physically present. They could not get any explanation from the elders too because they also had no idea too.

Reckoning of Passage of Time — Days, Months and Years

Clocks were not available in the settlement in which the author grew up. Everyone used the position of the sun in the sky for appointments and time estimates. Months are reckoned using the new moon. If a child is born today in daylight, for instance, and the new moon appeared later that evening at dusk, the child is one month old! Similarly, years were counted from the New Year celebrations after Christmas. If a child is born say on December 31st, that child would be one year old the next day because that day is the New Year! There were therefore many children that were one year old without ever being one week or one month old!

In the author's culture and language, a week consists of 8 days because in counting days either forwards or backwards, a number is skipped. Yesterday has a word in Igala; the day before yesterday is called '3 days ago' in the language; three days ago is called '4 days ago' in the language, etc. When counting days forwards also, there are words in Igala for tomorrow and next tomorrow, but the next day that would be 3 days hence, instead of being called '3 days time' is called '4 days time', etc. There is absolutely no standard time keeping either in hours, days, weeks, months or years.

As an illustration, the author's first child was born at 0830 hours on September 16, 1976. When the author took him home to his village in December 1982, a furious argument ensued about the kid's age. The author watched them in bouts of laughter. Their estimates of the boy's age ranged from 15 to 35 years! The boy was just over 6 years old. When the author told them so, they all rebuked him for not having an idea about even his own son's age! For him to try and educate his people about time frames, the author asked them how long it was since he married. Their answer varied from 20 to 40 years. The author was only 34 at that time! He married on December 28, 1974 (Figure 18-3). And there we were in December 1982, just 8 years later and his community was seriously convinced that the author had married 20 to 40 years earlier! Imagine the span of their estimates, 20 years range!

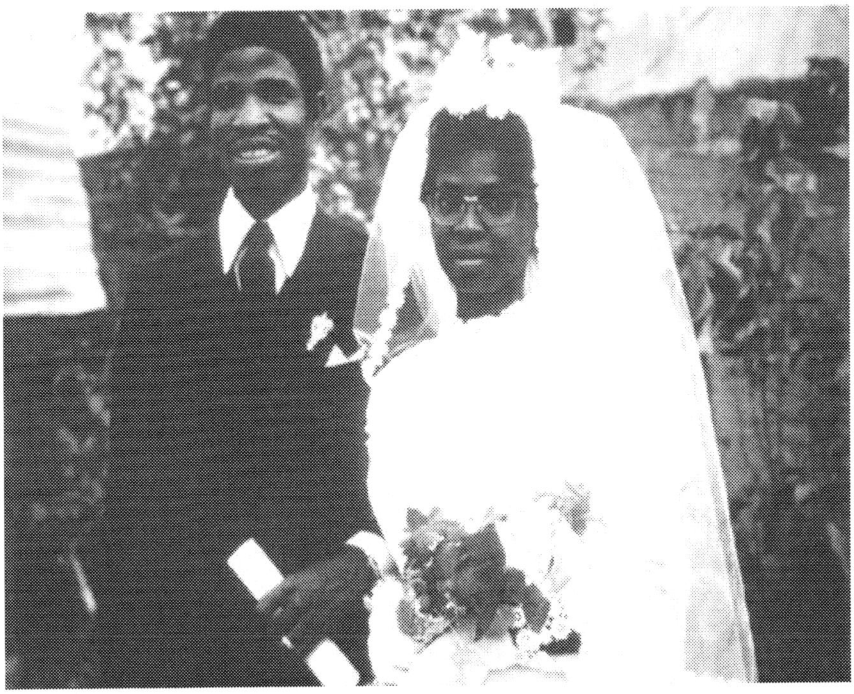

Figure 18-3. Esther and the author on their wedding day, December 28, 1974 at the ECWA Church, Zaria.

Christian Religious Instruction

In January 1954, a teacher was brought to the community to start Christian religious instruction for the children. Tom and the author were taken by their father to the Church to join other children for these studies that were carried out in the Igala language. Their father

(Figures 18-4 and 18-5) had to miss his farm work on that day because he did not want his children not to bear his name. Their mother (Figures 18-6 and 18-7) opposed the idea of sending Tom and Jeremiah to school, but her opposition was insignificant because the children did not belong to her but to her husband! The practice then was to give any child the surname of whoever brought him/her to school on the day the child first registered for school. Birthdays were not recorded in those days. How could they keep such records when writing was unknown to them? And to make matters worse, they could not even give a reasonable guess about even their children's ages or other events either! Most Igala people then would, at the best, relate any important event to the Attah of Igala that was on the throne when the event occurred.

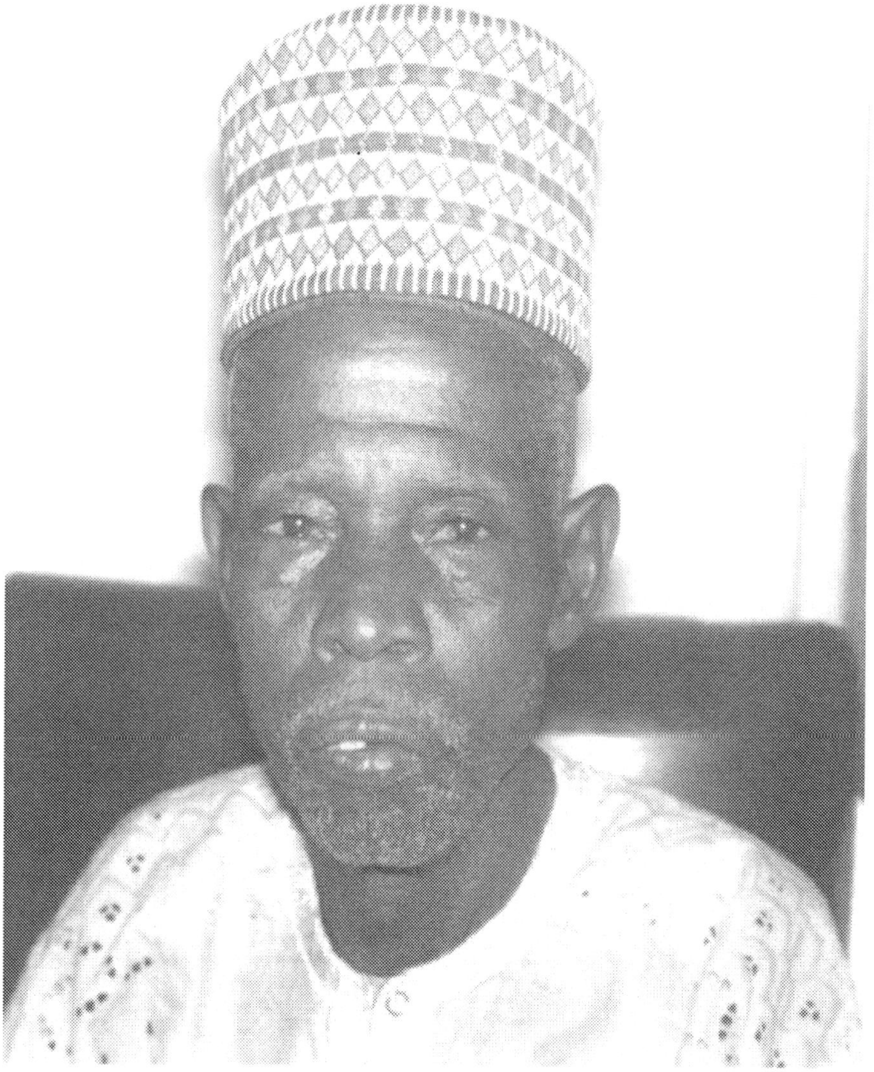

Figure 18-4. Daniel Alabi Abalaka, the author's dad, 8 Jan 2001.

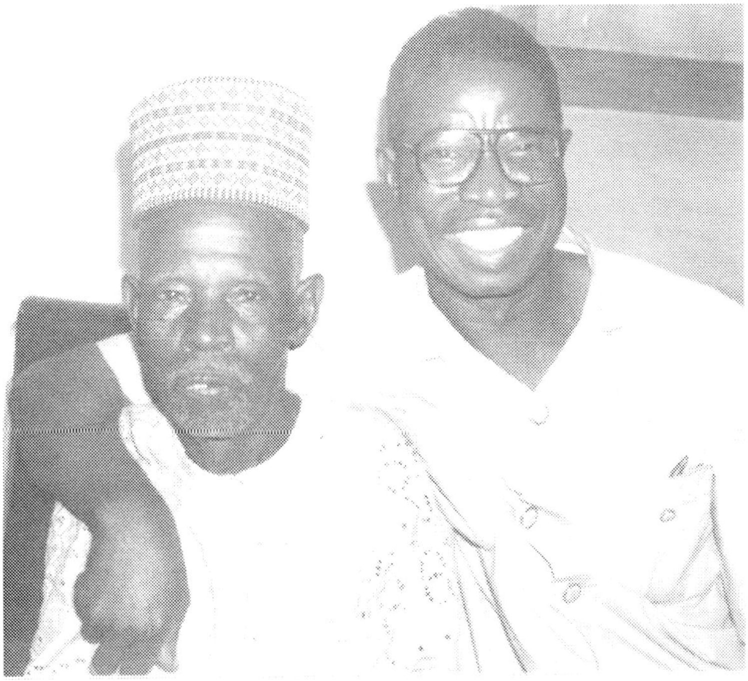

Figure 18-5. Daniel (left) with his second child and son Jeremiah, the author 8 Jan 2001.

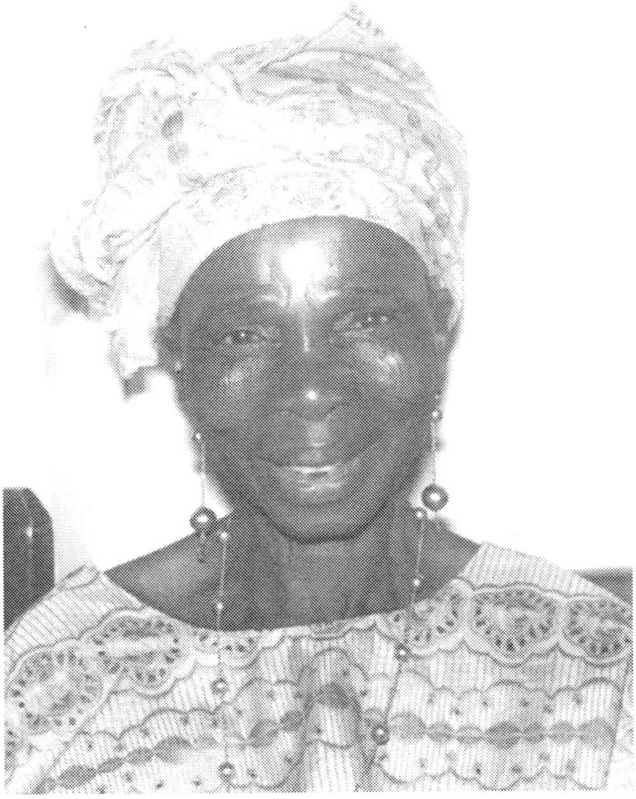

Figure 18-6. The author's mum Martha, 8 Jan 2001.

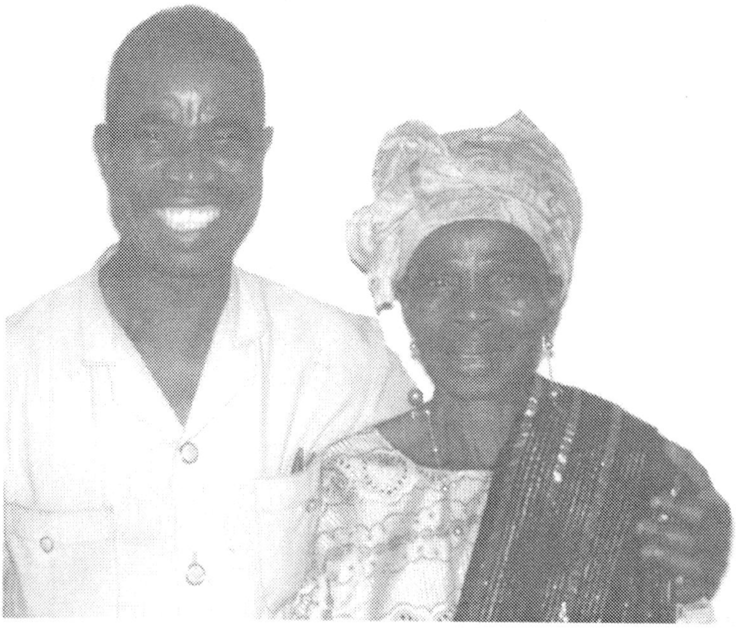

Figure 18-7. The author cuddles his mom Martha, 8 Jan 2001.

At the time Tom and Jeremiah were taken to start the Christian religious instruction class in their community, many in their class were grown up adults, some married. Tom and Jeremiah were tiny kids. Such small kids were asked to put one hand over the centre of their heads and touch the opposite ear. If the child could do that, he was old enough to start. If he could not, he was not old enough to join the class. The author imagines that a clever chap somewhere devised the technique for a society in which no one had any idea of ages of children. The author does not know even now how reliable the technique was!

As for educating female children, our father made it clear that he would never allow it for two reasons. He would not be stupid enough to train another man's wife! Secondly, girls would invariably end up with pregnancy as soon as they reached puberty, thereby putting an end to all the efforts to educate them! The man was so convinced about the issue that he never changed his mind throughout his life. Alabi's next five children after Jeremiah were all females, and he never put any of them in school.

Alabi's stand was a reflection of his culture. In his days, there was no western education. As soon as any female child reached puberty, she married, moved to her husband's family and started her own family. It was the ambition of any girl in those days to start procreation as soon as she was biologically ready for that role. Also, it was, and still is the culture that children belonged to fathers, not mothers. Female children, by culture, do not carry on the lineage of their fathers because her offspring would carry on the lineage of their fathers, not hers. In the Igala culture then and now, female children are regarded as temporarily belonging to their fathers; at puberty and marriage, they change over to their husband's family to have children to continue their husbands' lineages, not their mothers' lineages.

Readers should also bear in mind that human beings generally do not question their culture. Culture in that respect is similar to religion. One is not allowed to question religious beliefs. In some religions, one just has to accept it; some religions would not permit one to even change over to another religion; any one who attempts to leave such a religion is guilty of apostasy, and faces, in some cases, the death penalty from other adherents of that religion. Any person that questions religious beliefs and practices is an unbeliever or an apostate. Culture is at least as powerful as religion in determining the way of life and reasoning of most people.

Anyway, it was a very courageous decision by their father because he had literally deprived himself of the assistance of his children with his farming. The author recalls that many of his father's relations vehemently opposed his father's decision to take his first two sons to school, but the man refused on the ground that he had travelled to the Mission's Headquarters at Anyigba, 10 miles away, and consulted Mr. Paul Gross the missionary for advice on the issue. The reader may recall that this American missionary was more versed in Igala language and culture than the author's father, and he was far older than the author's dad.

The reckoning of the author's community was that if Paul the missionary and the author's dad had been children of the same parents, the author's dad would be, at best, the third child after Paul Gross! The author remembers clearly his dad telling all his relations that had gathered over the issue that Mr. Paul Gross had told him in clear terms that the worst thing he could to his children was to fail to let them go to school. On the strength of that, some of his relations sent one or two of their children to join us at the school, albeit for just a few days! As soon as the discussion ended, Alabi our dad summoned Tom and the author to the place they had just discussed. There and then, he publicly grabbed our ears, twisted them until they hurt us seriously, and declared that if we did not take our studies at school seriously, he would kill us. That was it!

In summary, the community into which the author was born was an atavistic society where every one did as their ancestors had done before them. No one ever thinks about making the environment better than he/she met it. It was a culture bristling with mental inactivity and laziness, like other cultures in Nigeria.

The Egyptians developed writing thousands of years before Christ. The Arabs, Europeans, Chinese, Romans, Japanese, Koreans, Russians etc independently developed their own writing and technology. No black tribe or culture or country has ever developed any form of writing, as far as the author knows.

When the Americans developed and dropped the atomic bomb on the Japanese cities of Hiroshima and Nagasaki in 1945, the rest of the world except the black race could not sleep. They were challenged to develop theirs except the black race. The Europeans, Chinese, Indians, Pakistanis, Israelis and South African whites subsequently developed their nuclear bombs. The black race remains unchallenged to this day.

Nigeria remains a consumer nation because the people there would not be challenged to use their own brains to develop any thing; it remains a country that exports raw materials for the industries of the developed world, like other sub-Saharan countries. The author is sad that his race has continued to live even in the 21st century with literally dormant brains.

The typical Nigerian, nay the typical black person wherever he may be is extremely lazy mentally as if his brain must not be involved in thinking out solutions to even very glaring problems like lack of water in the settlement, hygienic disposal of human waste in the community, provision of sources of light even for the natural hours of darkness after sunset, etc. Their ancestors had lived that way and no one would ever think of trying to improve. The author is sad about this state of affairs of the black person's brain. The black race would continue to be backward unless the black person decides to start using his brain to its capacity and is ready to face challenges by employing his brain to solve problems. The truth must be told even though it is bitter. As a race, the black has continued to be backward because of our unacceptable mental laziness in the name of culture.

The foregoing then encapsulates the circumstances of the author's birth and upbringing in a tropical country that was then colonized by Britain. The author plans to tell readers about his subsequent years in the coming chapters.

Conclusion

The reality that the author's surgical profession posed a real risk of his acquiring HIV propelled the author to consider various options for dealing with the desperate situation in which he found himself in the late 1980s and early 1990s. The author's desperate measures in response to the HIV threats facing him included a decision to join the many rookies worldwide in a solo adventure into HIV preventive vaccine development to try to protect himself against the ravaging, deadly and incurable HIV. That decision flew in the face of the culture and practice in his country and society.

Chapter XIX

Square Plug in a Round Socket?

Abstract

It is a truism that we are all the product of our genetic constitution and our environmental influence. The author is a trained general surgeon, but circumstances compelled him to become involved for the first time in his life in vaccine research and development against HIV. Generally, the field of vaccine research and development belongs to laboratory scientists, virologists, microbiologists and vaccinologists employed either in government institutions or in the pharmaceutical industry. Well, Edward Jenner was a surgeon when he developed the smallpox vaccination, but then surgeons in those days did not need to be doctors, and Jenner was not a doctor when he developed his vaccination. These days, all surgeons are doctors before specializing as surgeons. In our era, is it not a square plug in a round socket for a surgeon to involve himself in HIV vaccine research and development? Find out for yourself as you read this chapter.

Introduction

Readers may be wondering how a practicing general surgeon whose second home is the operating theatre could be involved in any vaccine research. They may therefore be asking, "Is this not a clear case of a square peg in a round hole?" The author wishes to address such concerns by providing the reader with the available facts so that the reader may decide for himself whether this is a clear case of a square peg in a round hole or not. More importantly, however, it is the author's opinion that what the world needs are safe and effective vaccines against HIV irrespective of where they originate. After all, neither square pegs in square holes nor round pegs in round holes have been able to develop such vaccines since 1984. And a peep into history tells us that so-called square pegs in round holes have made astonishing discoveries, like the English surgeon Edward Jenner who discovered a vaccination against smallpox or the Wright brothers, bicycle repairers who made the first aeroplane in 1903.

Medical School

As one would expect, the author's entire education was acquired under the British system because his country was a former British Colony until October 1, 1960 when Nigeria became independent. In that year, the author was a Primary 6 pupil.

In October 1967, the author was one of the 46 pioneer students of the Faculty of Medicine, Ahmadu Bello University in Zaria in the present-day Kaduna State of Nigeria. The University year then always started in October and ended in June the following year. The author had gained admission based on his December 1966 Advanced Level results in relevant science subjects. The medical training lasted five years. The author was one of twenty-nine medical graduates that formed the first batch of doctors turned out by the Ahmadu Bello University in Zaria in 1972. During the two years of pre-clinical studies (1967-69 academic years) in Medical School, the author was fortunate to be one of the four students in his class who was offered vacation jobs in the laboratory during the long summer holidays of three months (end of June to end of September). That was the first opportunity the author had of acquiring practical knowledge and experience in medical laboratory work. Each summer vacation job was rotational between Haematology, Microbiology and Chemical Pathology departments all of whom were headed by non-Nigerians from Britain and Egypt.

The following table contains the author's recollection from memory of the names and nationalities of his non-Nigerian teachers up to the time he graduated from Medical School in 1972. The author's reason for providing the reader with this detail would be apparent in subsequent chapters particularly the one dealing with Nigeria's Federal Ministry of Health (Chapter 36) and the Presidency (Chapter 49).

Immediate Post-Graduation Years

After graduation from Ahmadu Bello University's Faculty of Medicine in Zaria in June 1972, the author did his one-year internship (housemanship) at that University's Teaching Hospital. Nigeria had then not instituted the compulsory National Youth Service Corps, NYSC. In fact, it was at the author's Convocation in October 1972 that Nigeria's then Military Head of State, General Yakubu Gowon announced that his Government was going to introduce that Service, starting with the 1973 graduates.

After his internship, he took another year's contract appointment in Pathology, spending 3 months each in Haematology under one Prof. Allan Fleming, Microbiology under one Dr. Egler, Chemical Pathology under one Prof. Discombe, and Histopathology (Morbid Anatomy) under one Prof. Edington The author is sorry he has forgotten their first names). He then took another 1-year contract appointment in Histopathology under the said Prof. Edington who told him it was crucial for him to be trained 'in this new specialty of Immunology because no one would make any substantial progress in any field of medicine especially Pathology without a good training and knowledge of Immunology'. The author heeded his advice.

Non-Exclusive List of the Non-Nigerians who have Taught the Author from Primary School to Graduation from Medical School in 1972

Year	School	Name of Teacher	Teacher's Nationality	Subject or Department
1959/60	Native Authority Senior Primary School, Anyigba	Miss Newton	British	Religion
1961/64	Ochaja Secondary School	Mr. Johnston (First Principal)	British	Mathematics
		Miss Tector	British	English and Eng. Literature
		Miss Usher	British	Eng. Literature
		Miss Constantine Malpas	British	Mathematics and Biology
		Mr. W.J.R. Robinson (Principal)	British	Physics and Chemistry
1965/66	St. Paul's College. Zaria	Mr. Kerr	British	Zoology
		Mr. Leah	British	Chemistry
		Mr. Maltby	British	Physics
		Mr. Armitage*	British	Geography
		Mr. Ferry*	British	Mathematics
		Cannot remember (CR)	British	General Studies
1967/72	Ahmadu Bello University, Zaria	Prof. F. Nicholson (First Dean)	Canadian	Chemical Pathology
		Prof. Bunning	British	Anatomy
		Dr. Youssef	Egyptian	Anatomy
		Prof. Watson	Sri Lankan	Physiology
		Many in Veterinary Medicine but CR	Americans	Physiology
		CR	American	Biochemistry
		Prof. Meads	British	Genetics
		Many but CR	Cen. European	Microbiology
		CR	Cen. European	Parasitology
		Prof. Smith	British	Nigerian History
		Prof. E.H.O. Parry	British	Medicine
		Prof. Harold Scarborough (Dean)	British	Medicine
		Dr. B.M. Greenwood	British	Medicine
		Dr. Bryceson	British	Medicine
		Dr. H.C. Whittle	British	Medicine
		Dr. Davidson	British	Medicine
		Many but CR	British	Medicine
		Prof. J.H. Lawrie	British	Surgery
		Prof. Woods	British	Orthopaedics
		CR	Maltese	Surgery
		Many but CR	British	Surgery
		Many but CR	British and	Anaesthesia
			Indian	Morbid Anatomy
		Prof. Dawson	British	Morbid Anatomy
		Dr. Beckley	British	Haematology
		Prof. Alan Fleming	British	Medical Microbiology
		Dr. L.J. Egler	Cen. European	Ophthalmology
		CR	Pakistani	Obs and Gynae
		Prof. Una Lister	British	Obs and Gynae
		Prof. Jocelyn Moore	British	Obs and Gynae
		Many but CR	British	Paediatrics
		Prof. Dobbs	British	Paediatrics
		Dr. Werblinska	Polish	Paediatrics
		Many but CR	British	Community Medicine
		Dr. Schramm	British	Leprology
		Dr. Faltzgraff	American	

* Did not teach the author the subjects mentioned but had social and other interactions with the author when the teacher was on compound duties, during games or during Worship in the Chapel, etc.

Basic Training in Immunology

Professor Edington then arranged for the author to go and do a Postgraduate Certificate Course in Immunology under Prof. Osunkoya (the author is again sorry he has forgotten his first name) at the University College Hospital in Ibadan, about 600 km by road, south of Zaria.

WHO-Sponsored Immunopathological Conference in Geneva

While at that course, Prof Edington started making arrangements for the author to attend a WHO-sponsored Conference on the Immunopathology of Schistosomiasis in Geneva, Switzerland; the Conference was held at the WHO Immunopathology Research Unit.

In those days in Nigeria, the Nigerian Passport was issued from only Kakawa Street in Lagos, then Nigeria's capital city. The author made several journeys by road from Zaria or Ibadan to Lagos in pursuit of his first Nigerian Passport without which he would, of course be unable to attend the Geneva Conference. He finally collected the Passport No. 265138 "Given at LAGOS this 19TH day of SEPT. 1974." The author then raced across to the Swiss Embassy in Lagos for his visa. The Embassy had been waiting for him. Within a few minutes, he got his Swiss visa (written in French) No. 2370 issued on "19 Septembre 1974". And so, the author was able to attend the early October 1974 Geneva Conference for which he was completely sponsored by the WHO.

The author thoroughly enjoyed every aspect of the training in Immunology that he had received. The Geneva Conference was its practical peak as it gave him a good basis of the concept of immunogens for vaccine research and development. Despite his enjoyment of the training in Immunology and the far brighter future that laid ahead for the author in Histopathology, the author switched over to Surgery after the Geneva Conference because of deep-seated reasons that he would start to explain later in this Chapter.

Surgical Training

It took Jeremiah another 5 calendar years to complete his postgraduate training in General Surgery under Professor J. H. Lawrie, a Scot; at the end, he obtained his surgical Fellowship. During that training, he spent 18 months on Clinical attachment under one Professor Robert Shields, Head of Department of Surgery at the University of Liverpool in England. Jeremiah was attached to the Royal Infirmary and Broadgreen Hospitals in Liverpool. Jeremiah has continued to practice general surgery since he switched over to that discipline at the end of 1974.

The Author's Early Childhood

When Tom and Jeremiah started attending the Christian religious instructions class in January 1954, their dad told them that whenever they do not have to attend classes, they had to help him with his farm work. That was religiously obeyed by the two brothers throughout their schooling career.

The UNICEF Wonders of Injections and Rapid Prescriptions

During 1954, UNICEF came round, giving free injections to everyone. They came back a few weeks later for another round of injections. These injections cured and eradicated the then endemic yaws in central Nigeria. Tom and Jeremiah were suffering from yaws at the time of the mass campaign with the injections, and they were just overjoyed that their yaws ulcers had at last disappeared for ever. At about the same time (the author thinks it was in the same year) too, the same UNICEF came round vaccinating everyone in the left arm against smallpox. Tom and Jeremiah knew many sufferers of the disease, but as soon as the elders were sure someone had come down with the disease, they would cart Tom and Jeremiah and their peers away for quarantine. Fortunately for them, neither of them got the dreaded disease before the mass vaccination programme came. The disease was well known to the Igala people long before the British colonization of Nigeria. The Igala people knew that survivors did not get a second attack, but they had no preventive remedies.

The effectiveness of these two campaigns convinced every Igala person that injections are truly wonderful. Up till today, the average sick Nigerian who attends any hospital would not feel he has been adequately treated unless he has received an injection.

There was also fallout from the campaigns. Everyone came out, queued up, and rapidly received the injection or vaccination without any history taking or examination. When this is superimposed on the efficacy of these remedies, every one came to the conclusion that the more medically trained and efficient one is, the more rapidly he administers his remedy. It is unfortunate indeed. Up till now, the average Nigerian patient would not want a doctor to examine him /her. Their expectation is that the more the doctor is trained, the more rapidly he would administer his remedy without any wasting of time, just as UNICEF did in the 1950s. The average Nigerian patient would perhaps tolerate a little medical history taking and examination from the newly qualified doctors, but if they are referred to more senior colleagues, they expect no such things; they expect that on sighting them, the senior colleagues would know what is wrong with them and rapidly give them a prescription that would include an injection at least.

Learning Under Harsh Circumstances

Hitherto, Jeremiah had received all his education in his Igala mother tongue. By the end of 1955, he was very proficient in written Igala, an ability he has of course maintained up till today. The caning they received from the teacher during the Christian religious instructions class was terrible, so terrible that two of the pupils, Idachofo and Ali ran away into the forest for days without anyone sighting them. By the third day of their disappearance, it was assumed that some wild animals had devoured them.

Buffaloes and wild pigs sometimes appeared in the settlement in daylight, and these were wild ferocious animals. Fortunately for mankind, they would normally run away from humans, but if they were injured or nursing wounds, they were killers of whoever they sighted. The author recalls vividly the day a huge male buffalo just appeared in the settlement some hours after dawn. Most of the men had gone to their farms. It was wailing and crying from the women who were looking desperately for their children. Our mother succeeded in pushing Tom and Jeremiah into the nearest hut for safety.

The beast just continued its leisurely stroll through the community. Fortunately, there was a man at home called Ochalifu. He got his bow and poisoned arrow ready, stayed in his hut and waited for the buffalo to appear. As the animal strolled down close to his hut, he shot it with a poisoned arrow. The buffalo collapsed about 500 yards away and was killed. All the children went there to know the creature that featured prominently in the animal stories they had heard many times from the elders. The meat was shared by the whole community, as the culture was then. Ochalifu, as the person that killed the animal, had the head and neck for himself.

Anyway, after a week, Idachofo and Ali appeared from nowhere, and set the community agog with tears of joy. When the hullabaloo of joy settled down, they explained that they had run away because they could no longer tolerate the caning. Their parents ordered them out of school. Of course they remained uneducated. In response to this development, Tom and Jeremiah's father publicly pulled and twisted their ears till they were wailing in pain. He then repeated what he had told them before, that if ever they should do what Ali and Idachofo had done, that would be their death. Of course, Tom and Jeremiah never contemplated such a thing out of fear of their dad.

In December 1955, Jeremiah had to trek barefoot to Abocho, seven miles away to the west for an examination to continue his education at the Native Authority Junior Primary School there, the only such School for the District. That journey was the first time Jeremiah had stepped beyond a mile of his village along the granite road that passed through his community. Tom and he had been going to help their dad with his farm work during holidays. Though the farms were about 4 miles away from the settlement, they took forest paths to get there. Anyway, Jeremiah, to the delight of his dad, was successful.

In January 1956, Jeremiah had to move westwards out of his little world to the District headquarters at Abocho for his Junior Primary education. His father had arranged for him to stay with one of his relations called Omakwuchi; his house was just a stone's throw from the large market in the town.

All the 19 Districts that formed the Igala Division then had a bore hole cited in the District headquarters. The demand on these boreholes was so much that it was difficult to keep them running continuously; in fact, they were out of service most of the time. There was only one white 'Engineer', as he was called to maintain all the 19 boreholes, a really Herculean task. The borehole at Abocho was still out of function in January 1956 when Jeremiah landed there for his day schooling at the Junior Primary School. The natural source of water for Abocho was quite far, about 5 miles from the house of Omakwuchi.

Jeremiah's hostess bought an appropriate clay pot for him to use every morning to fetch water from the distant stream before going to School at 8 a.m. Of course, severe caning was the lot of the pupils that came late to school. On return from School, children had to go again to the stream to fetch water for the household. On Saturday, Jeremiah had to assist his guardian with his farm work, but his father had got his guardian to agree not to take Jeremiah to the farm on Sundays because of his religious belief – Christians then were not supposed to do any work on Sunday. Omakwuchi and his entire household were traditionalists, pagans.

Parents and guardians would wake children up at the first cockcrow (there were no clocks in general use then in the area) to start going to the stream to fetch water. This would be around 4 a.m. The evening trip to the distant stream would usually bring the children back home after dusk. At school, the teachers would ask some pupils to go to the stream and fetch water for them. This would be done on a rotational basis among the pupils. In effect, one went to the distant stream twice every day at least, with the occasional thrice a day when it was one's turn to fetch water for the teachers.

There were no lights for one to use to study at night. Unless there was moon light, the whole community would be in complete darkness after sunset, with specks of dim yellow light from the locally made by-product obtained during the extraction of red palm oil from the palm fruit. We would be given assignments from school especially the standard multiplication tables, starting with the 2 times table to learn.

Lessons began every morning with 10 mental arithmetic questions. As soon as the teacher finished his 10 oral questions, the pair of students on each bench would exchange their answers, and marking would be completed in a few minutes with the teacher announcing the answers to each of the questions in chronological order, starting from the first question. The best student escaped caning. If the best score in the morning exercise was, say 8 out of 10, those who scored 7 out of 10 received a good stroke of the cane. The caning was done by the pupil with the best score that morning.

Each class had its own permanent teacher that taught the class all the subjects. There were 40 – 50 pupils in each class. The Headmaster taught the students in Primary 4. Teachers were not transferred from one school to another during the school year which coincided with each calendar year.

The author noticed that illiterate people in his society would calculate accurately within a short time the cost of the items they buy or sell. In those days, the country used the British monetary system of pounds, shillings and pence. Twelve pence equalled one shilling, and twenty shillings equalled one pound. Even without the pressure from the teachers that pupils should know their multiplication tables thoroughly, Jeremiah decided on his own that he just had to be better and faster than the illiterates all around him in calculations, otherwise what would he have to demonstrate to them that he was better off than they? They had no idea of English or any of the other subjects that pupils were being taught at school.

Thirdly, Jeremiah weighed what he was going through – he was missing his mother's cooking, his environment at Ajiolo, his siblings and play mates because of getting educated. And here in this community 7 miles away from home, he had to be going to fetch water from a distant stream at least twice a day everyday, leaving him with little or no time to study. He decided he would not only enjoy it all, but would utilize the time spent on the way to and from the stream to learn his multiplication tables and other subjects thoroughly. That meant he would not be able to join his peers in story telling during these trips to the stream. He also decided that he would extend that to farm work that was just mechanical; while farming, he would be exercising his brain on improving his academic performance so that his studies would not suffer from the farm work that he could not avoid. This decision was to be his habit for the rest of his life, with very good dividends.

Jeremiah was in high spirits when his class teacher in Primary 2 in which he had been placed based on his performance at the entrance examination in December 1955 told the whole class that the first pupil to know his /her multiplication table would receive some cash prize (the author cannot remember how much the prize was). Any student who felt he was ready would be tested in front of the whole class. The test was not just repeating the multiplication tables parrot wise. The teacher would draw a large circle like the face of a clock on the blackboard, and put the numbers 1 to 12 in a circle round the circumference he had drawn. If he wrote 6 in the centre of the circle, the pupil was expected to churn out the product of 6 and whichever number on the clock face the teacher's stick touched. Multiplication tables 2 to 12 were those involved. If a pupil failed even just one, he had failed and would not get the prize. Besides, a failed attempt disqualified a pupil from the race for the money.

The Foundation for Easy Mathematics

The author was thrilled about the assignment. Before he returned from the stream that evening, he had mastered multiplication tables 2, 3, 4, 5, and 6, learning them along the road and testing himself in his imagination. He went to bed very pleased with himself. On the way to the stream the next morning, he realized that the remaining tables were easier than he had imagined. Since he had known the table up to the 6th multiplication table, the multiplication table of 7 that he needed to learn were from 7 x 7 down to 7 x 12 since 7 x 6 is the same as 6 x 7 that he already knew. Of course, the multiplication table for 10 was easy! For the multiplication table of 11, he had only to learn 11 x 11, and 11 x 12. For multiplication table of 12, he had only to learn 12 x 12 to complete the entire job. Before he returned from the stream that morning, he was perfectly confident he would not fail one. He rehearsed it as he hurried to school that morning.

After the usual mental arithmetic that morning, Jeremiah told the teacher he was ready for the multiplication table test. The teacher and the other pupils were taken by surprise. The teacher advised him to stop joking, but the lad stood his ground. Up went the teacher's clock face on the blackboard, and the author was summoned out for the drill. Of course, the lad had rehearsed everything thoroughly. To everyone's surprise, he made no single mistake. He not only won the cash prize, but the teacher decided to give him extra tips to entrench his multiplication table as his second nature. The teacher also told him in front of the class that with that knowledge, he would never have any problem with arithmetic in his life. He was correct; the author never had any problems with arithmetic or Mathematics throughout his educational career.

Jeremiah was always the youngest pupil in all his classes throughout his educational career. In his Primary School, he had many grown up adults as mates; some were even married with children. One of the subjects in those days was called 'Craft'. All male pupils had to produce something every term, but the item must be produced by the pupil himself. Female pupils would knit handkerchiefs, table covers or the like. The best the small kids like the author could produce was always the broom, made from palm leaves. The adult pupils always turned in something far superior such as special baskets, mortars and pestles made from the trunks of big trees, strong ropes made from special climbing plants obtained from the deep forests, etc. Craft carried 100 marks like other subjects. Jeremiah never had more than 10 per cent in Craft, whereas the adult pupils would get between 90 and 100 per cent in 'Craft'. One's position in the class would depend on the tally of his scores in all the subjects. Jeremiah's position would be 4th at the best, and 6th at the worst. If Craft were to be excluded, he would be first.

The Lad Who is Inquisitive Shall Surely Die

Jeremiah could not avoid learning more about traditionalists and idol worship while he was being brought up by one. They continued to hammer into his head that masquerades were their dead ancestors back to life. How Jeremiah missed Tom his elder brother with whom he would have discussed these issues but Tom was in far away Anyigba some 18 miles to the south east of Abocho! After days of debating with himself, Jeremiah was convinced that masquerades were more likely to be human beings dressed up to deceive women and children. How was he to confirm it? He would seize the next opportunity and move close to a masquerade to look into the mask over the face. If it is a normal person, he would see the eyes through the mask because the masquerades walked and ran about, not as blind beings but obviously with good sight.

The chance he had been looking for presented itself eventually. A masquerade that was, and still is feared throughout the District appeared at Abocho for a mission Jeremiah did not know about. By the market place, it stood with its stick, swaying and moving its head to the sound of sweet traditional flute music. The flute was locally made from a piece of wood but the player could bring out different tunes of sweet music from it as the player wished. Jeremiah knew about the flute at Ajiolo but he could not get any music out of it. It took strength and practice to play it. Children are not strong enough to play it. Poor child! Jeremiah did not know that the music from that flute is the bridle that controls the masquerade.

The flute player is a normal man by all standards; he is always some distance from the masquerade, bellowing out sweet music as far as children could hear and determine. However, that music tells the masquerade when to charge, when to hit with the stick, when to stand and show off its majesty, when not to take any step without further instructions from the flute player, etc.

Jeremiah walked close to the masquerade and peeped into the black net of a mask over the face, and saw human eyes clearly behind the mask. He also noticed that the flute had changed tune but he had no idea what it meant. Adult men around knew the tune and they ran, grabbed and pulled Jeremiah away from there. He was thoroughly beaten up by the traditionalists around, but Jeremiah was satisfied that he had accomplished his mission. Of course, the matter did not end there. It was intolerable sacrilege and an unacceptable insult to the deity!

The masquerade owners enquired and found that the culprit was a lad staying with Omakwuchi. Unknown to Jeremiah, they summoned Omakwuchi, one of them. They agreed the chap must not be allowed to live. Powerful poisons from leaves and insects were known to the tribe, but these were usually kept secret to privileged groups like the masquerades, traditional chiefs, etc. It was agreed that the masquerade would come back in 5 days on a mission to announce through the same flute music that the lad that dared to walk near the masquerade and look it in the face would be buried that afternoon. By agreement, Omakwuchi was to put the poison that would be given to him into the chap's food that afternoon. The deal was sealed while the ignorant boy went about his domestic chores, facing his studies quietly as he did so.

The day after the agreement with Omakwuchi was sealed, one of the masquerade owners (the masquerade comes from a community called 'Emewe Ogane', about 8 miles southwest of Abocho) asked who the father of the child was. In the Igala culture, as in most cultures in Nigeria, children belong to the father. They accept that mothers make some genetic contribution to children, but that contribution is not comparable to the father's at all. They received the correct answer – the lad is the son of Alabi Abalaka at Ajiolo. "What?" they exclaimed, "Alabi, our own child?" Quickly, they sent an emissary on a bicycle to call Alabi urgently.

In the Igala culture, one is not allowed to refuse a call from relations. One may refuse what is in a call, but not the call itself. Alabi left Ajiolo on his bike, rode through Abocho without calling on Omakwuchi because he was going on an urgent call, and reached Emewe Ogane. Alabi's mother is one of the daughters from the masquerade's family. Alabi, being a traditionalist before his conversion to Christianity, was well versed in the ways and culture of these deities. They told him everything. They ended up by telling Alabi to warn his son thoroughly. They all felt sad that they would have killed their own son unknowingly.

Let not the Lad Escape Both Death and Punishment

Alabi returned to Abocho on his way to Ajiolo, and called at Omakwuchi's house. Poor Jeremiah! He had no inkling of all that had been happening. He appeared before his dad to greet him and tell him how he was making good progress with his studies, and in response, he expected his father's approbation. This is not the time for such niceties, my lad! Alabi just grabbed him and gave him the beating of his life. A crowd gathered and eventually got Alabi's hands off Jeremiah. Some elders then called the angry Alabi aside to find out what the boy had done.

Alabi later told Jeremiah what transpired, but at Ajiolo. When the elders came out of the discussion, Alabi instructed Jeremiah to pack his items (his school uniform, grey khaki shorts and white shirt with some books) immediately and trek back to Ajiolo. In a few seconds, Jeremiah was on his way crying, thinking his education had come to an end. He had no idea what his offence was, stupid stubborn chap that he was! Alabi would not listen to entreaties from several people for him to pardon the chap.

Alabi reached Ajiolo long before Jeremiah. Jeremiah reached Ajiolo to meet wailing and bitter crying from his sisters, mother, and other relations. Everyone gathered. Alabi had poured the story to them all. It was then that Jeremiah knew it was his masquerade adventure that had caused all the trouble for him.

Alabi eventually declared that only death would interfere with Jeremiah's school. Accordingly, he decided that Jeremiah's punishment would be simple. He would no longer stay at Abocho. He would stay at Ajiolo and be going to school daily from there. Jerry's mother was happy with the decision, too.

Inwardly, Jeremiah was happy also. By his reckoning, walking 14 miles every day to go to school and back was shorter that trekking 5 miles to and fro twice a day to fetch water from the distant stream at Abocho. Besides, he could join moonlight games with his peers, and enjoy his mother's food. But it was a close shave with death, Jeremiah told himself. He analyzed and concluded that he had not lost much. He had confirmed for himself that masquerades are normal human beings, not the dead back to life! Looking back now, Jeremiah thinks this event happened around October/November 1956.

Jeremiah continued his education from his father's compound, and got a lot of opportunity to learn more about his culture. He received a lot of teachings from his father at almost every opportunity. One particular account he repeatedly got from his father was to change his life later.

The Triumvirate in Igala Division then

Under the colonial administration then, Nigeria was divided into 3 Regions, Eastern Region, Western Region and Northern Region. Each Region had a number of Provinces. Igala Division was the biggest of 4 Divisions that made up Kabba Province in Northern Region. Each Division had a Divisional Officer (DO) posted to it. Since the Igala Division had its headquarters at Idah, the DO was also based at Idah. Every Igala man knew about the DO, but very few knew what the letters stood for. Jeremiah's dad knew much about the DO.

Each Division had a General Hospital located at the Divisional Headquarters; Idah was therefore home also to the only Government Hospital in the Division. Every Igala man knew that. In fact, there was no other Hospital in the whole Division then. Each District headquarter in the Division had a police post, a Dispensary, a Native Authority (N.A) Junior Primary School, a Native Court presided over by the District head, and a borehole. The Igala Native Authority had three Senior Primary Schools, all Boarding Schools, located at Ofugo, Anyigba and Oguma. Entrance examinations and admissions into these boarding schools were the responsibility of the Idah headquarters of the NA.

Alabi repeatedly told his 2 sons either together or separately that the 3 most important people in Igala land were the Attah of Igala, the DO and the doctor all at Idah. According to the man, the Attah was a hereditary post that none of his children could ever occupy. The DO, he said, was a position meant for the Hausa/Fulani people, the tribe of all the DOs that had ever been posted to the Division. He therefore told his children to forget about ever being the DO at Idah since his children would never be able to change their tribe from Igala to any other tribe. As for the doctor at Idah, the man told his children that even though the doctor at

Idah had always been a white man, he had been enlightened by Mr. Paul Gross, the missionary that any intelligent person could study and be a doctor like the one at Idah; one did not have to belong to any tribe or family or race to achieve that in life. Alabi therefore told his children to always face their studies so that one of them at least would be a doctor like the white man at Idah and be performing operations. The man always concluded the account by stating that he would have lived a fulfilled life if one of his two sons at least ended up as a doctor, performing operations on the sick, as all the white doctors at Idah had been doing.

Finding Favour with the Chief

Things changed at the beginning of 1958 when the author was in Primary 4. The District Head visited the school, with cash gifts for the best 4 pupils in the last examinations in each class. When he got to Primary 4, Jeremiah had his bench on the front row nearest the blackboard. The back row of benches was for the biggest pupils while the smallest pupils occupied the front row of benches. The relevant result was the last examination in Primary 3 when Jeremiah was 4th. Impressed that the small pupil came 4th, the Chief asked who the boy's father was. When Jeremiah told him his father's name, the Chief asked him for his mother's name. Jeremiah told him. The Chief then explained that Jeremiah's mother was his daughter. He asked where Jeremiah was staying and was told that Jeremiah was coming from Ajiolo everyday for his education.

There and then, the Chief directed Jeremiah to come and stay with him for the rest of his school days at Abocho. The lad pleaded that his father would be angry. The Chief told Jeremiah not to bother, that before the school closed that day, he would send a messenger to inform his parents at Ajiolo. Jeremiah's parents were never angry; instead, they were very grateful to the Chief.

The Chief had 4 wives when Jeremiah came to stay with them. Jeremiah was able to learn at close quarters what life in a polygamous family was like. He enjoyed his stay there. The Chief on his part was pleased with Jeremiah, so pleased that he instructed Jeremiah's parents that whenever the boy was on holidays, they must allow him to spend part of his holidays with him. That was carried out to the letter. Jeremiah learnt how to ride a bicycle during the time he was with the Chief in 1958.

Chief Shaibu Ogbadu had a younger brother called Daniel Ogbadu; they were of the same parents. Daniel was a politician living and working in Kaduna (10 30N, 7 21E), the capital of Northern Nigeria. Daniel Ogbadu would come home in one or two cars to his political base at least once in two or three months with one or two of his wives and some of his children. Whenever he came, he would stay with his elder brother, the District Head. That gave Jeremiah the golden opportunity to hear stories from Daniel's children about Kaduna, the journey by car from and to such a distant place, the airport and aeroplanes in Kaduna, the train, etc.

For the first times in Jeremiah's life, he was able to sit inside the stationary cars, huge Pontiac or Cadillac beauties that Daniel and his family brought home. He was allowed to this because he had earned it by moving close to the driver who granted him his request. Who would have given the village boy that opportunity if not because of the great favour the Chief had bestowed on him by inviting him to stay with him in 1958? The opportunity to experience being in a moving car would not be Jeremiah's lot for several years to come though.

At Idah at Last

At the end of 1958, Jeremiah and many others from his class trekked to Dekina, 18 miles northeast of Abocho to take the common entrance examination to Senior Primary School. There was no 'Craft' subject for the examinations. 5 pupils, Jeremiah included, from the Primary 4 class at Abocho were invited for the oral interview scheduled for Idah. The Chief arranged for Jeremiah to go there. Jeremiah's joy was beyond imagination. The journey was partly by bike and the last 30 or so miles by road in a lorry.

At Idah, he saw a river for the first time in his life, the River Niger. He was thrilled to know canoes and small boats that were common sites by the river bank. He also knew and went near the Palace of the Attah of Igala and the Igala Division's office Headquarters. He visited the General Hospital and saw ceiling fans for the first time in his life. It was more than an interview, as far as Jeremiah was concerned. Jeremiah came back with a letter of admission to the Native Authority's Senior Primary School at Anyigba.

Back in Abocho, the Chief let him go to Ajiolo to tell his parents. Before he got there, they had heard the news that Jeremiah had gone to Idah. On his arrival, the young and the old gathered to hear from him about Idah. He told them all he saw and witnessed. It was very interesting indeed. Idachofo and Ali shed tears of regret for running away from school because they felt they too might have travelled to Idah if they had continued their schooling!

The reader may expect to read in subsequent chapters about what happened to Jeremiah at, and after the Senior Primary School.

Conclusion

The author, like most people was profoundly influenced by the circumstance of his birth, early life and upbringing in pre-Independence Nigeria. He received his early education under circumstances that amount to a fairy tale, but it is not. The author was greatly influenced not only by his own culture and immediate environment, but by other circumstances that started creeping into his life, directly or indirectly. This chapter has recounted them.

Chapter XX

Can Any Vaccine Legally Circumvent Nigeria's NAFDAC or Such Regulatory Agencies?

Abstract

The use of compatible whole human blood or its components as a medical remedy has been practised for decades. Similarly, autogenous whole human blood transfusions have been practised for a long time. These remedies do not require registration with any regulatory agencies in any country. Were a vaccine that is just a pure human blood extract or component developed today, such a vaccine would also not require registration with any regulatory agency before being used as a remedy; it would not have to undergo any clinical or other trials for safety because it would be as safe as the administration of human blood components or extracts, and if such a vaccine were to be an autogenous therapeutic vaccine, it would immediately be eligible for efficacy trials in infected persons who have given their written and informed consent to take it. The problem, however, is that such a vaccine is hitherto unknown to human medicine.

Introduction

In Chapter 8, we saw that vaccines are subjected to phased clinical trials before licensure or registration. All the vaccines in use in human medicine are produced in the laboratory. They are harvested and purified before packaging for clinical use. When the causative organism has to be cultured for vaccine preparation or when the toxins have to be converted to toxoids using formaldehyde, the purification removes as much of 'the contaminants' as possible. These vaccines therefore contain other substances that make them eligible for sanction by the Regulatory Agencies before clinical use. Must all vaccines undergo phased clinical trials and be registered with Regulatory Agencies before being used? This chapter will answer the question.

We All Know These Things Very Well

All of us know very well that all drugs and vaccines we use in human medical practice must be registered with a country's food and drug regulatory authority before such drugs and vaccines are used. Such regulatory agencies are the United States' Food and Drug Administration (FDA) and Nigeria's National Agency for Food and Drug Administration and Control, NAFDAC.

We also know that the manufacture and application for the registration of drugs fall within the professional responsibilities of pharmacists while the production and the application for the registration of vaccines are some of the responsibilities of vaccinologists, medical laboratory scientists and virologists.

Of course, we also know that medical practitioners are not trained at all to manufacture or produce drugs and vaccines; rather, they are trained to use them on their patients through prescriptions.

We all know, too, that some remedies we administer to patients in modern orthodox medical practice are exempt from registration with regulatory agencies like the FDA and NAFDAC. Universally, the transfusion or administration, usually by the intravenous route, of whole human blood and/or its components/extracts does not require registration with any country's drug regulatory agency. As the author's teachers taught him during his medical training, the use of whole human blood or its components is a private business involving four parties only: the donor of the blood, the person (patient) that receives the blood or blood product, the laboratory that stores the blood/blood product and performs the cross-matching to ensure compatibility if required, and the clinician in charge of the patient. The Pharmacist and the Regulatory Agencies have no hand in the business at all.

In other words, we all know that the transfusion or administration of whole human blood or any of its extracts/components (packed red cells, plasma, platelets, pooled platelet concentrates, cryoprecipitates, granulocyte transfusions, etc) does not require registration with any country's drug regulatory agency.

The author does not know of any vaccine that is just human blood product. If it were possible for one to successfully conceive and develop any vaccine that is just a human blood extract, one would not need to register it with NAFDAC or any other country's regulatory agency before using it.

Furthermore, the safety associated with the administration or transfusion of compatible whole human blood or its extracts has been established long ago by others, some were long before the author went to medical school. We all know that there would be no safety concerns for any such vaccine that is just a human blood extract; we all know that if such a vaccine were to be given to another person, one must ensure that it is free of known infectious agents like malaria, yellow fever, the hepatitis viruses especially Hepatitis B and C, Treponema pallidum, and HIV.

We all know, too, that autogenous whole blood transfusions have been practised for decades without any safety concern, e.g. in cases of ruptured spleen, lacerated mesentery or ruptured ectopic pregnancies with massive blood loss while undergoing surgery. In these instances, we all know that such transfusions do not even involve the medical laboratory scientist or another donor. Such autogenous whole blood transfusions involve only two parties: the clinician and the patient. We all know of course that such intra-operative autogenous whole blood transfusions are not registered with any regulatory agency at all. We all know that there is no need to screen the blood used for autogenous transfusions for any known blood-borne pathogens in the blood before it is auto transfused into the patient.

We all know therefore that if one could just develop any candidate autogenous therapeutic vaccine that is just a human blood product, one would not need to bother at all about its safety since such a vaccine would not only be derived from the infected person's own blood but it would eventually be given back to the same person. Such an autogenous therapeutic vaccine would not pose any danger to the patient from whom it was developed and to whom it would be given. Such an autogenous therapeutic HIV vaccine would only need to be assessed for efficacy in willing patients.

It is therefore not surprising that no orthodox medical practitioner has ever faced criminal charges for carrying out any compatible whole human blood transfusion or the administration of compatible human blood extract or component. This implies that there is no law that forbids this worldwide and common practice.

Nigeria's NAFDAC Statutes

As mentioned earlier, The National Agency for Food and Drug Administration and Control (NAFDAC) is Nigeria's regulatory Agency for foods and drugs. In other words, NAFDAC is Nigeria's equivalent of the FDA in the US. It is therefore created by Law; it is a creation of Statute(s). It was formerly Decree No. 19 of 1993. It was amended by Decree No. 15 of the Food and Drugs and Related Products (Registration etc.) Act 1999 and Decree No. 20 of 1999.

The words 'vaccine', 'blood transfusion' and 'blood components' are not mentioned at all in the entire NAFDAC Act. However, these issues are covered by the word 'drug' in the Act. Section 31 of the act says:

> 'Interpretation
> In this Act:-
>
> "cosmetic" includes any substance or mixture of substance intended to be rubbed, poured, sprinkled or sprayed, introduced into or otherwise applied to the human body or any part thereof for cleansing, beautifying, promoting attractiveness or altering the complexion, skin, hair or teeth and includes deodorants and detergent powder;
>
> "drug" includes any substance of vegetable, animal or mineral origin or any preparation or admixture thereof manufactured, sold or advertised for use in –
>
> the diagnosis, treatment, mitigation or prevention of any disease, disorder, abnormal physical state or the symptom thereof, in man or animal;
>
> restoring, correcting, or modifying organic functions in man or in animal;
>
> disinfection or the control of vermin, insects or pests; or
>
> contraception:
>
> "medical device" means any instrument, apparatus or contrivance (including components, parts and accessories thereof) manufactured, sold or advertised for internal or external use in the diagnosis, treatment, mitigation or prevention of any disease, disorder, abnormal physical state or the symptom thereof, in man or in animal;
>
> "regulated products" means food, drugs, cosmetics, medical devices, detergents, bottled water and chemicals.'

Readers would likely agree that from the definition of "drug" in the Act, vaccines being medical products used for the prevention or treatment of infectious diseases are covered by the Act. According to the Act, 'drug includes any substance of vegetable, animal or mineral origin or any preparation or admixture thereof manufactured, sold or advertised for use in ... It is therefore clear that according to the NAFDAC Act, human blood is not covered by the Act since it is not of vegetable, animal or mineral origin. Accordingly, if one were to develop any vaccine that is just a human blood product, such a vaccine would not come under the purview of NAFDAC. In other words, it would be perfectly legal for such a vaccine to be put immediately into clinical use on willing persons without any requirement for registration.

The only unfortunate problem however, is that such a vaccine is hitherto unknown to medicine.

The Author's Late Childhood

Senior Primary Education

In January 1959, Jeremiah trekked south eastward from Ajiolo to the Native Authority Boarding Senior Primary School at Anyigba to start Primary V. The School had just three classes, Primary V, VI and VII. Pupils were drawn from all over Kabba Province but the majority were from Igala Division. Jeremiah was shocked to find himself in a class of 21 females and 19 males.

When he later told his father about it during the first holiday, his father was unimpressed and would not alter his stand about educating his daughters, stating that those female pupils must have come from parents where the mothers too were educated (that was not true). According to Jeremiah's father, such men with educated wives owed it a duty to educate their daughters, but since he was not married to any educated woman, he would not educate other people's wives for them.

Again, Jeremiah was the smallest and youngest of all the pupils in his class. For the first time, Jeremiah had to take the Nigerian food called 'gari'. It is prepared from the cassava plant. It was part of the school menu. Until then, his community believed, albeit falsely that gari was poisonous to the Igala who regarded it as despised food that was consumed only by the Ibo people.

When he told his mother during the first term holidays about the gari meals he had been taking at the school, his mother broke down in tears. At the end, his mother made a fruitless appeal to her husband to let her children stop schooling because their lives were in danger from gari.

She therefore called Tom and Jeremiah and advised them never to take any hot drinks with or soon after taking gari soaked in water because the hot drink would turn the gari into 'eba' that would block the intestine and result in death! Eba is the cooked form of gari that is normally eaten as solid food taken with any type of soup (the soup known to Nigerians is nothing near the soup known to the Western world please).

This reminds the author of one of the first things he was taught in the community in which he was born and brought up. A child would be asked to sit down, bend his head backwards and open the mouth for other children to look far back into the back of the throat. Of course, they would all see the uvula moving about like a small short snake. After all the children around had seen it, they would all be told that the moving uvula performs a very important function – it separates the solids from the liquids during swallowing. The liquids and solids go to different places through two different channels, one for liquids and the other for solids!

Craft and Agriculture were still subjects at the Senior Primary School. The two subjects required sheer physical strength and Jeremiah did not possess it. Jeremiah's position throughout the three terms in Primary V was 6th.

The school fee at the Boarding school was just two shillings per term. We had Tilley lamps, bright lamps that used pressurized kerosene that burns in a net. We had afternoon and night 'prep' classes. We had three regular meals every day. All the teachers were Nigerians except a Missionary, an English lady called Miss Newton that taught us Protestant Christian religious studies. Jeremiah, like other Protestant pupils attended the Fellowship Church ran by Miss Newton. She made things very interesting for the pupils.

Meanwhile, all the adult Protestant Christians throughout Igala Division were levied one pound in 1959. The levy was for the building of a Secondary School at a small settlement called Ochaja. That School would be the first Secondary School in the Division. Everyone was told that Ochaja had been chosen because it was said to be the geographical Centre of the Division. Ochaja had a big flowing stream nearby, and it was located along the Trunk A road in the Division. The Trunk A road was a dusty granite road in those days. That Secondary School opened in 1960 with 30 students.

The ambition of every Senior Primary pupil interested in further studies those days was to pass The Common Entrance Examination, as it was called. Those that passed the examination would subsequently be invited for an oral interview. The pupils that succeeded in the interview would then be placed in the appropriate post-primary schools, Government Colleges, Secondary Schools, Teachers' Colleges, Technical Colleges and Schools, Craft Schools and Middle Schools that were scattered throughout Northern Nigeria. The Middle School those days had just Forms 1 and 2, meaning that students in Form 2 in a Middle School would have to take and pass another examination for Form 3 admission into other Schools.

Normally, only student in Primary 7 were eligible to take the Common Entrance Examination that was held throughout the Region about March or April every year. However, at the NA Senior Primary School at Anyigba, the Headmaster one Mr. Okonkwo announced at the end of 1959 that the first 5 students in Primary 5 would move temporarily to Primary 7 at the beginning of 1960 so that they would be prepared along with the Primary 7 students for the Common Entrance Examination that year. After the Common Entrance Examination, the 5 pupils would come back to join their own mates in Primary 6.

Jeremiah just missed the cut. During the first term examination in Primary 6 in 1960, Jeremiah opportunistically came first in the class for the first time since he started his Primary education; that was possible because the other 5 students that would have beaten him were away temporarily in Primary 7. During the second and third terms when the other 5 pupils returned to the class, he reverted to his usual position of 6th.

During the first term in Primary 6, Jeremiah's father paid him a visit at the School. It was not usual for the man to do so. Jeremiah was afraid and frightened, wondering if there had been a catastrophe at home. There was nothing of the sort. The man explained that he had just come from seeing Mr. Paul Gross for enlightenment. In a nutshell, the man told his son to sit for the entrance examination to Ochaja Secondary School because Paul had assured him that the School was the equivalent of Government College Keffi.

Father and son had discussed the issue during the 1959 Christmas holidays, and Jeremiah had told his father that Ochaja Secondary School was not the same as Government College Keffi because the name Secondary, to Jeremiah, must have been coined from the word second. To him, Ochaja was a sort of Senior Primary School education a second time. He clearly told his father so. Jeremiah was honest but completely wrong. The father believed his son Jeremiah was being dishonest on the matter. The man wanted his children to benefit from the levy he and his wife had struggled to pay for the school at Ochaja to be built.

The man departed, but before doing so, he left Jeremiah with three shillings to pay for the Ochaja Secondary School entrance examination fees with clear instruction that the lad must take that examination. The entrance examination for Ochaja Secondary School was open to Primary 6 and 7 pupils, unlike the Common Entrance Examination for Government post-Primary Secondary Schools and Colleges.

All the examinations into Secondary Schools were held around March/April but on different weekends. Jeremiah had the opportunity of taking just one, the one to Ochaja Secondary School. He succeeded. For the interview held later at Ochaja, 14 miles away to the east from the NA Senior Primary School at Anyigba, Jeremiah and another classmate of his called Alilu Agbaji trekked the distance. The interview again had written papers in English, Arithmetic and General Intelligence followed by an oral session.

During Jeremiah's oral interview, the white man that interviewed him was the first Principal of the School, one Mr. Johnston. He had a huge fearful left upper limb but a weak dangling right upper limb. We learnt later that his deformed right upper limb that had no bone in the arm was a result of a motor accident in his country some years before he came to Nigeria.

The white man started by telling Jeremiah that they would like him to come to Ochaja Secondary School. Jeremiah recalls that he told the man that he wanted to finish his Primary School so that he would try and go to Government College Keffi. Asked why, Jeremiah gave several reasons. First, he said Ochaja Secondary School was a sort of repetition of the Primary School because of the word 'Secondary' that was derived from 'second'. Secondly, he said his father was just a peasant who would not be able to pay the fees at Ochaja, £35 per annum, way beyond his father's means. Thirdly, he said that he had an elder brother Tom who was in Primary 7. He therefore expected his father would wish to ensure that Tom went to College before him. And there was no way their father would be able to cope with the education of both children unless Jeremiah went to Government College Keffi where children of peasants like him do not pay any school fees.

In response, the white man explained to Jeremiah that Ochaja Secondary School and Government College Keffi would be teaching students the same things and that at the end, students from both Schools would be taking the same examinations. Jeremiah then realized that he had been wrong all along, and that his illiterate dad had been correct. As for the fees, the man told Jeremiah that the Igala NA had agreed to give every Igala pupil that gained admission an automatic scholarship of £25, leaving all Igala students just £10 to pay per annum. After checking Jeremiah's results for the entrance examination, the man told Jeremiah they would be giving him another scholarship of £3 per annum if he agreed to come to the School. His father would therefore be paying just £7 per annum for his school at Ochaja.

Jeremiah thanked the man, but still told him that his father's yearly income from his farming was not up to £7, and the man had another child, Tom to educate. The interview ended after the white man told Jeremiah that if he came to the School, he would see if he would be able to source for other scholarships for him. After the interview at Ochaja, the two friends, Alilu and Jeremiah trekked back to their Senior Primary School at Anyigba.

At about that time, it was announced in 1960 that the Northern Nigerian Government had agreed to upgrade Dekina Middle School in Igala Division to a full Secondary School with effect from 1962. In other words, Form 1 students in that School that year would be able to continue their Secondary School education there, thereby giving Igala Division another Secondary School.

In 1960, Tom was in Primary 7 in a CMML Senior Primary School at Alloma, somewhere in Igala land too, and so he qualified to take the Common Entrance Examination that year. He was successful, and at his interview, he was given admission to Dekina Secondary School. He also had admission to Ochaja Secondary School. Jeremiah had admission to just Ochaja Secondary School.

When both lads were at home for the summer holiday in 1960 and told their father these facts, their father again went to Anyigba to consult Mr. Paul Gross. He returned with his decision. Tom would go to Dekina Secondary School that would be upgraded to a full Secondary School. Jeremiah would proceed to Ochaja and not wait to take the Common Entrance examination the following year. The man promised his two sons that he would struggle and do his best to pay their fees provided the boys would do their part by making good progress with their studies. He reiterated that during the holidays, Tom and Jeremiah would have no option but to be helping him with his farm work.

In one of Mr. Paul Gross's visits to Ajiolo in 1960, Jeremiah was one of those that had passed and qualified to be baptized. We all went to our stream for the immersion in water for the baptism. When we returned to the village, Paul issued those baptized with their Baptismal Certificates. No one in the village knew the age of their children, but Paul would routinely ask the parents anyway. As the parents of every child grossly inflated the age of their child, it would elicit a lot of infectious laughter mixed with ridicule from Paul. When Paul asked Alabi for Jeremiah's age, Alabi said Jeremiah was well over 30 years! Everyone joined Paul in the laughter that followed. On a serious note, Paul then asked Alabi whether Jeremiah was his first or second son. When Alabi told him Jeremiah was the second son. Paul thought for some time and said Jeremiah was born around 1948. In the Baptismal Certificate he issued to Jeremiah, he wrote, 'Jeremiah Alabi born about 1948'. The episode sparked some interest in birthdays in Jeremiah, but the matter went away from his consideration soon afterwards.

October till April is Nigeria's rainy dry season when there are hardly any rains. Instead, there are winds blowing in from the northeast, bringing cold and dust from the Sahara Desert.

The other months of the year constitute the wet or rainy season when south westerly winds bring rains from the Atlantic Ocean.

Nigeria was granted her Independence from British Colonial rule on 1st October 1960. The National anthem changed from 'God bless our gracious Queen' to 'Nigeria, we hail Thee'. Jeremiah and the other pupils took part in the events marking the country's Independence even though many of the pupils including Jeremiah did not understand the event well then. In spite of the Independence, the British influence was all over the place as readers would readily notice from accounts involving the author after Independence.

In the list of things for students to bring to the School at Ochaja, they were optionally allowed to bring and use sandals. Alabi ruled out any footwear for Jeremiah because of lack of funds. The man however provided all the things that were compulsory. In January 1961, the peak of the cold, dry, dusty season in Igala land, Jeremiah found his way from Ajiolo to Ochaja by foot with his wooden box on his head, a distance of 21 miles to the southeast. Tom, on his part, found his way to Dekina, 10 miles north from Ajiolo.

The author would let readers know how he fared at Ochaja in the next chapter.

Conclusion

The transfusion of whole human blood or the administration of its components /extracts has been known to medicine for many decades. The safety associated with these remedies is also well established. These remedies are not registered with any country's food and drug regulatory agencies before they are administered to patients. Similarly, autogenous whole blood transfusions are well recognized procedures in human medical practice worldwide. If there were to be any vaccines that are pure human blood products or extracts, such vaccines would not require registration with any regulatory agencies in any country, and there would be no need to establish the safety of such vaccines especially if they are autogenous therapeutic vaccines. The problem, however, is that such vaccines are hitherto unknown to human medicine.

Chapter XXI

The Crucial Issue of the Appropriate Immunogen(s) for Candidate Safe, Effective HIV Vaccines

Abstract

The author was taught at a WHO-sponsored Immunopathological Conference/ Workshop in Geneva in October 1974 that when thinking of any vaccine against anything, the most important fundamental issue is the concept, design and development of the appropriate immunogen and its effective delivery. The author is of the opinion that those well trained and experienced in vaccine production know far more than him not only about this fundamental issue of the appropriate immunogen and its delivery, but they are also far more knowledgeable and experienced than him on all other aspects of vaccine development and production. In fact, the fundamental fact is that the author is a nondescript nonentity in all facets of vaccine development, design, production and marketing. Why and how then did the author succeed in developing safe and effective (sae) HIV vaccines when others still claim that such vaccines, if ever they would be developed at all, are at least a decade away? The author will attempt to answer such questions in this chapter.

Introduction

In the foregoing chapters, especially Chapters 13 and 14, we looked at what the experts called the daunting problems facing HIV vaccine development. The experts have come out with various reasons for failure. However, the author is convinced that the more extraordinary, novel and daunting any problem is, the more important it is for anyone interested in providing a solution to keep an open and receptive approach at all times, ready to alter his approach the moment new facts calling for such a change emerge.

Let us get our bearings correct. Since 1984 when it was announced that the virus that caused AIDS had been identified, the race for its vaccine began. Before then, mankind had not developed safe and effective curative and preventive drugs against most, if not all, human viral diseases, but vaccines had been particularly effective in preventing most of them and even curing a few viral infections like rabies and hepatitis B in the newborn. The advent of the HIV/AIDS pandemic called for universal efforts at developing HIV vaccines using pragmatic and empirical approaches that had resulted in many successes in the past. The world wide hunt was not, and it still is not a race to:

- determine who has the best modern technological techniques for HIV vaccine production;
- identify the first person to come out with a recipe or formula for HIV vaccine production;
- understand how and why such a vaccine would act;
- condemn other approaches for such vaccines by others;
- abandon humanity at the mercy of the ravaging HIV/AIDS while researchers keep trying for decades to understand more about the correlates needed for protection against HIV;
- organize annual or bi-annual jamborees called World HIV/AIDS Conferences in various cities around the world while millions keep on perishing from the HIV/AIDS scourge;
- legislate and enforce obnoxious policies that ban HIV-infected persons from other countries from visiting any particular country even for one day even though the first cases of AIDS known to mankind occurred among citizens of that country who were living in that country;
- deprive mankind of benefitting from safe and effective HIV vaccines developed outside the developed countries, etc.

The worldwide hunt has always been a race for safe and effective HIV vaccines, no more and no less. In this chapter, the author will attempt to put readers in the correct frame of mind about his approach at developing saeHIV vaccines. The only justification the author thinks he has for attempting to do so is his success at developing these vaccines in 1998/99.

The Established Knowledge of Our Days

The details of the position of the HIV vaccines experts, researchers and developers of our generation may be found in Chapters 13 and 14 of this book. For the reader's convenience, the author will reproduce here some relevant excerpts.

Excerpts from Chapter 13:

(On April 23, 1984) Robert Gallo, who had never made a vaccine against anything, went on to detail a recipe for an AIDS vaccine that, instead of relying on the entire virus like the traditional live and killed approaches, only called for using a piece of the agent that had been produced with genetic engineering techniques. Just such a hepatitis B vaccine was then being engineered that contained the surface protein, or envelope, of that virus. When it came to AIDS, said Gallo, the same logic would apply. "In my view, you'd vaccinate with the envelope protein of the virus," said Gallo. "We'll go to recombinant technology, we are doing that now, and we will produce the protein that way. That protein, I would certainly be willing to take if I were a high-risk person, and I'd do it voluntarily. . . . That's the direction we're kind of thinking about."

Question: And 20 years later (in 2005) we have no vaccine yet. How close are we?

Prof. Gallo: Vaccine has been the most significant failure of the scientific quest. In our institute there has been some important progress. I don't want to say breakthrough, I don't even want to say milestone yet, but the progress that has been made is proving that you can get a vaccine candidate that will make an immune response of the type we believe to be what's needed to block HIV from entering the cell. A type which raises neutralizing antibodies and can do it against the majority of strains of HIV. But we don't have other technical problems solved yet; we can't make that vaccine last a long time. We want to get it to the right levels; those are problems we are still working on with collaborators. While I'm here in Israel it's important for me to point out that intellectually the contributions for this vaccine came from one of my colleagues Dr. Devito, but also from an Israeli scientist, a young guy from the Weizmann institute then, he's now in Tel-Aviv, John Gershoni, who made important intellectual contributions to this pathway.

The following excerpts are from Chapter 14.

Unlike most other viruses, the singular properties of HIV make it a uniquely difficult target for vaccine design and development. First, the HIV virus particles coat their surface proteins with sugar-like molecules, so that antibodies have difficulty binding to appropriate protein sites on them. At the same time, HIV constantly alters its outer coat through genetic mutations, thus staying one step ahead of the immune response to any given vaccine preparation. The HIV mutates every time it replicates, and it replicated every 6 to 8 hours!

As Nobel laureate, Dr. David Baltimore remarked in an article in *The Chronicle of Higher Education* (May 28, 1999):

"Antibodies are the first line of defence against most viruses, and [HIV] has breached that line."

Indeed, it is doubtful whether antibodies alone can protect against HIV. Virtually all HIV-infected individuals produce measurable amounts of antibodies to HIV, but studies have shown that high levels of HIV-neutralizing antibodies – levels at least 200-fold greater than those found in HIV infection – would be required to probably protect against HIV infection.

Also, one of the defining characteristics of HIV is that it can be transmitted not only through free-floating virus particles in blood and other body fluids, but directly through cell-to-cell contact in the mucosal linings of the vaginal and gastrointestinal (including oral and anal) tracts. *Most traditional vaccine preparations elicit only the production of antibodies in blood and body fluids and do not stimulate a cellular immune response*. But because HIV can be transmitted sexually – and possibly directly from cell to cell without entering the blood – a successful HIV vaccine might need to elicit cell-mediated immunity in order to prevent infection. Additional studies suggest that other, as yet undefined, immune responses might also be needed for an HIV vaccine to be successful.

HIV poses other obstacles to designing an effective vaccine. In addition to the two major types of HIV (HIV-1 and HIV-2), there are already at least nine known strains or clades, of HIV-1 circulating worldwide and many genetic variants within each clade. It is considered unlikely that a single vaccine preparation will protect against all of them. Furthermore, HIV often remains hidden inside some body cells and tissues for long periods of time, thus evading antibodies. And, of course, HIV attacks and destroys the very immune cells that are supposed to learn how to recognize and respond to both an HIV vaccine preparation and a real HIV infection. *It is claimed that to date, there is no evidence that the immune system of any HIV-infected person has been able to destroy or eliminate the human immunodeficiency virus on its own.*

Lack of an Ideal Animal Model

Another clinical challenge in the development of an HIV vaccine is the lack of an ideal animal model to test candidate vaccines. Chimpanzees, man's closest genetic relative, are the only animals that can be infected with HIV-1, but they do not usually develop clinical AIDS from the virus. Monkeys develop an AIDS-like syndrome from an HIV-related monkey retrovirus, the simian immunodeficiency virus (SIV), but the virus differs from HIV-1 in important ways. Researchers have created hybrid viruses called SHIV viruses that combine SIV with HIV's outer coat, and will make it easier to test HIV candidate vaccines in monkeys. But such experiments cannot fully predict the safety or efficacy of a vaccine designed for use against HIV in humans.

In 1984, after the confirmation of the aetiological agent of AIDS by scientists at the U.S. National Institutes of Health and the Pasteur Institute, the United States Health and Human Services Secretary Margaret Heckler declared that a vaccine would be available within two years (Associated Press, 1984).

However, the classical vaccination approaches that have been successful in the control of various viral diseases by priming the adaptive immunity to recognize the viral envelope proteins have failed in the case of HIV-1, as the epitopes of the viral envelope are too variable. Furthermore, the functionally important epitopes of the gp120 protein are masked by glycosylation, trimerisation and receptor-induced conformational changes making it difficult to block with neutralizing antibodies. In February 2003, Vaxgen announced that their AIDSVAX vaccine was a failure in North America as there was not a statistically significant reduction of HIV infection within the study population (Francis et al., 2003). In November 2003, it also failed clinical trials in Thailand for the same reason. These vaccines both targeted gp120 and were specific for the geographical regions (Billich et al., 2001).

The ineffectiveness of previously developed vaccines primarily stems from two related factors. First, HIV is highly mutable. Because of the virus' ability to rapidly respond to selective pressures imposed by the immune system, the population of virus in an infected individual typically evolves so that it can evade the two major arms of the adaptive immune system; humoral (antibody-mediated) and cellular (mediated by T cells) immunity. Second, HIV isolates are themselves highly variable. HIV can be categorized into multiple clades and subtypes with a high degree of genetic divergence.

Therefore, the immune responses raised by any vaccine need to be broad enough to account for this variability. Any vaccine that lacks this breadth is unlikely to be effective.

The typical animal model for vaccine research is the monkey, often the macaque. The monkeys can be infected with SIV or the chimeric SHIV for research purposes. However, the well-proven route of trying to induce neutralizing antibodies by vaccination has stalled because of the great difficulty in stimulating antibodies that neutralize heterologous primary HIV isolates (Poignard et al., 1999). Some vaccines based on the virus envelope have protected chimpanzees or macaques from homologous virus challenge (Berman et al., 1990), but in clinical trials, individuals who were immunized with similar constructs became infected after later exposure to HIV-1 (Connor et al., 1998).

A website carried the following editorial. The author has put his comments in parenthesis and italics please.

Editorial

Aids and the Next 25 Years

Later this month, researchers will gather at the Institut Pasteur in Paris to mark the quarter century since human immunodeficiency virus (HIV) was discovered as the cause of acquired immunodeficiency syndrome (AIDS). Since then, over 60 million people have been infected with the virus and over 25 million people have died. These numbers make the results of two "proof of concept" vaccine efficacy trials-the STEP and Phambili trials-extremely disappointing. Indeed, these results have raised questions about whether investments in HIV vaccine research are misplaced and whether a vaccine is even achievable. Those views are misguided. *(They are misguided indeed because safe and effective vaccines have already been developed since 1998/99. The so-called search for safe and effective HIV vaccines is analogous to crying when one's head is off)*

The failure of candidate vaccines or drugs is to be expected. More than ever, investigations in humans are essential to explore concepts, test hypotheses, and delineate the human immune response to HIV immunogens. *(Humanity is not looking for concepts, hypothesis or the delineation of anything. With the scourge, humanity is in dire need of safe and effective HIV vaccines irrespective of who produced them, irrespective of how they are produced, irrespective of anything else.)*. The STEP and Phambili trials, cosponsored by the pharmaceutical company Merck and Co. and the U.S. National Institutes of Health were designed to test the efficacy of a recombinant adenovirus vector cocktail expressing three HIV genes.

The vaccine candidate failed to limit viral replication in people who became infected with HIV and failed to prevent the acquisition of HIV. Most disconcertingly, a subset of volunteers appeared to show an increased probability of acquiring HIV (see the Perspective by Moore et al., p. 753). These results reflect our still-limited knowledge of HIV, its interactions with the human immune system, and the formidable, unprecedented challenges that it poses. *(The author thinks the results are telling you very loudly that the immunogen concept, design and delivery are not correct.)*

Why Has Developing an HIV Vaccine Been So Difficult?

One reason is that HIV has evolved highly sophisticated ways to evade the immune system. Its extraordinarily high degree of sequence diversity, caused by mutation and recombination, makes it especially challenging to design neutralizing antibodies that recognize the broad range of epitopes needed for effective immune protection. *(The author maintains that researchers have put the cart before the horse by outlining recipes for the vaccine before the vaccine is developed. A recipe is a methodology. It should follow discovery, not precede it.)*

Moreover, HIV wipes out some of the very cells needed to mount an effective immune response. Despite progress in characterizing cellular and humoral immune responses to the virus, we still don't know enough about the magnitude, breadth, or types of immune responses necessary for effective vaccine protection, in part because of the lack of a robust animal model that recapitulates critical features of both HIV and the human immune system.

Indeed, these are major challenges, but evidence of immunological protection in certain experimental models of HIV in nonhuman primates, and the intriguing observation that a small proportion of HIV-infected individuals ("elite controllers") can completely suppress the virus for years, suggest that a vaccine may be achievable (see the Review by Walker and Burton, p. 760). *(Safe and effective HIV vaccines were achieved since 1998/99)*

Furthermore, new technologies in structural and computational biology are providing novel approaches for designing immunogens that might elicit broadly reactive neutralizing antibodies, and new insights into innate and mucosal immunity are expanding vaccine design strategies. *(There goes the wrong approach again, putting the cart before the horse. Get the safe and effective vaccine first before trying to find out how it works if you are keen on that. Instead of doing that, they are looking for immunogens that fit into their pre-suppositions.)*

At meetings over the past few months, including an international workshop convened last week by the Global HIV Vaccine Enterprise, there was broad agreement on many points, particularly that more, not less, basic and early-stage clinical research is needed. *(The broad agreement was irrelevant and unnecessary. The author developed these vaccines without any such agreement.)*

Understanding the human immune response to HIV remains a priority. *(The author disagrees. The priority should be getting safe and effective vaccines, not any understanding.)* We need to understand the role of both the innate and adaptive immune responses during HIV infection. Better assays are needed that reflect the functional biology of cellular immune responses and incorporate a systems biology approach - that is; encompass the integrative functioning of gene, protein, and biochemical networks - to monitor the immune system. We need to make it much more attractive for young researchers, including those from other fields, to enter the HIV vaccine field. And the continued engagement of industry is essential if we are ever to have a vaccine. *(There goes the cart before the horse again! How did they know it is essential? Since 1984, they have engaged industry and not succeeded. The author did not engage any industry and he succeeded.)*

Laboratory research has led to effective drugs against HIV that have prolonged the lives of infected individuals, and epidemiological studies have shown that interventions such as circumcision (see the Policy Forum by Potts et al., page 749) can reduce viral acquisition. However, we know from experience with other pathogens that a vaccine is the best way to stop a virus.

The only end for a journey that began 25 years ago should be the development of a safe and effective HIV vaccine. *(If the development of a safe and effective HIV vaccine is the only end for the journey that began 25 years ago, it means of course that the journey ended in 1998/99, the time the author developed his safe and effective HIV vaccines!)*

– Alan Bernstein

10.1126/science.1159797

Alan Bernstein is executive director of the Global HIV Vaccine Enterprise, New York.

Published by AAAS

The Author's View of the Appropriate HIV Vaccine Immunogen(s)

It is generally believed and accepted that safe and effective HIV vaccines have been difficult to achieve not only because of the extensive genetic variability of the virus and the problem of how to eliminate the provirus but also because of the problem of conceiving the appropriate immunogen(s) delivered appropriately. Accordingly, most candidate HIV vaccine concepts and strategies involve the use of immunogen(s) specific for the predominant subtypes found within a country or geographic region.

The HIV is very immunogenic. HIV infection is associated with humoral and cell-mediated immune responses but these are unable to clear the infection. As mentioned earlier, the outpouring of anti-HIV antibodies after HIV infection is massive and extensive. The relentless progression of HIV infection to AIDS and death after, on the average, 10 years from initial HIV infection occurs in spite of these immune responses to the virus. In the author's view, any candidate HIV vaccines that aim to stimulate anti-HIV antibody production would likely be ineffective just as happens in natural HIV infection.

Besides, the author still cannot see how such a vaccine would ever cure HIV infection as he earlier explained when dealing with the meaning of cure of HIV infection. Even if such a vaccine were efficacious, how would one confirm such efficacy? How would one differentiate between vaccinated persons and those infected with the HIV when the universal method of screening for HIV infection is by the detection of anti-HIV antibodies in the blood? Recipients of such vaccines would also be as stigmatized as those with HIV infection.

In a nutshell, the author thinks it is unscientific and naïve to consider developing any candidate HIV vaccines that involve the production of anti-HIV antibodies. Such vaccines would not only fail efficacy trials, but they would stigmatize the recipients, as they have been doing.

In the light of our present knowledge of the immunopathology of HIV infection, the author is better off discarding the possibility of such vaccines. Until we realize that anti-HIV antibodies do not, and cannot provide cure of, or effective protection against HIV infection, we are likely to continue to harvest failure in our attempt to successfully develop safe and effective HIV vaccines. After all, a person already infected with one type or strain of HIV is not protected against infection by another HIV type or strain even though that person already has massive quantities of binding anti-HIV antibodies against various HIV proteins/peptides. The new HIV strain proceeds and successfully establishes itself in the person already infected with the HIV. In other words, the adage, 'He who is down needs not fear a fall' does not apply to HIV infection; any HIV-infected person is at risk of picking other strains of HIV infection

It is trite immunology that any successful vaccine must contain the appropriate immunogen delivered appropriately. An appropriate immunogen is one that stimulates the necessary appropriate specific immune responses when administered. How would one get an immunogen that would tackle all the millions of mutants of the HIV when in any infected person, there are millions of such mutants?

Besides that problem, how would one conceive an immunogen that would eliminate the HIV provirus covalently incorporated in the infected cell's DNA? This appears really formidable because immune responses take place extracellularly, not intracellularly. Is it possible to think of an immunogen that would eliminate the provirus from its sequestrated and protected position in the nucleus of the infected cell, a position that very effectively shields it from the host's immune responses? Unless and until one conceives and develops a vaccine that eliminates the provirus, one would just be wasting his time thinking of getting an effective HIV therapeutic vaccine. And even an HIV preventive vaccine would fail if any HIV virion succeeds in entering any CD4+ target cell because the subsequent provirus would not be eliminated.

If the reader agrees with the foregoing analysis, then the stage is set for the next phase of intense intellectual exercise and activity to work out possible candidate HIV vaccine immunogens that would

- Not trigger the production of anti-HIV antibodies in the recipient;
- Induce an effective immune response that would get rid of the provirus; and
- Induce an effective immune response against all the HIV types, clades and mutants.

The author thinks it is not only interesting and challenging but it is very possible that several candidate HIV vaccine immunogens may be developed by different readers out of those that decide to be involved in this intellectual exercise. The author believes that some of those who involve themselves in this intellectual activity may likely arrive at independent and better concepts than he did. Readers may notice that the author has not suggested any specific recipe or formula for candidate HIV vaccine immunogens or development. The author has only utilised the known features of the HIV to work out the characteristics of the appropriate immunogens that would likely result in a safe and effective vaccine against the virus. The criteria that such immunogens must meet are dictated by the extraordinarily novel and peculiar problems of the HIV, particularly its extensive mutation, the fact that anti-HIV antibodies in HIV infection do not carry the good news that we normally associate with antibodies in other viral infections, and the provirus phenomenon in HIV infection. All these peculiar attributes of the HIV are radical departures from our established knowledge of immunology and must be matched with equally radical departures from our established knowledge of vaccine concept and development if we are to make real our dream of successful development of safe and effective HIV vaccines.

The Author's Secondary School Days

When Jeremiah started his secondary school education at Ochaja in January 1961, he was the youngest and smallest in the school. His class of thirty students was the second set in the new school. It was a boarding school for the 60 students. The school itself was under heavy construction. A white man, Mr. Cook from Britain was the one in charge of Works in the School. He was a very hard working Briton, always in his shorts and sweating away at various jobs. His wife was the one that attended to students who were sick. They had 2 or 3 small kids. Students only encountered Mr. Cook either during the course of construction or maintenance, or on Sundays during Service especially if he was the one that preached, but he did not teach any subjects. The buildings he put up are still standing there up till today, as if they had been built just a month ago. This is remarkable in a society whose local buildings last for a maximum period of a year, and in a country in which some urban houses even in the capital city of Abuja and other major towns are still collapsing while under construction!

Students had to fetch firewood for the cooks to use to prepare their meals. They also had to fetch water from the nearby stream to be used for cooking their meals. They also had to go to the same stream morning and evening to take their baths and fetch water in their buckets on their return. They were provided with double deck 'Vono' 8-spring iron beds.

In the cold harmattan winds especially at night, Jeremiah had more than he could chew. He had no other clothes other than his school uniforms, so he could not afford to wear them at night. The iron springs of their beds were particularly cold at night. He had no mat or mattress for the beds, but he had one wrapper, popularly called covering clothe when used by men. The cotton wrapper he had was given to him by his mother when he left for Ochaja. He would put the wrapper on the bed, but on lying on it, the iron springs would not let him sleep, and worse, he was exposed to the biting cold. In Nigeria, a temperature of 28 degrees Celsius is biting cold especially if it is windy and dry as it usually is in the dry season.

He was brought up sleeping on the bear ground in his mother's hut, and had been accustomed to sleeping in that way all his life. When he was in the Chief's palace at Abocho, he had the luxury of sleeping with others on mats on the smooth cemented floor in small rooms. His present problem was worse though. The dormitory was a large open room for about 20 students; it had large window pane glass windows that would not shut out gusts of harmattan wind. He had to sleep alone unlike in the past, when he would sleep with peers. It was against the school rule for any student to sleep on the cement floor. He decided he would sneak out of the dormitory, go to the deserted kitchen and sleep beside the hot ashes left behind by the cooks. That solved his problem. He would lie on the ground close to the hot fire place and cover himself with his wrapper.

This worked for about a fortnight before trouble came knocking. One of the prefects noticed in the night that Jeremiah's bed was empty. He waited for some time, thinking the little boy had gone out to ease himself, but the lad never showed up. He then raised an alarm because there were many wild animals around including some hippos in the nearby stream. The noise woke Jeremiah up and he ran to meet the others. He had to explain where he had been and why. They all came and confirmed indeed that someone had been lying down close to the still hot fireplace. In the morning, the head boy warned him of the danger in going there to sleep at night, but there was no punishment. Of course, the lad could not avoid going back there to sleep. When the other students realized that the lad continued to sleep out there alone at night, they reached their conclusion that Jeremiah had been given much charms by his parents, hence he was not even afraid of wild beasts!

Jeremiah recalls Messrs Odoh and Nwosu, Nigerians that taught him in Form 1 in 1960 along with British Teachers particularly Miss Tector. Miss Tector encouraged all the pupils to use the holidays to try and find out their birthdays, or birth years at least. All the British teachers and workers around told us they know their birthdays and those of their parents and other relations. Mr. Johnston, the Principal, was of particular interest to Jeremiah because of his mathematical knowledge. Jeremiah always strived, though unsuccessfully to get 100 per cent in Algebra, Geometry, Trigonometry and Arithmetic that were separate subjects in Form 1.

Throughout his four years of Secondary education at Ochaja, Jeremiah had an Igala nickname that he himself had to accept. Literally translated, the nickname *Jeremiah odi* meant 'Jeremiah the dwarf' Then and now, anyone who gets irritated or angry or upset at being called a nickname by his peers would be acting stupidly because the name would then stick on him and continue to be widely used. Jeremiah answered his nickname happily every time any student called it. That meant the nickname would be used less and less. By the time he left Ochaja, the nickname was not rampantly used since everyone found that it did not evoke an unpleasant response from Jeremiah.

In Form 1 in 1961, Jeremiah decided to enquire as much as possible from the elders in his community about the circumstances or events surrounding his time of birth that they could remember. After extensive investigation, he obtained the most helpful information from his mother. She recalled clearly that Jeremiah was born on a Sunday thirteen days to Christmas. She could not give Jeremiah any hint about the year. Jeremiah eventually pinned the year down. There is another child in the village that had a relation then working in Kaduna, the capital of Northern Region. He came home about the time that chap was born, and he wrote down the year for the father of that boy, 1949. Every one agreed that Jeremiah was three months older than that boy. Even though the three months could be anything from two to four lunar months, Jeremiah had successfully worked out his birthday, 12th December 1948 (Figures 21-1 to 21-6).

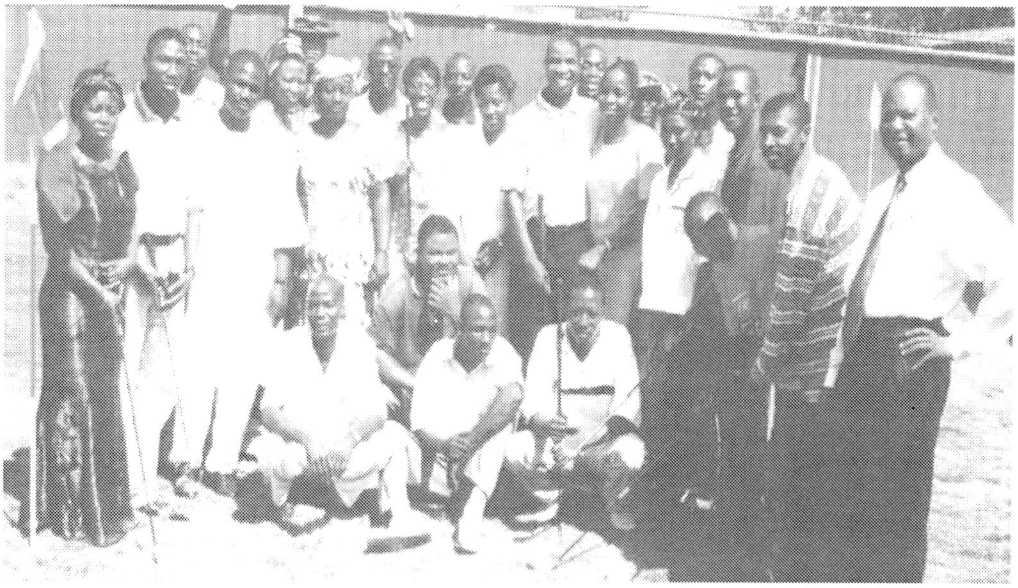

Figure 21-1. The staff of Medicrest Specialist Hospital including security personnel in a group photograph with the author on the 'green' in the Hospital's premises on 12 December 2002 celebrating the author's birthday,.

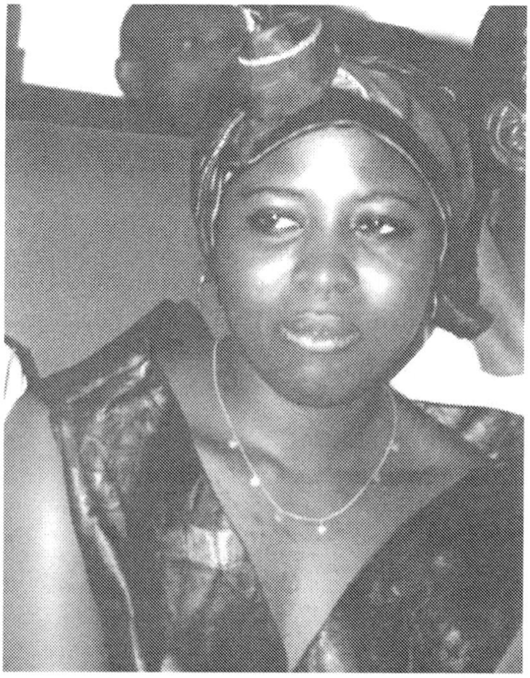

Figure 21-2. Angela, a staff member of the author's Hospital on 12 Dec 2002during celebration of the author's birthday.

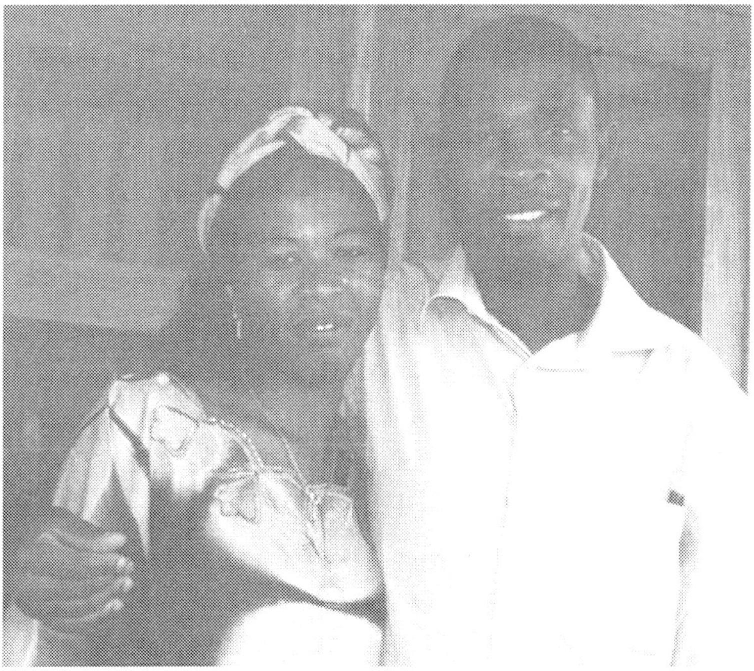

Figure 21-3. Salamatu (left), a staff member of the author's Hospital poses with the author's younger brother Akogu on 12 Dec 2002 during celebrations of the author's birthday.

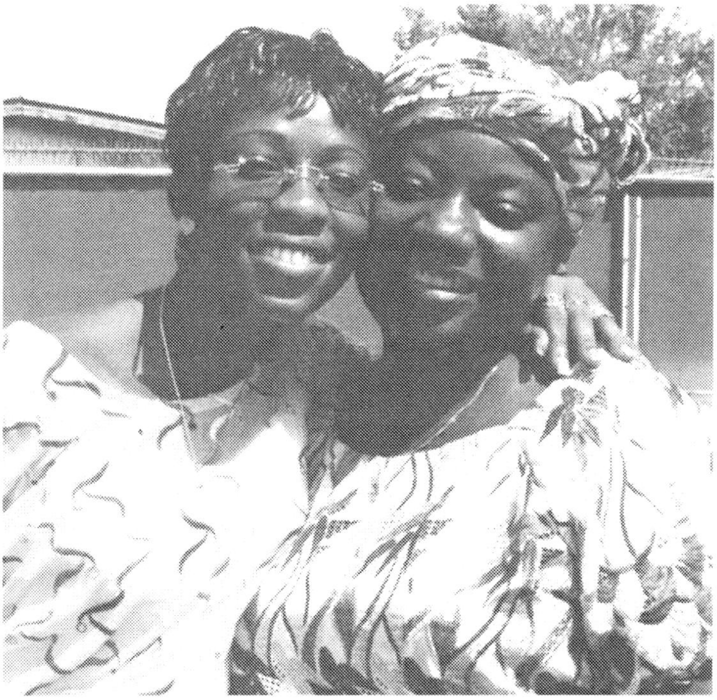

Figure 21-4. Vera (left) and Rachel, both staff members of the author's Hospital on 12 Dec 2002 in the Hospital's premises during celebrations of the author's birthday.

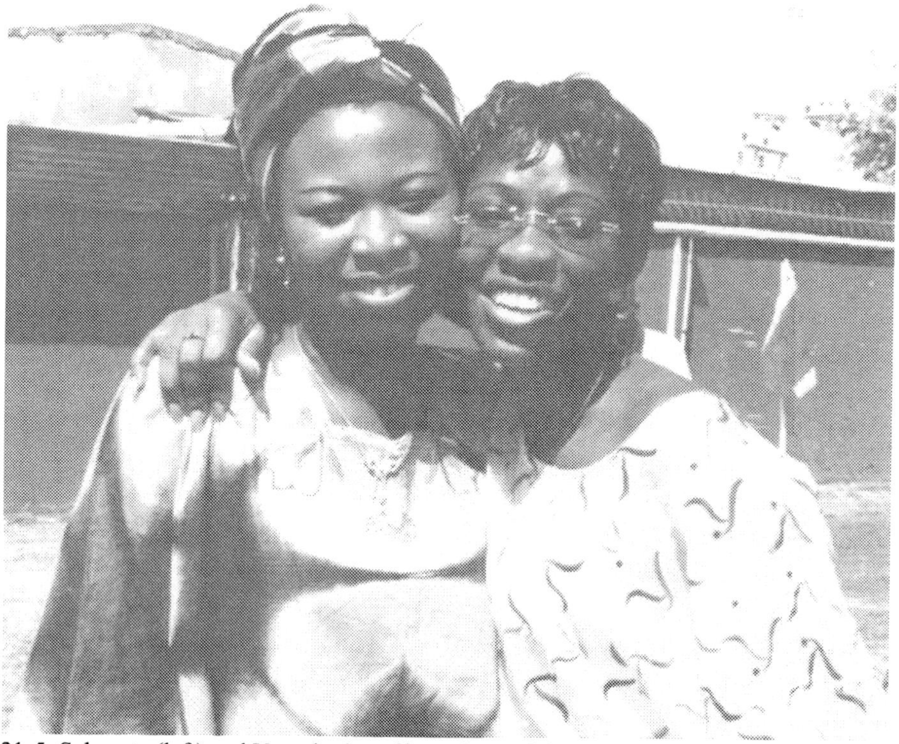

Figure 21-5. Salamatu (left) and Vera, both staff members of the author's Hospital on the 'green' in the premises of the Hospital on 12 Dec 2002 during celebrations of the author's birthday.

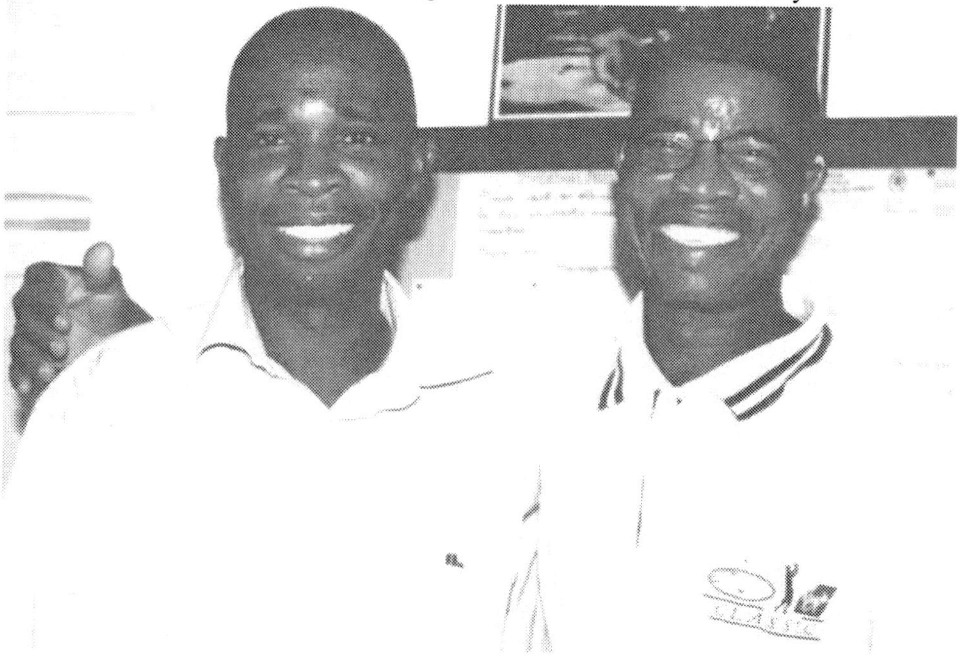

Figure 21-6. Akogu (left) and his elder brother Jeremiah on the premises of the author's Hospital on 12 Dec 2002 during celebrations of the author's birthday.

True to the Principal's promise at Jeremiah's oral interview for admission into the Secondary School at Ochaja in 1960, Jeremiah was given an additional scholarship of £2 at the end of his Form 1. Just a few days into the first term in 1962, the Principal summoned Jeremiah to his office in the afternoon around 5 p.m. during the games period. Jeremiah went shaking with fear from head to toe. He had never been so summoned since he came to the school. What offence might he have committed to cause that frightful afternoon development? As soon as Jeremiah entered the Principal's office, the Principal allayed his fears. He offered Jeremiah the opportunity of joining Form 3 to see if he could cope, adding that if he found out that he could not cope with his new class, he could return to Form 2. Jeremiah accepted the offer on the spot. Mr. Johnston immediately gave the student the books for Form 3 and asked Jeremiah to bring the Form 2 books back to him immediately. Jeremiah returned the Form 2 books as instructed, and moved over to Form 3.

Jeremiah put in his best. Two weeks later, he had caught up with the rest of the class in Maths and the other science subjects. A month further on, he was reasonably okay with the other subjects. He never remembered for a second that the option of going back to Form 2 existed; all that concerned the chap was how to progress as a Form 3 student. He worked hard and obtained commensurate results. Alabi and Tom especially were happy with his performance.

In 1962, Nigeria had a national census. Jeremiah took part as an enumerator. He received about £10 for the job. Without taking a penny for himself, he turned every penny over to his father to assist the man in paying his fees. At the time he did that, Jeremiah did not have any footwear of any kind.

Sometime in 1962 also, Jeremiah had some painful swellings in his right groin. Mr. Cook's wife that was responsible for attending to sick students recommended he be taken to the Mission's Medical Centre at Ochadamu, some 25 miles west of Ochaja. All the whites working then at Ochaja used Volkswagen Beetle cars. Jeremiah started wishing he should not improve so that the Principal would take him and two other sick students to Ochadamu. That would be his first opportunity of entering a moving car in his life, and he did not want to miss it. The three sick students were taken to Ochadamu, Jeremiah inclusive. Jeremiah was so elated that by the time he got out of the car at Ochadamu, he was much better.

The white doctor at Ochadamu saw the three sick students and treated them. He placed Jeremiah on daily injections for seven days. Thinking back now, Jeremiah thinks it was Procaine Penicillin injections he had. While there, Jeremiah discussed as much as possible with the attendants there and tried to know more about putting someone to sleep for operations. Communications were so bad in those days in the author's area that his father received the news of his son's illness three days after Jeremiah had been discharged from Ochadamu. To get back to Ochaja, he had to trek about 5 miles from Ochadamu to Umomi before he boarded a lorry to Ochaja. The Ochadamu experience stimulated Jeremiah the more to try and be a doctor that would perform operations.

In 1962, Mr. Cook successfully electrified the School using a diesel generator. In that same year too, he provided pipe borne water that was pumped up from the big stream near by. Students though were not allowed to take their baths with the tap water. They still had to go to the stream twice a day for that purpose. The author recalls that some time in that year, his entire class did not know that ice was lighter than water. None of them had ever seen ice. The

British teacher had to bring some ice blocks from her house to demonstrate to the class that ice indeed was, and still is lighter than water.

Nigeria cancelled the 1962 census results and repeated the exercise in 1963. Jeremiah again took part as an enumerator, and was paid about £10 again for the work he did. As in the previous year, he turned everything over to his dad. This time, his father decided to buy for him spare shorts and shirts so that he would no longer need to go about naked in the village during his holidays. In both censuses, enumerators went to their place of assignment with an estimate of the population of the area they were to cover. The first census was fairly accurate because each enumerator turned in what he/she actually counted, irrespective of whether it was more or less than the projected population and the superiors accepted the returns for collation. The 1963 census was radically different. The projected population figures the enumerators were given before the exercise were invariably grossly inflated. They were instructed that unless the enumerator produced at least his projected population, his return would not be accepted. They therefore compelled all the enumerators to sit down and make up the numbers with fictitious names and their particulars. It was very sad and unfortunate.

At the beginning of 1964, the Principal announced that the nineteen Form 5 students would be taking their external West African Schools Certificate (WASC) examinations at the end of that year. Jeremiah was one of the 15 students in that class that had never heard of WASC! Quickly, the School arranged and got the past mock WASC and WASC papers for 10 years and made them available to the class so that students would have an idea of the standard expected of them.

At the WASC level, the students obtained Ordinary level (O level) in various subjects. Until 1963, Form 5 students in Northern Region took an external exam called Mock WASC examinations during the 2nd term to determine those that would be selected to go for their 2-year Higher School Certificate (HSC) course for Advanced Level (A Level). This was changed in 1964. From then on, each school organized its own Mock WASC exams, and the results would still be used to select students for the HSC course. The School of course had to put in each student's choice of 3 Principal subjects for the HSC course because the course was designed then for 3 A Level subjects, no more and no less.

During the 1964 Easter holidays, Alabi had again brought up the issue of his wish that one or both of his sons should train to be a doctor that would be performing operations. On issues like this, it is the culture for the more senior of the sons to declare his position; he had the choice. Tom explained that he was not even studying Biology, and as such he would never qualify to study medicine even if he wanted to be a doctor. Alabi then instructed Jeremiah that he should study to be a doctor and a surgeon; otherwise he (Alabi) would live with regret for the rest of his life for sending the two of them to school. Maths, Physics, Chemistry and Biology were the science subjects Jeremiah was studying at Ochaja; out of these four subjects, Biology was his worst while Maths, Chemistry and Physics were his best in that order.

For the HSC combination, the School recommended that Jeremiah put in for Maths, Physics and Chemistry, but Jeremiah told them he had to choose a combination that would allow him study Medicine, that is, Physics, Chemistry and Zoology. The School, in fairness, contacted Jeremiah's father on the issue; of course, the man confirmed to them that Jeremiah should study to be a doctor and a surgeon. And so, the School put Jeremiah in to study Physics Chemistry and Zoology for his HSC course.

Jeremiah was selected to go to St. Paul's College in Zaria (11 0N, 7 40E) for his HSC course. After the WASC exams in December 1964, he took his admission papers for HSC to his dad. The man was elated even though Zaria was so far away from Igala land. Jeremiah too had never stepped out of his Igala area since his birth. This offered him the opportunity to see the world beyond his tribal area. The School listed out things that each HSC student should come with. These included sandals and games shoes. Alabi had to buy them for Jeremiah. December 1964 marked the time Jeremiah's feet were having the luxury of being in any form of foot wear. It took over a week before the chap could learn to walk fairly normally with shoes. At the time Jeremiah completed his education at Ochaja, he was only sixty-three inches tall. He himself had reached the same conclusion as everybody else - he would be a dwarf for the rest of his life.

The Northern Region would be responsible for all the expenses for the HSC course. In addition, they would provide each HSC student a weekly stipend of five shillings. They would also pay the to and fro transport expenses for each student during all the holidays. Of course, it was a pre-requisite that each student selected for HSC passed the WASC exam with an O level in the English Language and also obtained O levels in his three principal subjects for the HSC.

In the next chapter, Jeremiah would let the reader know what happened to him during his HSC course at St. Paul's College, Zaria.

Conclusion

The author has laid bare his unbiased analysis of the peculiarities of the HIV that he believes should be matched with commensurate and appropriate approaches in candidate HIV vaccine immunogen concept and development. In doing so, the author has not put the cart before the horse; he has not allowed established knowledge and entrenched immunological dogmas to sway him from the path of objectivity; he has not suggested any recipe or formula for HIV vaccine research and development; he has not suggested that any person, group of persons, institutions, countries or class has the monopoly of knowledge to try and develop the concept of appropriate candidate HIV vaccine immunogens that would likely be effective. It is an open field that may eventually result in the availability of many candidate HIV vaccine immunogens.

Chapter XXII

Which HIV Vaccine to Tackle First, the Preventive or the Therapeutic?

Abstract

The author is a beneficiary of the principle of not being rigid in one's stand on any issue. One should always be ready to alter his approach or position whenever new facts emerge. The appearance of the disease AIDS in 1981 and the subsequent isolation of its causative agent, HIV, were a new development in man's battle with viral diseases. HIV is not a conventional virus from many angles. The successful development of vaccines against it would likely involve the adoption of non-conventional methods. This chapter deals with how the author eventually succeeded in finding an opening that might lead him eventually to the development of a saeHIV preventive vaccine that he very desperately needed for his own protection.

Introduction

When the author finally decided at the end of 1991 to involve himself quietly and secretly in HIV vaccine research and development, his first assignment was to educate himself as fast and as much as possible on this new disease, HIV/AIDS. Some basic facts about HIV/AIDS that he had learnt include the following:

The HIV is an enveloped RNA virus unaffected by freezing but inactivated (killed) by heat, desiccation, oxidizing agents, formaldehyde, etc., reminding the author that it is like most human pathogenic viruses. Its infective genome includes the reverse transcriptase enzyme for transcribing a double-stranded DNA template from its RNA when its infective genome enters the cell's cytoplasm. The viral DNA template so produced is moved across into the nucleus where it is permanently incorporated into the host cell's DNA as the provirus.

The HIV targets, infects and destroys CD4 helper T-lymphocytes, resulting in acquired immune deficiency syndrome (AIDS) after several years. When the virus infects a cell, it leaves its envelope permanently attached to the cell membrane of the infected cell. The virus mutates very rapidly and extensively. HIV infection progresses relentlessly to AIDS and death; it is incurable.

HIV infection is diagnosed by confirming the presence of antibodies against various HIV viral proteins in a person's blood, reminding the author that this indirect method of diagnosing HIV not only confirms that the virus is immunogenic but differs very significantly from other viral infections where antibodies are protective.

It takes about 2-3 months for an infected person to produce detectable anti-HIV IgG antibodies in the blood. After infection, it takes, on the average, about 10 years for AIDS to develop. In other words, HIV is very unlike most human viral infections that cause acute infections.

Man is the only known natural host of the virus, reminding the author of smallpox. Laboratory cultures of the virus are available in the developed countries.

Its routes of transmission are through blood-to-blood contact, coitus, the placenta from mother to offspring, and breast feeding. Tests to detect the virus directly are costly and difficult to perform.

Attempts at producing a vaccine using inactivated virus and modern genetic engineering techniques had been unsuccessful so far. Around 1996, antiretroviral drugs had been introduced in the developed countries to try and reduce the progression of the disease to AIDS but such drugs were costly, toxic and non-curative.

Armed with these facts, the author felt in June 1992 that time had come for him to start tackling his secret, self-assigned and daunting task of trying to conceive and develop, for his personal protection, a safe and effective HIV preventive vaccine. While engaged in that assignment, he would of course continue learning about HIV/AIDS from all possible sources within his reach so as to continuously modify his approach in the light of new facts about or related to his assignment.

The author wishes to emphasize that he contributed absolutely nothing to the entire scientific researches world wide that unravelled all these facts that he learnt about the HIV. Other researchers laboured and toiled to elucidate these facts about the HIV, and the author just had the simple task of merely learning the facts. The author very sincerely acknowledges with deep gratitude the work and efforts of all the researchers that led to the elucidation of these facts about the HIV. The foundation for the author's attempt at developing HIV vaccines was laid by all these other researchers. The author profoundly, gratefully and wholeheartedly acknowledges their contributions wherever they may be.

Is the Gate of Progress Closed?

The author admitted to himself that he had embarked on a very difficult assignment indeed. He had, and still has

- no training or experience in any vaccine development,
- no experience in virology,
- no access to HIV viral cultures or any other viral cultures for that matter,

- no training in, experience of or facilities for modern genetic engineering techniques or recombinant technology and
- no source of funds.

All the same, he had no alternative but to continue to encourage himself by reminding himself that because those without these handicaps had not succeeded, he had at least a chance, even if infinitesimal, of success even with the handicaps.

In 1992, his country had neither internet nor GSM communication facilities. As a result, he had very limited access to current medical literature and current developments on HIV and its vaccine development efforts elsewhere.

On the encouraging side, he told himself not to surrender, that the roadblock may be temporary or by-passable. He should consider himself very lucky to even know the few facts he had known about the causative agent of AIDS, which is HIV. He recalled that other people such as Edward Jenner and Louis Pasteur who developed effective human viral vaccines in the past were not as lucky. He reminded himself of his father's persistent words to him right from his childhood that it is more honourable and rewarding to attempt to solve any problem than to do nothing and end up a victim of that problem. He also reminded himself of the adage, 'When things get tough, the tough get going'. He would not be chicken-hearted in the face of this extant danger of his picking up the virus during his surgical practice. He was determined to proceed. He would continue to rattle his brain even when doing other things. He might be lucky to get an opening. Would he?

The Gate Opener Is Identified

While searching for an opener for him to proceed, the author continued to look at the features of HIV/AIDS that he knew to seek out any possible openers. When he took up the chronicity of HIVAIDS for the umpteenth time, he reminded himself that this was an uncommon feature in man's viral diseases that he knew. 'Look at it again closely, Jerry', he told himself. 'Is there anything in the chronicity of HIV infection that you can capitalize on to help you in your assignment?'

Eventually, he realized that common sense dictated that he should start by trying to develop an HIV therapeutic vaccine first, unlike what is done for other human viral diseases that are almost invariably acute infections. With an average incubation period of 10 years for HIV infection to develop into AIDS, he was elated indeed to see that there was actually ample time to try to develop a safe candidate therapeutic vaccine for use in those already infected, and to test the efficacy of such a vaccine on such people.

Instead of trying to develop a preventive vaccine for himself, he had to alter his priorities and tackle the therapeutic vaccine first. If he succeeded in developing such a vaccine, he was optimistic that he would then be just a stone's throw away from getting the preventive vaccine that he very much needed. He felt that if he took this full sea tide, so to say, it might lead him to his target but if he missed it, he might end up in miserable failure. He recalled the words of Shakespeare in *Julius Caesar* Act IV Scene III,

> "There is a tide in the affairs of men
> Which, taken at the floods,
> Leads on to fortune;
> Omitted, all the voyage of their life
> Is bound in shallows and in miseries.
> On such a full sea are we now afloat;
> And we must take the current when it serves,
> Or lose our ventures."

He believed, and still believes that the key for optimism in his HIV preventive vaccine research effort was the realization that the chronicity of HIV infection could be cheaply, conveniently, safely and effectively harnessed for the development of safe and effective HIV therapeutic vaccines.

The handicaps that seriously bothered him initially, namely,

- no experience in virology,
- no training or experience in any vaccine development,
- no access to HIV viral cultures or any other viral cultures for that matter,
- no training in, experience of or facilities for modern genetic engineering techniques and recombinant technology,
- no animal models with which to experiment, and
- no source of funds suddenly vaporized into irrelevance and insignificance.

After all, he could as well imitate HIV's reverse transcriptase enzyme: he would tackle his problem in reverse gear – try and get the therapeutic vaccine first. Prevention is easier and cheaper and better than cure, but in this case with this strange virus, it may be better indeed to try the therapeutic vaccine first before the preventive one. Even though that would likely be a more difficult approach, he was satisfied that this 'reverse' approach for a virus that transcripts in reverse was pragmatic, had fewer problems and might be what the virus required. All this prodded him to proceed with much joy, optimism, satisfaction and enthusiasm.

The Author's Higher School Certificate Course

In January 1965, the author still had his wooden box as he took off for Enugu (6 30N, 7 30E), the capital of Eastern Region. There, he got into an Express passenger train from Port Harcourt (4 40N, 7 10E) to Lagos (6 25N, 3 27E) through Kaduna (10 30N, 7 21E). The author had never seen a train before in his life. Throughout the journey that lasted about forty hours, he would come down at stations and examine the rail tracks because he had been taught in Physics lessons about the allowance made between iron rail bars to allow for expansion as the temperature varies during the day and seasons, but he had never seen it. In the English Essay paper in the WASC examination he had just taken, one of the questions was 'Describe an interesting train journey you have made'. No one in his class had attempted that question because they had never travelled by train.

About forty hours after leaving Enugu, the train reached Kaduna junction. There the author disembarked, and found his way by road to Zaria, 50 miles further north from Kaduna. He found his way to St. Paul's College in Wusasa, a western suburb of Zaria. The College lay near a huge rocky mountain called 'kufena' in Hausa (Zaria is a Hausa town). The local lad called Jeremiah was the only one that had a wooden box in that College that year. All the other students had portmanteaus.

Zaria then was truly the educational Centre of Northern Region. The Ahmadu Bello University (ABU), School of Pharmacy, Advanced Teachers' College (ATC), School of Agriculture, Nigerian Military School, Government College, Government Secondary School, Government Teachers' College and St. Paul's College were all located in the town. ABU was the only University in the huge Northern Region. There were two hospitals in the town, the Government's General Hospital and a Mission Hospital at Wusasa. Wusasa Hospital and St. Paul's College were both owned by the Anglican Mission. Many Primary Schools were located in the town.

As at Ochaja, Jeremiah was placed in Johnston House at St. Paul's College. The College just lay west of the Kaduna-Zaria rail line. Wells provided the College with its source of water, and students used rope to fetch water from the wells for their needs. It had electricity supply from the country's National Electric Power Authority (NEPA).

Jeremiah had noticed from the notice board allocating new students to dormitories that there were Upper Six Arts students in the College, but that his Lower Six Science class was the first in the College. "You are in another class that is the first in the College, just as in Ochaja", Jeremiah told himself.

As the dwarf was carrying his wooden box and his new iron bucket to his new dormitory Johnston House, a tall Form 2 student noticed him, and reckoned that he was definitely a new Form 1 student. As soon as Jeremiah put his things down in the dormitory and was trying to get his bearings correct, this gangling student summoned him, gave him a bucket and ordered him to fetch water for him from the well. Jeremiah thought about it briefly. It was possible that the student sending him was an Upper Six student. At Ochaja, fagging was not allowed, but he did not know if his new College allowed it.

He obeyed and fetched water from a well for the first time in his life for the student. In fact, he had never seen a well before, but he just observed how the other students fetched water from it and imitated them. When he appeared with the bucket of water, the boy was not through with him. He ordered him to take the bucket of water to the bathroom for him. He led Jeremiah to the bathroom since the boy was smart enough to realize that this new Form 1 student would not know where the bathroom was located.

At the House roll call later that evening, the tall boy that had sent Jeremiah to fetch water for him was there. The House Captain, an Upper Six Arts student started calling the students' names class by class, from Form 1 up to Upper Six. Jeremiah noticed that the student that had sent him answered his name under Form 2. The boy too looked bewildered when he noticed Jeremiah did not answer when all the Form 1 boys were called. Of course, all the old students of the College knew all the other students except Form 1 students and Lower Six students from other Schools. Jeremiah answered his name when Lower Six students were called.

As soon as the meeting ended, the Form 2 student came to apologise profusely to Jeremiah in the HSC students' section of the dormitory. The other HSC students witnessed it, and before long it was the talk of all the students even in other dormitories. When other students met Jeremiah, they would jokingly say something like this, "You should be in Form 1, and not Lower Six!"

Anyway, Jeremiah rapidly settled down like the other students. Studies began in earnest. Almost all the teachers in the College were expatriates especially British. All Jeremiah's teachers were British.

Jeremiah had never been exposed in his life to the Anglican form of worship until he reached St. Paul's College. It was a very strange form of Christianity to him. He had never heard of prayers being read. He had never heard of written prayers for all occasions that are recited throughout the year including Marriages, etc. He had never seen Christians praying with their eyes wide open, looking around and reading from any book even though in the case he was encountering at St. Paul's College, the reading was from a Prayer Book. He had never heard Psalms being sung during worship services and sung in such a way that it looked more of a recital that a sung to him.

He wondered if these recited prayers and routine observances could be genuine at all since they were not the words of the person praying or reciting them. Christianity, to Jeremiah, had taken on a new and bizarre turn at St. Paul's College. He was convinced that these recitals and readings were being done routinely, and not as a result of any conviction or belief of the person or congregation involved. He could not bring himself round to take part in these recitals throughout the two years he spent at St. Paul's College. To Jeremiah, the Anglican form of worship had taken faith and belief to the cleaners whereas all his life before then, he expected Christianity and Christian worship to be founded on faith or belief, not recitals.

At Ochaja, the students used to be given free American-produced powdered milk from time to time. Two students would share a packet. Every student struggled to be paired with Jeremiah for the powdered milk because Jeremiah would not take the milk. He was not used to taking milk. The first time he took milk was when the British wife of one of his teachers brought it to him to take while sick from malaria. The drink caused him severe nausea and vomiting. Since that episode, the mere sight or smell of milk nauseated him.

Jeremiah was surprised that during the first term in Lower Six at St. Paul's College, he developed an insatiable appetite for milk and other foods. He would use his weekly stipend of five shillings on tinned Peak milk, consuming it without any sugar. Milk suddenly became appetising and sweet to him, unlike the nausea that milk caused him at Ochaja. Jeremiah did not know that he was undergoing his puberty growth spur! By August 1965, he was sixty eight inches tall whereas he started the year at sixty three inches. Of course, that meant he had outgrown most of his clothes and footwear. Fortunately for him, the College agreed to give him larger sizes of the uniforms he had been given. He only had to replace his footwear from his weekly allowance.

During the first term holidays in 1965, Jeremiah received his WASC results by post from Ochaja. He had done very well. Maths in which he scored 'Excellent' grade was of course his best subject. In Chemistry, he scored 'Very Good'. In each of the remaining five subjects he offered for WASC, he scored 'Good' grade. Jeremiah had met the O level requirements for University admission; at least six O levels in relevant subjects that must include English Language and in some Universities, Maths.

He therefore had to concentrate on his HSC course and pass with good grades all his three Principal subjects at A Level if he was to have a chance of doing Medicine. At that time in Nigeria, only the Universities at Ibadan and Lagos offered courses in Human Medicine and each of them did not only require three A levels in the three subjects Jeremiah was studying but the average A level score for the three subjects for Northern Region students must be at least grade D. There were grades A down to E for the A levels, A being the highest and E the lowest grade.

We were made to understand that there were political considerations in the admissions to study Medicine in these Universities. These two Universities that offered Medicine courses were located in Western Region in Yoruba land. We were told they would give admissions to their own students that have just two good A levels in any two of those three subjects or to those with three A levels in the three subjects even if the grades were just three Es, but students from Northern Region would not be considered for admission unless they had three A levels with the average being at least the D grade.

Jeremiah decided to travel home to Ajiolo for the 1965 summer holidays. He had really become home sick after eight months. Three months was the longest he had ever stayed without seeing his family and his community since he was born. The journey took three days, partly by road and partly by rail. As he trekked westwards through his village towards his father's compound with his wooden box on his head, he passed several groups of people gathered for various discussions in the community. He expected some children to come to his aid, welcoming him home and helping to carry his box but no such thing happened. It was when he turned towards his father's compound that he was recognized and welcomed.

News soon spread round that Jeremiah had come home. His father quickly rushed home. He was elated at seeing his son. He then revealed that they had been arguing about the man that passed with a box on his head. Some said that it was Jeremiah, but many including him disagreed on the ground that Jeremiah could never be that tall. Everyone laughed that Alabi had failed to recognize his own son. "What have you been eating, Jeremiah?" "What have white doctors done to you in Zaria that you have turned from a dwarf to a giant, Jeremiah?" that marked the end of anyone in the community calling Jeremiah a dwarf. Even in St. Paul's College, Jeremiah had metamorphosed from being the smallest student in the class at the beginning of Lower Six to being above the average class height just two terms later.

During that summer holiday, Tom and Jeremiah helped their father with his farm work. When Jeremiah's time to return to Zaria came, his father still offered him transport money but Jeremiah refused on the ground that he already had the money for that purpose. Instead, he suggested to his father to use the money to put one of his daughters in school, but the man refused. The elders in the community gathered over that last minute disagreement between father and son. At the end, it was resolved that Alabi should not send any of his daughters to school against his wish, and that Jeremiah had no right to refuse money from his dad. Jeremiah thanked them all, collected the money with the usual traditional way of showing appreciation to one's father, and left for Zaria.

Back at school in Zaria, Jeremiah noticed that he continued to grow taller. By the beginning of Upper Six in 1966, he had reached 71 inches in height. The simmering political crisis in Nigeria took an unexpected downhill plunge on January 15, 1966 when the first military coup in the country took place. The following account of the coup comes from the author's memory. It is therefore possible that there may be a few errors in his account that he is writing now, 42 years after the event.

In that coup, two allies and friends the Premiers of Northern and Western Regions, Sir Ahmadu Bello The Sardauna of Sokoto (his traditional title) and Chief Samuel Akintola respectively were killed, but the Premier of Eastern Region Chief Michael Okpara, an Ibo man and the one for Mid-Western Region Chief Denis Osadebay were left unharmed. The Premier of Northern Region had been killed by an Ibo officer, Major Chukwuma Nzeogu. At the Federal level, the Prime Minister who was from Northern Region was also assassinated along with his Finance Minister from Mid-Western Region. The ceremonial President of the country, Dr. Nnamdi Azikiwe, an Ibo man, had travelled abroad two weeks or so before the coup, ostensibly for medical treatment.

The Nigerian Army then had Major-General J.T.U. Aguiyi-Ironsi as its head; he was from the Ibo tribe too. Under him were three Brigadiers and a number of Colonels. The three Brigadiers were Ogundipe a Yoruba man from Western Region, Ademulegun a Yoruba man also from the same Region, and Maimalari from Northern Region. In that mid-January night coup, Ibo officers assassinated Brigadier Maimalari in Lagos, then the country's capital. Brigadier Ademulegun in Kaduna was shot dead along with his pregnant wife. The author cannot recall the circumstances of Brigadier Ogundipe, but he escaped death.

Furthermore, there was one Colonel Pam from Northern Region. He was said to be on leave and was in a hotel room on the night of the coup. The Ibo officers that carried out the coup traced him to his hotel room and killed him there in cold blood. In addition, it was said that a few days before that coup, one Lt Colonel Yakubu Gowon from the North had just returned to Lagos from a military training in the UK. It was said that the Ibo coup plotters had earmarked him for elimination that night but good luck smiled on him. How he escaped was interesting to us in those days, and even now.

Gowon was then unmarried. On the night of the coup, he was with his Ibo girl friend in the lady's apartment, completely oblivious of any coup de tat. Listening to the early morning news on Radio Nigeria that morning, the lady heard martial music. She immediately woke Gowon up, and quickly packed foods and drinks for Gowon to go and hide under a culvert not too far away. In a twinkle of an eye, Gowon had gone into his hiding sanctuary. Shortly afterwards, the Ibo coup plotters came to her and asked of Gowon. She said she had not seen him. They pleaded and begged her in their Ibo mother tongue to help them locate him, but the lady insisted she did not know his whereabouts. Unsatisfied, they ransacked her apartment but found no trace of Gowon. The lady continued to provide Gowon's needs under the culvert for several days until the hunt for him had died down and there was little risk of his being killed. Gowon then surfaced in the Barracks and survived.

That coup brought Major-General Aguiyi-Ironsi to power. He abolished the Regions and replaced them with Western Group of Provinces, Northern Group of Provinces, Eastern Group of Provinces and Mid-Western Group of Provinces. (During the politicians' rule from Independence Day in October 1966, a fourth Region, the Mid-Western Region had been created out of the former Western Region.) Dissatisfaction in Northern Nigeria with his Government and policies was palpable every where. As a student, the author listened to other students discussing the pros and cons of where the General should be killed in retaliation for the January coup that targeted politicians and soldiers from the North.

General Aguiyi-Ironsi went on a tour of the different Groups of Provinces in the country around June/July 1966. While he was in the North, the author heard from other students that it had been decided to leave him in peace while he was in the North but that he would be assassinated in Ibadan when he would be touring the Western Group of Provinces. At the same time, less open but definitely not secret conversations were going around about the plan to involve civilians in paying back the Ibos for the January massacre of Northerners during the coup. The author was dazed about all that was going on, the lack of respect or regard for human life especially by soldiers and what the future for his country was. He would ponder over these issues for days on end, and that is why he still remembers the events up till today.

Just as students had been discussing at St. Paul's College Zaria for the author with poor hearing to hear, General Aguiyi-Ironsi left the North for the Western Group of Provinces where he was hosted by one Colonel Fajuyi, the Governor of the Western Group of Provinces. Both officers were kidnapped there and have never been seen alive up till today. For five days or so, Nigeria had no Head of State. Eventually, it was announced that Lt Colonel Yakubu Gowon had been appointed the Head of State at the age of 32. Shortly afterwards, there were mass civilian reprisal attacks on Ibos in many parts of Northern Nigeria. Many were killed. Civilian murder gangs went about hunting for Ibos. Many such gangs came to St. Paul's College hunting for Ibos that had fled and come to the College for safety. The College did its best to keep them alive and away from the murderous gangs until they were put on trains to take them south to their own Region. We later learnt at the College that some made it safely but that some lost their lives on the way to the same marauders.

One Colonel Chukwuemeka Odumegwu Ojukwu (he is still alive) was the Governor of the Eastern Group of Provinces then. He refused to accept Gowon's leadership and was daily steering his Region towards secession from the rest of the country. It was under this political instability that the author took his HSC exams in December 1966. Before leaving St. Paul's College, he had routinely completed all the necessary forms for the College to forward to both the University of Ibadan and the University of Lagos for possible admission to study Medicine. He had also completed the application form for Northern Nigerian Scholarship for University studies. All the Upper Six students from the North completed the Scholarship form before leaving the College.

Barclays Bank DCO (Dominion Colonial Overseas) had employed him as a Bank Clerk before he even started his HSC exams. The appointment followed written and oral examinations the bank had conducted on Upper Six and Form V students. Many jobs abounded then because the Ibos had fled and abandoned their jobs of course. While the author was sitting for his last paper, the Bank, after prior agreement with the College authorities, had sent its bus to collect those it had employed! The Bank started paying them that same day. The author was successfully trained by the Bank at Kaduna for about two weeks. After that training, the author was posted to the Bank's Branch at Makurdi (7 43N, 8 28E), the capital of Benue Province in Northern Nigeria. The author arrived in Makurdi on January 1, 1967 to begin his life as a bank clerk.

In the next chapter, the author would tell readers about the next phase of his life before he gained admission to study Medicine in October 1967.

Conclusion

To the author, dealing with an unconventional virus like HIV meant thinking of unconventional approaches for its vaccine development. After all, when a virus is smart enough to transcribe nucleic acids reversely, one may as well think of reverse methods of developing effective vaccines against it. Is it not said that when one is in Rome, he should behave like the Romans? In the next chapter, the author will narrate how he battled to proceed along his reverse approach.

Chapter XXIII

Establishment Beyond Reasonable Doubt of the Safety of the Author's Candidate HIV Therapeutic Vaccine

Abstract

The author has covered some ground in his quest, after changing gears to reverse, for a saeHIV therapeutic vaccine. He had designed what he hoped and expected would be an appropriate immunogen, studied it theoretically and concluded that it ought to be safe. The problem though was that many times, there might be a world of difference between expectation and what eventually happens. He decided he would have to carry out a human trial at least to confirm the safety. Since he had opted to try to develop an autogenous HIV therapeutic vaccine first, he was still far away from efficacy trials of any sort. He needed to confirm the safety of the methodology he had chosen. This chapter tells the reader how he went about it and his reasons for so doing.

Introduction

Basically, the author had decided on an autogenous HIV therapeutic vaccine approach first. That approach was his best option with the numerous handicaps he faced. If it proved to be safe, then he could readily look for willing HIV-infected persons to assess the efficacy of the approach. He would not be exposing such persons to any danger since he would be giving them their own blood that had been processed into, hopefully, an effective therapeutic vaccine. At the end of the process he had worked out, his final product, the vaccine would be just pure human blood extract. The administration of an autogenous blood extract is devoid of any danger to the recipient of the product.

More Details of the Candidate HIV Therapeutic Vaccine

After several months of further and extensive intellectual exercise and self criticism, the author selected a method that he believed would give him an effective immunogen for an autogenous HIV therapeutic vaccine. In processing the blood sample into a vaccine, he had to come out with a final product that is just pure human blood product, i.e. the only additive to the blood should be the CPD-A anticoagulant used universally in collecting human blood used either for whole blood transfusion or for the preparation of human blood components.

Since his candidate HIV therapeutic vaccine would eventually come from the blood of HIV-infected persons, the blood sample that would be processed into the candidate vaccine would naturally contain live and infective HIV. After processing the raw material, it would be necessary for him to inactivate the HIV in the blood without using chemicals.

The non-chemical method the author chose to use for inactivating the HIV in the final product was one of the already established physical means for HIV inactivation. The author knew about this method during the 1969/70 academic year when he was in the third year of medical school. It was during Microbiology lessons that they were taught about the physical methods used to sterilize autogenous bacterial vaccines. If he used any chemical for inactivating the HIV, he would no longer have pure human blood extract. If he could achieve these objectives, he would not need to register such a candidate vaccine with any regulatory body before human administration.

The author's further and repeated criticisms over several months of his proposed approach convinced him that the methodology he had conceived should be safe. But that was obviously not enough. He had to confirm its presumed safety beyond reasonable doubt. Simultaneously, he had to bear in mind that time was of the essence since many infected persons were dying daily in his country and elsewhere. He therefore decided to use himself for the needed safety confirmation. The author did not, and still does not see anything unethical about his decision to carry out the safety trial on himself particularly when his approach did not involve asking anybody to physically assist him in the experimentation. After all, the *Nuremberg Code (1947)* says:

> "No experiment should be conducted where there is a priori reason to believe that death or disabling injury will occur, except perhaps in those experiments where the experimental physicians also serve as subjects"

Safety of the Candidate Autogenous HIV Therapeutic Vaccine Is Confirmed

The author knows that rabies vaccines used in man are usually therapeutic vaccines given over a period of 14–30 days (depending on the type of vaccine one is using) to persons bitten by rabid or suspected rabid animals. He therefore decided empirically that if the method he had chosen eventually reached the stage of testing its efficacy on HIV-infected persons, the dosage regimen would consist of initial daily outpatient injections for thirty days followed by monthly boosters.

He began the safety experimentation on himself on January 1, 1996. He took twenty millilitres of his peripheral venous blood, processed it exactly as he had designed for the candidate therapeutic vaccine he had conceived, and injected himself with the product using the intradermal, subcutaneous, intramuscular and intravenous routes every time. He continued the daily injections until the end of March 1996, a period of ninety-one days. The author arbitrarily decided that a dose of his vaccine would be the final product he obtained from 20 mls of his peripheral venous blood.

Over that period of ninety-one days therefore, he had had 364 jabs to take the ninety-one 'doses' since he used four injection routes each day for each dose. While taking these injections, he watched for any symptoms or signs of toxicity. He also carried out weekly haematological examinations (full blood count with reticulocyte counts and ESR) and renal and hepatic function tests. He did not observe any evidence of toxicity.

For the next eighteen months (April 1996 to the end of September 1997), he reduced the dose to once a week but still using the four injection routes every time. During those eighteen months, he had received an additional seventy-eight weekly 'doses' through 312 injections. He still did not have any evidence of toxicity. He stopped at that point, convinced that the method was indeed very safe for the 91 + 78, i.e. 169 'doses' he had taken continuously over twenty-one calendar months. If there were to be any toxicity, he expected that such toxicity should have been enhanced or amplified by his taking the 169 doses over the compressed period of just twenty-one months.

If he went ahead and gave the treatment by daily intramuscular injection for the first thirty days to HIV-infected patients followed by monthly boosters, it would take 140 months (eleven years and eight months) for any patient to take the 169 doses he had taken. He felt, and still feels that a new candidate autogenous HIV therapeutic vaccine with an established safety for a period of eleven years and eight months was good enough for HIV infection that takes, on the average, ten years to progress to AIDS.

He was very satisfied that he had a candidate HIV vaccine recipe whose safety he had established beyond reasonable doubt. After taking stock of his approach to that point, he was satisfied that the time had come for him to embark on efficacy trials of the very safe candidate vaccine in willing HIV-infected persons.

Nine Months as a Bank Clerk

Since it was the dry cold harmattan season, January 1967 was quite cold in Makurdi, though not as cold as in other parts of the Middle Belt because the town lies on the banks of River Benue, Nigeria's second biggest river. The Barclays Bank in which the author worked as a Clerk for the next nine months was the only bank within a 150-200 mile radius. It was therefore a busy branch. Like all the other institutions in Nigeria then, the Branch Manager and the Accountant were Britons.

Jeremiah enjoyed the work in the bank very much but the hours of work were demanding. It was open to the public six days a week. Sometimes, the work would not allow the Clerks to close until 11.30 p.m. Around March 1967, Jeremiah received his Higher School Certificate (HSC) results. At the advanced level, he had scored grades B, A and E in

Physics, Chemistry and Zoology respectively. He had also passed the General Paper. He was happy because he had scored an average of better than C for the three subjects. With that, it was almost certain that he would be offered admission to both Ibadan and Lagos Universities to study Medicine. He forwarded his results to them, and awaited their decision on his application.

Meanwhile, the Northern Region's Scholarship Board arranged an interview at far away Kaduna for all its students wishing to enter the Universities in the 1967/68 academic year. With the Bank's reluctant permission, he went to Kaduna for the exercise. There, the Board told all the students wishing to study Medicine and who had qualified for admission to forget about going to Ibadan or Lagos. They announced to them that ABU Zaria would start its Faculty of Medicine in October that year. Those involved like Jeremiah were shocked because none of them had applied to ABU. The Board told them not to worry because they would take care of all that at the interview.

Apparently using a copy of the HSC master result for the whole Region, the Board identified those that had qualified for admission to ABU's new Faculty of Medicine, called them out and gave each of them ABU's application form to complete there and then. Jeremiah along with the others did so. When Jeremiah went in for the oral interview, he was first of all given his copy of ABU's Admission letter to study Medicine for five years starting in October 1967. Neither Ibadan nor Lagos had issued any letters of Admissions at that time. The Board agreed that Jeremiah would be given admission to study Medicine but only at ABU Zaria. Jeremiah and the other students from the North that qualified for University Admission that year received their Scholarship letters at the interview, unlike in the past when it would take the Board some time to issue such letters. Those students that requested to be considered to go and study Medicine at Ibadan or Lagos were told point blank that the Board would consider their wish only if they produced their Admission letters from those Universities. Of course, they could not produce any such letters. The political developments in the country a few weeks later meant that Jeremiah's batch would be the last students to be sponsored by Northern Nigeria as a geopolitical entity.

Back in Makurdi, the British Manager and Accountant at the Bank called Jeremiah and advised him to take to Banking as a career, telling him that whoever went to study Medicine for five years as he planned to do would "never meet you in life". The chap from the local settlement of Ajiolo did not have enough general knowledge then to understand the Britons. Besides, the boy had to do Medicine in order to be a surgeon to satisfy his dad. Anyway, he continued to enjoy his work at the Bank.

The political crisis in Nigeria under General Yakubu Gowon (he had been promoted from Lt Colonel to General shortly after being made the Head of State) continued to escalate with Colonel Chukwuemeka Odumegwu Ojukwu in Eastern Region threatening secession. Suddenly, the Federal Government announced in May 1967 that it had abolished Regions or Groups of Provinces and had created just twelve States, six from the former Northern Region and six from the other three Regions. Two States were created out of the former Western Region, three from the former Eastern Region and the former Mid-Western Region became a State. A few days later, Ojukwu announced the secession of the former Eastern Region from Nigeria; he called his new country Biafra. The secession led to a civil war that raged from then till 1970.

The political crisis caused the Bank at Makurdi to lose the services of its female typist who came from the Eastern Region even though she was not Ibo by tribe. She fled to her Province out of fear for her life in the North. That caused trouble for the Bank. There were no typists available for employment. The Manager and the Accountant immediately summoned all the six Clerks and told them about the crisis. They then asked the clerks to choose one from among themselves who would have to go and learn typing within a week and return to duty combining typing with other clerical duties at the Bank as circumstances dictated.

All the clerks were aware of the heavy typing work that the lady had been doing before she ran away for dear life, and as such they could not get any one to agree to going to learn typing. The following morning when the Branch Manager and the Accountant enquired from the clerks, they were not surprised that none of the clerks had volunteered for the job. The Manager said laughingly. "All of you are running away from the heavy typing duties, eh? Don't worry. The Accountant and I will think about it and let you know in a few minutes our choice for the job."

The clerks waited anxiously for their decision. After a few minutes indeed, they called the Clerks to tell them their decision. Jeremiah had been chosen to get off work immediately, and return a week later to start typing the backlog of letters. A miserable and dejected Jeremiah had to leave the Bank immediately. Even though he had been offered the use of the Bank's typewriter, he did not take it away, promising the Manager and Accountant that he would come back for it after he would have got somewhere to learn the typing. They agreed.

He went right away to the General Hospital in misery to tell his friend Mr. Andrew Adaji what had befallen him. Andrew was then the Hospital's Chief Clerk and was good at typing. Andrew changed Jeremiah's misery and dejection to joy, telling Jeremiah that he was very lucky to have been selected because he would never regret for the rest of his life for learning how to type. Moreover, he told Jeremiah that he was certain that he would be able to start typing well within 48 hours and therefore, the seven days the Bank had given him was much too long. He therefore told Jeremiah to shock the Bank by returning to work three days later at the latest and start typing the backlog. Jeremiah changed to a happy mood and was ready to start learning.

Andrew immediately made a typewriter available to Jeremiah and told him the functions of the different keys on the board. He then taught him which keys are for the different fingers. After some minutes for Jeremiah to learn the keys for each finger, practice started.

In less than 24 hours, Jeremiah started typing slowly without looking at the keyboard. With Andrew constantly encouraging him and teaching him useful tips when typing, Jeremiah was happy and satisfied with his progress after 48 hours. Andrew told him to report at work after 72 hours so as to give the Manager some pleasant surprise.

When the Manager and the Accountant saw Jeremiah in the Bank on the third day after they had asked him to take a week off and learn typing, they were cross with him for showing his face. After venting their anger and disappointment, they asked the chap why he had come back. Jeremiah told them he had finished his learning. They looked at each other in bewilderment. They gave him a letter to type for a test. They were delighted that he had done it without any mistake. "We knew we made the correct choice!" said the elated Manager.

Jeremiah happily and enjoyably combined clerical banking duties with typing as and when required. The Manager and the Accountant kept trying to convince him to make a career out of banking, but Jeremiah just could not because of his dad's wishes.

In mid-September 1967, he ended his banking career when the resignation notice he had given expired. He had to leave then so that he would do the two weeks orientation for fresh students at ABU Zaria. Jeremiah was again going to be in another class that would be the first set in the University's Faculty of Medicine! The author intends to let the reader know how he faired at ABU Zaria for five years in order to qualify as a doctor.

Conclusion

The author had conceived a candidate autogenous HIV therapeutic vaccine that was just pure human blood product. On theoretical grounds, that candidate vaccine ought to be safe. The author however, did not want to depend on any presumed safety. Over a period of twenty-one months, he subjected himself to his autogenous recipe, taking the finished product each time through four different parental routes. The dosage he took over twenty-one months would take an HIV-infected person 140 months to receive. The author did not observe any toxic effects of the autogenous recipe. Of course, the author was on a secret assignment, so he kept his work to himself. It was known only to members of his family. He was ready to move on to the next stage of efficacy trials of the candidate autogenous HIV therapeutic vaccine on HIV-infected persons with their informed and written consent.

Chapter XXIV

Efficacy Assessment of the Author's Safe Autogenous Candidate HIV Therapeutic Vaccine

Abstract

Working at that time with only the Physician's Oath to guide him, the author decided that the time had come for him to look for willing HIV-infected persons to undergo the definitely safe autogenous HIV therapeutic remedy he had developed. That would be the best, fastest and most convenient method for him to assess the efficacy of his remedy. Would he need controls? He decided that there was absolutely no need for any controls of any kind or description. HIV infection had been established as incurable. If he succeeded in curing even one single case of HIV infection with his safe autogenous therapeutic remedy, he would have achieved what had not been achieved before, and he would be in a position to build on it in order to get an HIV preventive vaccine for himself. This short chapter deals with the initial findings of the efficacy trials of the author's autogenous HIV therapeutic remedy.

Introduction

The author had made some progress on his self-imposed but secret assignment. He had confirmed beyond reasonable doubt that his autogenous candidate HIV therapeutic remedy was safe. He had then reached the important stage of testing the safe remedy on willing HIV-infected persons. He was not sure the remedy would be efficacious, and as such he did not consider it proper to ask the patients willing to take the remedy to pay anything at that stage. Since he was dealing with a very chronic infection, he did not expect any quick results from the efficacy trial, and he told the patients so. He would have to meticulously follow their symptoms and signs for any changes as those might be likely pointers to the usefulness or or worthlessness or otherwise of the remedy.

Efficacy Trials of the Author's Safe Autogenous Candidate HIV Therapeutic Vaccine

The author started the efficacy trial on willing HIV-infected persons with their informed and written consent in October 1997. The remedy was an autogenous extract of each patient's own blood. Each person received a daily 'dose' of the remedy by deep intramuscular injection for a month followed by monthly boosters of a 'dose'. The reader may wish to read Chapter 23 again for more details of the dose and dosage regimen.

Clinical Effects of the Candidate Therapy

The author was very pleased with the effects of the vaccine on his patients' health, their well-being, symptoms and signs. There was rapid improvement in the symptoms of many patients within days of commencement of therapy. Weight that had been lost was regained rapidly. Health and vitality were rapidly restored. Skin lesions like recurrent carbuncles and itching that were common in some of them disappeared rapidly with the treatment. Anorexia, oral leukoplakia, vaginal discharge, thrush (oral, oesophageal or vaginal), diarrhoea and hyperpigmentation of fingernails, where present, responded rapidly in many cases to the therapy /vaccinations combined, as necessary, with specific chemotherapeutic agents.

'Dirty lung' appearances reported by radiologists on chest radiographs responded to the vaccinations with radiological evidence of improvement within a few weeks of therapy. Severe anaemia was treated by blood transfusions that were usually carried out by other clinicians looking after the patient since his therapy was an outpatient procedure. Any other identified and treatable disease was aggressively managed. In many cases also, initial (pre-treatment) blood pictures of abnormal morphology of erythrocytes and leucocytes especially atypical lymphocytes reverted to normal rapidly with therapy while elevated pre-treatment ESR fell drastically with therapy.

As the author had expected from the extensive and intense safety experimentation he had carried out on himself, there were no cases of any significant adverse reactions or side effects. Of course, there was some discomfort from the jabs just as happens with all injections given without anaesthesia.

The Author in Medical School

The author was one of the forty-six students admitted by the Ahmadu Bello University in Zaria to start its Faculty of Medicine in October 1967. The Vice-Chancellor of that University throughout the five years the author spent there was Prof. Ishaya Audu, a Paediatrician.

Being the first set of medical students, the author's class had to dissect the cadavers used for Anatomy. It was a unique experience that most medical students in all parts of the world do not have. Virtually all the lecturers that taught the author in Medical School were non-Nigerians, expatriates from various countries with British nationals forming the overwhelming majority. The reader may wish to look again at the Table in Chapter 19 that shows the names and nationalities of his University lecturers that he recollected from memory in 2008.

The author's Northern Nigeria Scholarship was able to meet all his needs in the Medical School. The reader may recall that the author was in the last batch of students to enjoy that Scholarship because General Gowon had abolished Regions in May 1967. If the author had been even a year behind, he would have had to depend on his new State's Scholarship for his medical training. His elder brother Tom got such a Scholarship to study Mechanical Engineering at ABU in October 1968. Tom abandoned the study because he could not see how he would be able to cope with the meagre Scholarship. Instead, he went and trained as an Air Traffic Controller at the School of Aviation in Zaria.

When Jeremiah looked back over his circumstances, he was particularly grateful to his father for forcing him to skip Primary 7 when he instructed him against his wish to take the Ochaja Secondary School entrance examination from Primary 6; when Jeremiah was admitted into that School, his father also insisted the boy had to go there. That paved the way for the golden opportunity Jeremiah had there of skipping Form 2. If he had missed any of these opportunities, he would have missed the Northern Nigeria Scholarship, and would subsequently have found it extremely difficult, if not impossible, to study Medicine. Jeremiah knows many University graduates who lost their lives during the compulsory NYSC that General Gowon introduced in 1973. Jeremiah just missed the Scheme. That was some luck for him, too, because the allowance given to graduates during the NYSC was, and still is, pea nuts.

Nigeria was involved in a civil war until 1970. Nigeria's bachelor Head of State General Yakubu Gowon eventually got married to one Victoria Zakari in 1970. Every one heard that it took many years before Gowon married because he had a terrible dilemma. It was said that he wanted to marry the Ibo lady who saved his life in January 1966 when the first coup took place. In fact, it was said that the lady had born him a child. Unfortunately for Gowon, he had become Nigeria's Head of State and Nigeria was fighting a civil war with the lady's Ibo tribe. Under these circumstances, Gowon was advised to forget about marrying the Ibo lady because the leader of any country at war would never be allowed to marry a lady from the enemy camp. The author knew all this just like all his colleagues in Nigeria's universities then.

At the beginning of his clinical years as a medical student in October 1969, a cholera epidemic raged in Northern Nigeria, affecting Zaria and its environs. There were so many cases that the 'new' Teaching Hospital in Tudun Wada, Zaria could not cope with the number of cases. Actually, the former General Hospital at Tudun Wada, Zaria had been renovated and upgraded to become the Teaching Hospital for the two-year old Faculty of Medicine of Ahmadu Bello University. With lightening speed, the authorities decided to use the Infectious Disease Hospital located about a kilometre from the Teaching Hospital for treating the numerous cases of cholera that continued to pour in. There was shortage of manpower to handle the epidemic.

One of the measures worked out by the authorities was to immediately teach the first batch of clinical students how to set up life-saving IV lines, and to administer and monitor IV fluids in cholera victims. Duty rosters were quickly worked out for the 29 pioneer medical students to provide 24 hours coverage seven days a week for the cholera epidemic. The author was one of these pioneer medical students that took part in the ad hoc arrangements to handle the epidemic.

Suddenly, the Hospital ran out of IV fluids: normal saline, Darrow's solution and Dextrose solution. Of course, it was impossible to effectively manage a cholera epidemic without these life-saving intravenous remedies. As medical students, we were highly worried. A solution was worked out overnight, so to say.

Some of our British lecturers in Medicine put their heads together and started producing IV fluids in the garage of one of them. Like the medical students then, most of the lecturers were staying in the University staff quarters in the University's Institute of Administration campus located in Kongo area of Tudun Wada (the medical students were also staying in the students' hostels at the campus). The Kongo campus was just about 3 kilometres from the Teaching Hospital by road but there were shorter routes by foot.

The author's recollection is that these IV fluids were prepared by Drs. Anthony Bryceson, David Warrell and Brian Greenwood overnight in the garage and brought down every morning for use on the patients. Using their personal cars every morning, they would bring down enough supplies of IV fluids to last till the following morning. As medical students, we wondered about the source of these morning supplies of 'manna from heaven'. The author recalls vividly the explanation from Dr. Bryceson, then a Senior Lecturer in Medicine. We arranged to go to the garage to see for ourselves the production outfit for these IV fluids. We were impressed with the ingenuity of these lecturers, and tried to learn as much as we could from the solution they had worked out.

Consequently, the mortality from that cholera epidemic was very low. The IV fluids from Kongo were not registered with any drug-regulatory body. They were fluids produced under a dire emergency to save lives endangered by the cholera epidemic. The author later recalled this episode when he learnt a few years later that a missionary doctor some where in the West Indies used the fluid in immature coconut fruits as source of IV fluids to save human lives endangered by dehydration! The coconut fluid did not require any form of sterilization; it was not registered with any drug regulatory body but it saved many lives too!

When the cholera epidemic abated, these lecturers continued working in their garage and eventually turned it into an immunology research unit with funds they told us they had received from the Medical Research Council in Britain.

The first set of forty-six medical students that started ABU's Faculty of Medicine in October 1967 graduated in June 1972, but only twenty-nine of them made the course in the regulation time of five years. Fortunately for the local boy from Ajiolo, Jeremiah was one of the twenty-nine who graduated.

At the author's Convocation at the Ahmadu Bello University in Zaria in October 1972, General Gowon announced to the country that his Government would start a National Youth Service Corps for all University graduates, and that the graduates of the 1972/73 academic year would be the first to kick off the Scheme.

Conclusion

In the efficacy trials of the safe autogenous candidate therapeutic HIV remedy the author had conceived and developed, the remedy had promising clinical effects on the symptoms and signs that patients had before receiving the remedy. Would that be the best the remedy would achieve? Find out in the next chapter.

Section V: The Birth and Infancy of Safe and Effective HIV Vaccines (1999)

Chapter XXV

The Initial Efficacy Results of the Author's Safe Candidate HIV Therapeutic Vaccine

Abstract

In this challenging hobby that the author embarked upon at the beginning of 1992, he had no idea where it would lead him to or what should mark the end of the journey. He embarked on the adventure in the hope that he would be able to develop a preventive vaccine that he would take. It was along the route that he discovered that the circumstances dictated he reverse gears and tackle the therapeutic vaccine first. He had observed the rapid improvement the remedy produced in the presenting symptoms and signs of some of the patients, but that of course might not mean much. Would he ever be able to get any of them to reverse to HIV antibody negative status? That would be the great news to him and the world at large because such a development would mean that HIV-infection had become curable; it would no longer be uniformly fatal, and the stigmatization and ostracization of HIV-infected persons would start a rapid plunge in the journey toward extinction or annihilation.

Introduction

In the last Chapter, the author reported that his safe autogenous candidate HIV therapeutic vaccine had caused rapid improvement in the symptoms and signs of the recipients. Unfortunately, the author practises medicine in a third world country where most patients have no regard for their health, and as such do not keep medical appointments. In addition, most patients would just disappear as soon as their presenting symptoms disappear. Almost everyone knows that HIV, being incurable and fatal is greatly stigmatized. Those who are HIV-infected do not wish to let anyone know of their positive status. Ironically, patients' disregard for medical appointments in the author's country is more pronounced if the medical management being given to the patient is free. The author thinks that the combination of these factors was responsible for the failure of many patients to keep their follow-up appointments. This chapter deals with the initial efficacy results that the author eventually got.

The Tidings of 28 December 1998

The author had continued his efficacy trials on the few willing patients who had chosen to take the author's candidate HIV therapeutic vaccine. Many on whom he was planning to do 6-monthly HIV screening tests had been lost to follow-up. The GSM was not available in the author's country then. Most of the patients in the author's country have no address that one would be able to locate readily. Many, too, gave fictitious names and addresses. The author had at his own expense of course, travelled to several of the addresses he had been given only to find that they were fictitious addresses, probably given out of fear of stigmatization and ostracization if it were to be known in their vicinity that they were HIV-positive.

One of the early persons to undergo the efficacy trial started taking the remedy in December 1997. Three HIV screening tests from two different laboratories had been positive, and the patient had bilateral cervical and axillary lymphadenopathy. He had come to see the author because he was worried about his recent febrile illness that failed to respond to antimalarials and antibiotics. He agreed to undergo HIV screening using a pseudonym. The result was positive. Another sample from him was sent to that same laboratory under a different pseudonym; it was again positive. A third sample using a pseudonym was sent to a different laboratory for HIV screening; it was also positive. Western Blot and other HIV antibody confirmation kits were then not available in the vicinity where the author was practising. After these three positive results, the man agreed to take part in the author's efficacy trial using the author's innovative autogenous vaccine.

The point of this story is the following. The patient explained that he would not be able to take the remedy in the daytime. Instead, he pleaded with the author to treat him between 3 a.m. and 6 a.m. every night to avoid prying eyes. The author agreed. Throughout the 1997 Christmas and 1998 New Year nights, the author would get up at 2 a.m., prepare his things ready for the man who promptly appeared at 3 a.m. and process the man's blood for the autogenous product. The author usually finished with the patient around 5.30 a.m.

After a few days, the patient's children had noticed that their daddy went out every night around midnight. They confronted their dad what the problem was. He could not tell them, but as a compromise he told them he was seeing the author for medical attention every night that he went out. The patient alerted me about his children's enquiries. Soon after, two of his children came to find out from the author what the problem with their dad was. Fortunately for their dad, the author was doing this exercise secretly, so people did not know. As the author is a surgeon, the children were worried that perhaps he was planning to operate on their dad. The author told the children that he was monitoring some things in their father every night for a month in the hope that his observations would assist him in reaching a diagnosis. They were satisfied and left. At the end, that patient ended up well and cured even though he too failed to keep to his follow-up appointments regularly.

Four patients who had received the author's autogenous remedy but who had been lost to follow-up came one by one on different days to see the author at his Clinic in December 1998. They all said they had come to thank the author for the treatment they had received. When the author asked them why they failed to keep their appointments, they said they felt so well that they did not consider it necessary to come and bother him any longer! Anyway, they agreed to the author taking their blood samples for HIV screening. They author separated their serum and kept them frozen. When he realized that he had the serum samples of four such patients, he sent the samples on 28 December 1998 for HIV screening at his expense of course.

Before they started taking the remedy, that laboratory had performed their HIV screening tests and reported that they were HIV seropositive. The four samples that the author sent for HIV screening on 28 December 1998 all tested negative. The author's joy at this development was indescribable. His family joined him to celebrate into the New Year. The author's family naively told him the world would be extremely happy at the development.

Did the Tidings Carry Good or Bad Omen?

The author told them that the contrary would likely be his reward and portion, that in history such discoveries have never received the sort of treatment they were thinking about. He reminded them about Edward Jenner and his smallpox vaccine, about Louis Pasteur and his rabies vaccine, about the Wright brothers and their aeroplane, and about Einstein and his Theories of Relativity. The author told them that even though all these discoverers were whites born and brought up in their countries, the experts in their days received and welcomed them not.

He therefore asked them to imagine what his lot would likely be, an unknown Nigerian black surgeon practising in a developing country that had used only his family's resources to successfully develop a safe and effective therapeutic vaccine against HIV that the experts of the day have already declared incurable and invariably fatal. Hmm! The author told his shocked family that if he did not proceed carefully and cautiously, the development might cost him his life in record time. His family severely chided him for his pessimism. The author would not allow his family's optimism to becloud his sense of reasoning. He told them that time would tell who was correct.

Conclusion

December 28, 1998 brought great tidings of joy and fulfilment for the author's labour of seven years. On that day, he had negative HIV screening results on the serum samples of four of his patients that had undergone his innovative, safe and autogenous candidate HIV therapeutic vaccine. The author and his family celebrated the development into the first few days of 1999. His family was optimistic that the world would welcome the news heartily. From the lessons of history on new discoveries, however, the author was of a different view. He knew he had to proceed with serious caution and care because the development might cost him his life. After the reader would have gone through the remaining Chapters of this book, he would hopefully be in a reasonable position to adjudicate and decide whether it was the author's family or the author that was correct.

Chapter XXVI

Ask Not What Your Country and the World Can Do for You; Let Them Know What You Have Done for Them

Abstract

What the author had been doing secretly for seven years had, by January 1999, reached a stage where, if he was to make further meaningful progress, he had to try and recruit others especially a reliable and experienced medical laboratory scientist to help him perform critical laboratory tests as he decided to proceed by systematically collecting more data to confirm or refute these unique results from the therapy. The secrecy with which the author had carried out his assignment would have to be abandoned more and more in the days ahead.

He had just had four cases of cured HIV infection but who would believe that tale? When was science reduced to just story telling followed by unquestioning belief? Jeremiah knew he needed to do more work on the matter. He got the services of a laboratory scientist to help him perform necessary tests. He also informed his country's Head of State, and other interested establishments in his country to inform them. He expected to be given further directives or receive some referred HIV-positive patients at least from these sources for treatment so that others would be able to confirm or refute his claims. He was daydreaming because his efforts were not good enough for any response, not even an acknowledgement.

Introduction

The reader may recall that on 28 December 1998, the author was delighted to high heavens to receive a lab report of negative HIV antibody screening result on the four serum samples he had sent. The four samples were taken from four different HIV-positive patients who had received the author's innovative, autogenous HIV therapeutic vaccine. It was a unique family celebration for the author's family, indeed for the unexpected result they had obtained. Could this indeed be an indication that HIV was tameable? The author definitely needed to do more scientific work on the development.

After the celebrations, Jeremiah took stock of the situation objectively, and reached the conclusion that very serious and formidable problems and dangers indeed lay ahead. He informed his family of them including the risk to his life if he did not handle the matter with caution and maturity. His family did not see things as he did then.

Fully aware of the dangers, criticisms and antagonism that lay ahead, the author decided to handle the keg of explosive on his hand with great caution. This chapter describes the early steps he took and the outcome.

Involving a Reliable Medical Lab Scientist

First, he went in early January 1999 to visit one Mr. Manason Rubainu (Figures 26-1 to 26-3), the best medical laboratory scientist known to the author in the vicinity. After the usual exchange of pleasantries, the author told the lab scientist about the secret assignment he had been doing since 1992 and the recent result of serodeconversion to HIV negative in four patients who were previously HIV-positive. He asked his friend to join him to carry out further investigations into the matter by performing relevant lab investigations.

The man exploded in fury! In the past, the man and the author had worked together for almost four years in the same hospital. The author was stunned because he had never seen the man in such a mood before. Mr. Manason Rubainu fumed and said something like this: "What are you up to, sir? You think I know nothing about HIV? There is no cure for HIV infection for many reasons that I appreciate and can teach you as a lab scientist? What has a surgeon got to do with HIV vaccine development? Please do not involve me with your 419. How dare you come to me at the beginning of this New Year to do this to me? You may leave my house please."

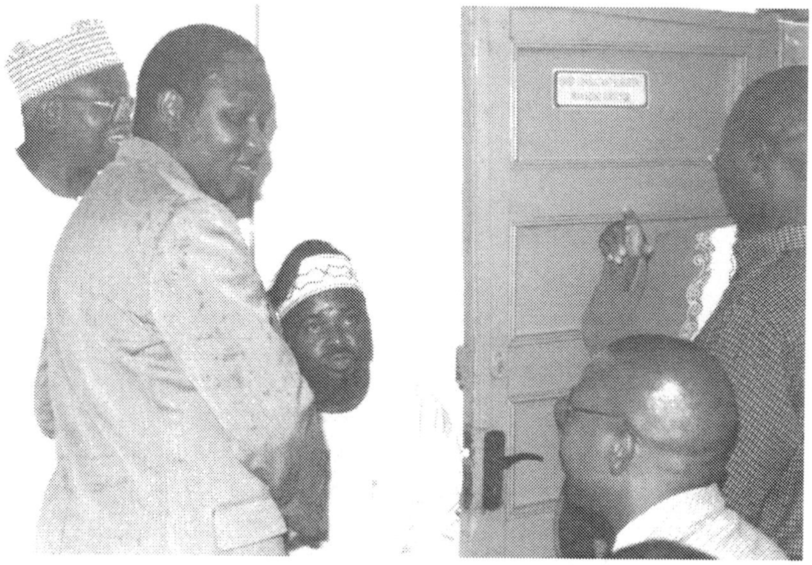

Figure 26-1. Mr. Manason Rubainu (left, foreground) in the author's office during the visit of Miss Nigeria 2000, 15 Jun 2000.

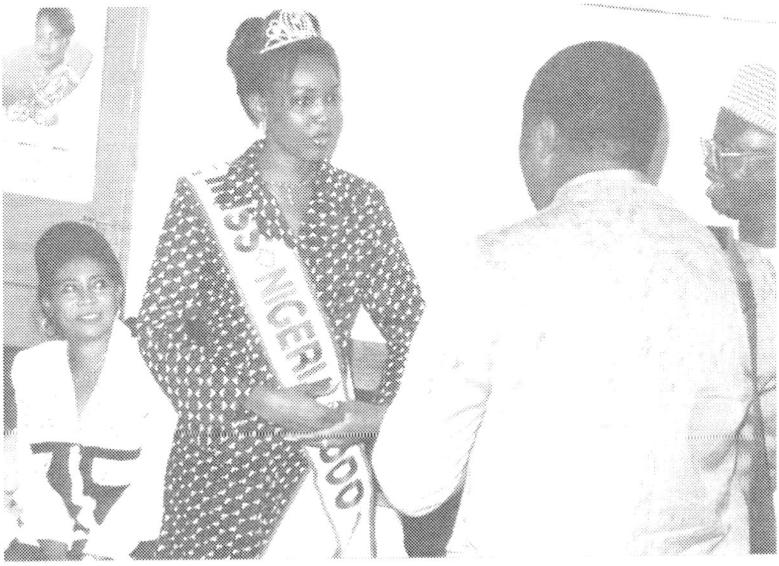

Figure 26-2. Miss Nigeria 2000 speaks with Mr. Manason Rubainu, Chief Medical Laboratory Scientist during her visit to the author's Hospital, 15 Jun 2000.

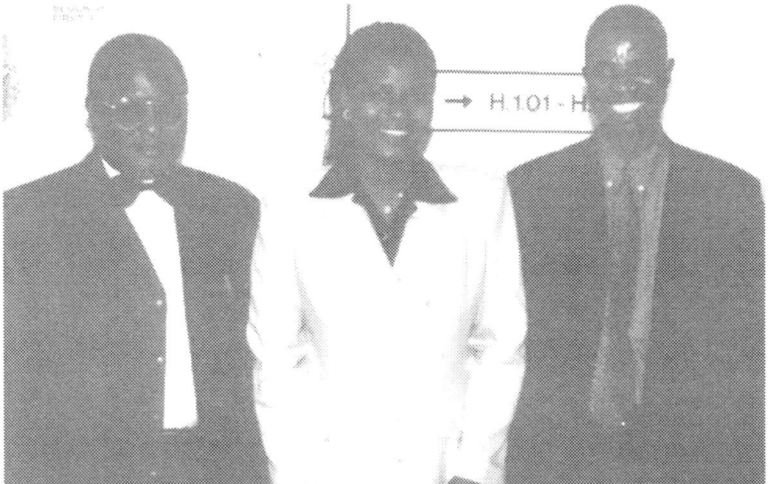

Figure 26-3. From left, Mr. Manason Rubainu Chief medical Laboratory Scientist, Mrs. Shade Aturamu, Medical Laboratory Scientist and the author during the Blood Management Training Programme Workshop at the National Hospital, Abuja, 13 Sep 2000.

The author patiently explained to his friend that he would never be involved in 419, and would never think of involving him in any 419. The author then appealed to his common sense by asking him if he was no longer interested in scientific investigation even if he thought it was 419. Would he not grab the opportunity and investigate to expose the 419? For the benefit of readers who may not know, '419' is used in Nigeria to refer to criminal fraud or deceit. As the author was made to understand, it became popular because there is a section 419 in the country's criminal laws that deals with criminal fraud or deceit.

The man's anger reduced significantly. "Ok, sir. If you are serious on this matter, come back to see me tomorrow", he responded. The author thanked him and left.

On returning home, the author told his family about the development. They were dumbfounded. Anyway, they eventually agreed he should go back to the man the following day. He did.

The following morning, the author was back to see the man in the man's house. Their discussion was more pleasant than the one on the previous day. Eventually, the author convinced his friend to help him perform toxicological and other relevant assays like IgM, IgG, IgA, CD4 counts, and viral load as part of a more thorough scientific study to see if the results he had recorded in December 1998 were indeed reproducible.

That lab scientist has really lived up to the author's expectations. He developed his own private laboratory to a standard that made mockery of the Nigerian Government's so-called 'Centres of Excellence' for HIV research. His Peak Medical Laboratory started performing CD4 counts and viral loads using the quantitative p24 HIV-1 antigen assay, a technique that some claim is more sensitive than the polymerase chain reaction (PCR). Of course, the assays performed by the lab scientist confirmed that the author's HIV therapeutic vaccine was a reality. In August 2008, Mr. Manason Rubainu was elected President of the Association of Medical Laboratory Scientists of Nigeria.

Informing Nigeria's Head of State

Next, the author decided on 3rd February, 1999 to write and inform Nigeria's then Military Head of State General Abdulsalami Abubakar of the development, bearing in mind the political, economic and diplomatic advantages that Nigeria stood to reap from his discovery. The author specifically asked him for whatever directives he deemed necessary on the matter. The author has not received any response till today.

Informing a Physician Colleague

The author was privileged to refer a patient about that time to one Professor John Idoko, a Physician with the Jos University Teaching Hospital, a colleague he had known for several years right from their medical student days when he was a year or two behind the author at the Ahmadu Bello University, Zaria. They had also worked together at that University's Teaching Hospital in Zaria for many years; he was in the Medicine Department while Jeremiah was in the Surgery Department. In the letter that the author wrote referring the patient to him, the author told him of his outpatient HIV therapeutic vaccine breakthrough, and asked him to send some HIV-infected patients to him to enable him to confirm the author's claim. He never responded even though he acknowledged when they met almost a year later that he got the author's letter but regretted he could neither reply nor send him any patient.

Informing the West

The industrialized nations of the world have never hidden the fact that they will always protect their economic interest anywhere in the world. Have they got any economic interests in the quest to develop safe and effective HIV/AIDS vaccines?

They author had no doubt in his mind that they definitely had, and still have huge financial interests in the matter. Since the global race for HIV vaccines began in April 1984, Britain, France and the United States invest at least millions of US dollars each year on HIV/AIDS vaccine research. Since 1984 when the Americans announced that they had isolated the virus that caused AIDS, these three super powers alone had, by 1999, invested at least 180 billion dollars in HIV/AIDS vaccine research.

Furthermore, the author had heard that these three countries have a gentleman's agreement among themselves that irrespective of whichever of their researchers first developed the elusive vaccine, the other two would partake in sharing the economic benefits of the discovery. The author could see that the agreement was a plausible development.

The author reminded himself that it took three years — and the intercession of the French and U.S. Presidents — to smooth the ruffled scientific feathers and work out a settlement in which the two researchers, Dr. Robert Gallo (American) and Dr. Luc Montagnier (French), call themselves co-discoverers of the virus that causes AIDS and shared the profits of the blood tests for the HIV that were developed after the isolation of the virus! The profits were shared between the United States Human and Health Services Department and Luc Montagnier's Pasteur Institute in Paris. This 1987 agreement was announced at a ceremony at the White House attended by then US president Ronald Reagan.

The author found it more interesting because these two superpowers, the US and France, have been allies for several centuries, yet they dragged themselves to court for three years in a bitter dispute over the issue of who first isolated the virus that caused AIDS! Naturally, would they not be prepared and very willing to do worse to any person who dared to proclaim he had developed the elusive HIV vaccine for the deadly virus that is responsible for the worst pandemic so far in the history of man's occupation of this terrestrial ball, especially if such a development emanated from a nonentity from the third world? The author's answer was in the affirmative.

The author later knew that the West was likely instrumental in fashioning out the UNAIDS guidelines on HIV preventive vaccine research. The West likely used its great influence in the United Nations to produce the UNAIDS guidelines. One of the guidelines makes it clear that only sponsor countries in the developed world may conceive and manufacture HIV candidate vaccines for trial in the developing countries.

Anyway, a prepublication version of that document was faxed to Nigeria in March 2000 when UNAIDS Executive Director Dr. Peter Piot (he is from Belgium in Western Europe) was visiting Nigeria. The prepublication version was faxed from the Institute of Human Virology (IHV) in Baltimore, Maryland. Readers would likely recall that Robert Gallo is based at that Institute. Ordinarily, would UNAIDS and /or IHV send a prepublication version of any document to Nigeria? They had to do so in this case because UNAIDS and the IHV knew or feared that the author's discovery of HIV vaccines might be genuine, but the economic interest of the Western world must be protected by all means. Why does Jeremiah say UNAIDS and /or IHV knew or feared that his discoveries on HIV vaccines might be real?

As far back as February 25, 1999, he wrote to the British and French Embassies in Nigeria as well as the United States Information Service (USIS) in Nigeria just to inform them he had developed an effective and safe outpatient curative vaccination therapy against the rampaging HIV. On March 3, 1999, he followed the matter up by sending each of them a copy of his Curriculum Vitae (BIODATA) to fully introduce himself to them.

On March 5, 1999, he wrote to the Coordinator of the World Health Organization (WHO) in Nigeria to inform him of his curative HIV vaccines. In that letter, the author concluded in these words,

> "I believe you would be interested in this development, and that you would like to let others know about it so that those who wish may avail themselves of this golden opportunity of ridding themselves of the dreaded HIV infection."

More details are in Chapter 32. There has been no response from the French Embassy, the USIS and the WHO up till today.

When the *Vaccine* Journal published a report of the author's work in September 2004 accompanied by an Editorial, the author sent copies of the published report and the preceding Editorial to several people and Institutions including the British and French Embassies in Nigeria, the USIS in Nigeria and the WHO in Nigeria (see more details in Chapter 48). Neither the British Embassy nor the French Embassy nor the USIS nor the WHO in Nigeria extended even the basic courtesy of an acknowledgement to the author!

Conclusion

Soon after the author's HIV vaccine research efforts yielded four cases of serode conversion to HIV-negative status at the end of 1998, he informed a medical laboratory scientist Mr. Manason Rubainu and succeeded in getting him to help with further and independent laboratory assays on the patients taking his innovative therapy. He also wrote and informed his country's Head of State, and asked for further directives. He never even got an acknowledgement. He also wrote and informed the French and British Embassies in Nigeria, the USIS in Nigeria and the WHO in Nigeria to all of whom he later sent his Curriculum Vitae. The author has not received any response up till today from the French Embassy in Nigeria, the USIS in Nigeria and the WHO in Nigeria. None of the four (British Embassy, French Embassy, USIS and WHO in Nigeria) sent even the basic courtesy of an acknowledgement to the author when in October 2004 the author sent copies of the *Vaccine* Journal's Editorial and the *Vaccine* Journal's publication of a report of the author's HIV vaccines work to each of them.

Chapter XXVII

Informing Other Stakeholders

Abstract

The first months of 1999 showed clearly that the author's safe autogenous HIV therapeutic vaccine was indeed efficacious as confirmed by the lab results from Peak Medical Laboratories (PML) and by the clinical observations on the patients taking the remedy. The author decided to tell many other relevant parties and institutions about the development. In doing this, the author's first consideration, focus and target were the HIV-infected persons. His patient's life and health had always been his first consideration, target and focus since he qualified as a doctor in 1972, and he had no intention on changing it for any reason because he had pledged himself to the Physician's Oath. The lack of response from those he contacted forced the author to think that perhaps all those he had contacted had other issues that were their first consideration, focus and target.

Introduction

One General Olusegun Obasanjo was Nigeria's Military Head of State from February 1976 to 1st October 1976 when he handed power over to a democratically elected President called Alhaji Shehu Shagari. The General retired from the Nigerian Army on the day he handed over power to Alhaji Shehu Shagari.

Around 1994/95, Nigeria's then Military Head of State General Sani Abacha set up a Military Tribunal that tried Retired General Olusegun Obasanjo for coup plotting. Obasanjo was found guilty. Before then, all those found guilty for coup plotting in Nigeria had, without exception, been executed even under Obasanjo's military dictatorship. Because of national and international appeals and pressures however, General Abacha eventually jailed Obasanjo for twenty-five years. While in office, General Abacha died suddenly on a Sunday/Monday night around June 1998, and General Abdulsalami Abubakar came to power. General Abubakar released Obasanjo from jail and granted him a State pardon. Subsequently, he entered the contest for the country's Presidency in the early 1993 elections and won.

In the last chapter, we saw that the author wrote on 3rd February 1999 to Nigeria's Military Head of State, General Abdulsalami Abubakar, about his HIV vaccines but the General did not respond in any way to the author's letter. On 29 May, 1999, a democratically elected government headed by President Olusegun Obasanjo, the retired Military General, came to power in Nigeria.

With the change to democratic rule in Nigeria, did the author do anything about the HIV vaccines he had developed? If he acted, what actions did he take? Before answering these questions in this chapter, the author would like to recall from his memory Nigeria's coups d'état to show the reader that he was of age when the events occurred.

Nigeria's Coups D'état

January 1966 (Author was a Lower Sixth Science student studying for his Advanced Level)

The first Military coup in Nigeria took place. Many politicians and military officers died in that bloody coup that brought Major-General JTU Aguiyi-Ironsi to power.

July 1966

Another very bloody coup took place; many military officers died in that coup. Then Lt Colonel Yakubu Gowon (later promoted General Gowon) became the Military Head of State. During his tenure, Nigeria fought a civil war from 1967 to 1970.

July 1975 (Author was a Registrar in Surgery)

A bloodless military coup ousted General Gowon from power while he was attending the Organization of African Unity (OAU) meeting of Heads of State in Addis Ababa. Gowon was granted asylum by the British Government. While in Britain, General Gowon enrolled for studies there and obtained a Ph.D in Political Science. Meanwhile, the coup that removed him from power brought General Murtala Muhammed to power with then Lt. General Olusegun Obasanjo as his Chief of Staff, Supreme Headquarters. In that capacity, Obasanjo was next in command to Murtala Muhammed.

February 1976

A failed but bloody attempted coup led by one Lt. Colonel Bukar Suka Dimka on Friday 13 February 1976 killed General Murtala Muhammed, but Lt General Olusegun Obasanjo who escaped unhurt took over the leadership of the country "much against my personal wish and desire". All the many military officers and some civilians who were found guilty by a Military Tribunal in the attempted coup were publicly executed by firing squads. Retired

General Gowon was said to be involved in that coup. Obasanjo's Government desperately sought his extradition from Britain for trial but Britain refused.

December 1983

A military coup ended the civilian (elected) Government of President Shehu Shagari to whom Obasanjo had handed over on 1st October 1979. One Brigadier Bako was said to be the only casualty in that coup that brought Major General Muhammed Buhari to power.

August 1985

A bloodless palace coup by then Major General Ibrahim Badamosi Babangida removed Buhari from power. Babangida took over. After annulling the Presidential election held on June 12, 1993, Babangida stepped aside and handed the Government to his handpicked lame-duck civilian Ernest Shonekan who headed an Interim National Government.

December 1993

General Sani Abacha kicked out the Interim National Government of Earnest Shonekan and took over the Government late in 1993. In 1994/95, General Abacha tried Retired General Olusegun Obasanjo and others for an attempted coup. Obasanjo and some others were found guilty. Abacha considered national and international appeals for leniency for the convicted coup plotters, and sentenced all those involved to various terms of imprisonment. Obasanjo was jailed for 25 years. That was the first time in Nigeria's history that convicted coup plotters escaped death. In August 1998, General Sani Abacha died suddenly on a Sunday/Monday night amidst signs that he planned to drop his military uniform and become a civilian President. General Abdulsalami Abubakar took over as Military Head of State.

Informing President Olusegun Obasanjo

At his inauguration on 29th May, 1999, President Olusegun Obasanjo told his country and the world that his Government would encourage scientific research and reward those who excel therein. The author was sceptical because he had known from the days of the man as Nigeria's Military Head of State that the man had no regard or respect for any scientific issue even though he himself was said to be an Engineer. After thinking about the man's inauguration pledge and media reports that the man had become a different person since his prison experience under General Abacha, the author said to himself, "Could it be true that the leopard had changed its spots?" He decided to give his country's new President the benefit of the doubt.

And so, by letter Ref MSH-99681-POO dated 18th June, 1999, the author wrote to Nigeria's President Olusegun Obasanjo in these words:

"President Olusegun Obasanjo
President of the Federal Republic of Nigeria
The Presidency
Aso Rock
Abuja FCT

Your Excellency,

Development of a Safe, Effective and Curative Outpatient Treatment for HIV Infection

I am one of the June 1972 pioneer medical graduates of the Ahmadu Bello University, Zaria. While working as a Senior House Officer (Pathology) at that University's Teaching Hospital in Zaria in 1974, I successfully completed a postgraduate course in Immunology at the University of Ibadan in October 1974. In November 1976, I specialised as a Surgeon. In November 1979, I obtained the Fellowship of the Nigeria Medical Council in Surgery. I have been in continuous clinical practice since 1972. I enclose a copy of my CV for more detailed information about me, sir.

Using my own human and material resources, I decided in 1992 to join others worldwide to conduct my own research to try and develop an effective treatment for infection with the dreaded human immunodeficiency virus, HIV, the causative agent of the AIDS pandemic that has remained mankind's albatross since the virus was discovered around 1983. It is universally accepted and acknowledged that there is yet no cure for HIV infection which is particularly very common in Nigeria and other sub-Saharan countries. From my years of research, however, I have successfully developed a safe, effective and curative outpatient treatment for the notorious HIV infection (se the pamphlet attached).

Out of patriotism, I wrote on 3rd February 1999 to your predecessor General Abdulsalami Abubakar (now retired) about this momentous development, and despatched the letter to him by DHL (copy attached), but I have not received any response.

I believe you would not only be interested about the discovery, but may wish to take further action as Your Excellency deems fit on the matter, sir. Thank you indeed for sparing your precious time to read this letter.

Yours truly

(Signed)
Dr. JOA Abalaka, MB.BS (ABU 1972), FMCS (1979), Cert. Immunol (Unibadan 1974),
Chief Consultant Surgeon /Chief Medical Director."

The four-page folded pamphlet attached to the author's letter to President Olusegun Obasanjo was captioned "*THE HIV/AIDS PANDEMIC* A STITCH IN TIME SAVES NINE, AND YOUR LIFE, TOO" on the front page. Its second and third pages carried these words:

"*THE HIV/AIDS PANDEMIC* – A Stitch in Time Saves Nine, and Your Life, Too!!!

The causative agent of AIDS (Acquired Immunodeficiency Syndrome) is a retrovirus called HIV (Human Immunodeficiency Virus). HIV infection occurs all over the world, but it is extremely common in Nigeria and in other sub-Saharan African countries. By the CDC classification, there are 9 categories of HIV infection, AIDS being the most advanced stage and the worst. It takes about 5-10 years for HIV infection to progress to AIDS.

HIV infection spreads like the wild harmattan fire because it is transmitted through sexual intercourse, blood, breast-feeding, etc. Early HIV infection may be completely asymptomatic, or it may mimic febrile diseases like malaria or typhoid fever.

It takes about 3-6 months of HIV infection before seroconversion occurs i.e. before detectable anti-HIV antibodies appear in the person's blood. It is the presence of such antibodies in the blood that is used to diagnose HIV infection. During the months before seroconversion, an HIV infected person will have a false negative test for HIV even though such a person is infective i.e. he/she can, and does transmit the virus to others.

The CD4 T-lymphocytes which perform a central function in our immune system are the major targets of the HIV which multiplies in the CD4 cell with consequent death of the infected CD4 cell. Eventually the virus depletes a substantial proportion of the person's CD4 cell population, whereupon the person acquires immunodeficiency syndrome (AIDS). Opportunistic infections then become rampant because of the immunodeficiency, and death usually occurs before long from such opportunistic infections.

In early HIV infection, about 200 million CD4 cells are destroyed per day by the virus, but in AIDS, the virus destroys about 20 billion CD4 cells per day. In other words, an HIV infected person would have lost 20 billion CD4 cells by the time he/she seroconverts, and by the time AIDS supervenes, such a person would have lost about 500-1000 billion CD4 cells to the deadly virus which has about 1-100 million mutants (variants) in any infected person.

For over 2 decades now, the whole world has been battling in vain to develop an effective treatment for HIV infection. Medicrest Specialist Hospital Gwagwalada, after several years of research, has now developed a safe and effective curative treatment for HIV infection. However, it is extremely difficult and costly to attempt to cure advanced HIV infection (AIDS), just as applies to the advanced stages of other diseases/infections.

Therefore, be prudent and frugal! Go for HIV screening today, and every 6 months thereafter if you are negative!! With an early HIV infection, Medicrest Specialist Hospital Gwagwalada offers you a safe and effective curative treatment.

For further information or enquiry, contact *MEDICREST SPECIALIST HOSPITAL,* near NEPA Substation, Gwagwalada, Abuja FCT, Nigeria.

Produced by MSH, Gwagwalada. June 3, 1999."

The pamphlet's back page had these words:

"NOW THAT YOU KNOW ABOUT THE GOOD NEWS OF CURATIVE TREATMENT FOR HIV INFECTION, HELP MANKIND AND THE SOCIETY BY TELLING OTHERS ABOUT THE CHEEERFUL NEWS"

Like his predecessor General Abdulsalami Abubakar (Retired), President (Retired General) Olusegun Obasanjo has, till today, not responded in any way to this letter, not even an acknowledgement. Since the author had told him that he "may wish to take further action as Your Excellency deems fit on the matter", the leopard apparently decided he would use it to show that the spots he had up to October 1979 had not changed. The action he deemed fit was to ignore the letter that was obviously worthless to the leopard then occupying Aso Rock, the residence of Nigeria's President.

Informing Other Stakeholders in Nigeria

On the same June 18, 1999, the author wrote the following letter:

"Dear sir/madam,

Availability of a Safe and Effective Curative Outpatient Therapy for HIV Infection

Using my own human and material resources, I have, since early 1992, been involved in research to try and find a safe and effective treatment for HIV infection. My research led to the development of an innovatory treatment which I started administering on some HIV infected persons about the end of 1997, with their free and informed consent. By the end of 1998, some of them had seroreverted to anti-HIV antibody negative.

Since then, another patient who had the treatment has shown up. He too has seroreverted, and has normal haematological and biochemical profiles. Presently, there are a number of HIV positive patients currently receiving the treatment; they are doing well clinically, with marked improvements in their general well-being, weight gain, rise in CD4 counts, and other monitoring profiles, just like those who had seroreverted. I expect these people to serorevert after 18-24 months of treatment.

The findings from my research so far show that a safe, effective, and curative outpatient treatment for HIV infection has indeed been developed (see a copy of the pamphlet attached). You may therefore, wish, in the greater interest of humanity and HIV infected persons, to take action as you deem appropriate.

With best wishes and kind regards indeed.

Yours sincerely,
(Signed)
JOA Abalaka, MB.BS (ABU 1972), FMCS (1979), Cert. Immunol (Unibadan 1974),
Chief Consultant Surgeon/Chief Medical Director."

The pamphlet attached to the letter was the same as the one that was attached to President Olusegun Obasanjo's letter of even date.

The author sent the letter with its attached pamphlet to, amongst others, the following:

- Nigeria's Federal Ministries of Health, Science and Technology, Information, and Defence
- The Medical and Dental Council of Nigeria
- The Chief Physician to President Olusegun Obasanjo, one Dr. Ajuwon, a Physician
- The Nigeria Medical Association
- The Chief Medical Directors of all the University Teaching Hospitals in Nigeria
- The Chief Medical Directors of all the Federal Medical Centres in Nigeria
- The Guild of Medical Directors in Nigeria
- The Pharmaceutical Society of Nigeria
- The National Institute for Pharmaceutical Research and Development (NIPRD)
- The Institute of Medical Laboratory Scientists of Nigeria
- The Nursing and Midwifery Council of Nigeria
- The World Health Organisation (WHO) in Nigeria
- The President of Nigeria's Senate
- The Speaker of Nigeria's House of Representatives
- The British and French Embassies in Nigeria
- The United States Information Service in Nigeria
- The Chief Justice of Nigeria
- Some multinational companies in Nigeria involved in the marketing and distribution of antiretroviral drugs, GlaxoWellcome, Roche, and Neimeth (formerly called Pfizer)
- The Chief of Defence Staff and the Service Chiefs
- The Inspector General of Police
- Many professional colleagues of the author
- The Guild of Editors and
- The Nigeria Television Authority and other media institutions in Nigeria.

The overwhelming majority of them did not respond in any way to the letter

AmFAR Informed

The author sent an email in March 2000 to inform the American Foundation for AIDS Research (AmFAR) about his HIV vaccines. Here is the email he sent:

From: Dr. Jeremiah Alabi Abalaka <Medicrest @nova.net.nq>
Date: 21 March 2000 20:15
To: donors@amfar.org<donors @amfar.org>;
Subject: Preventive and Curative Vaccines Against the HIV

We have just stumbled into your website, and wish to seize the opportunity to thank you for all your highly commendable efforts to fight HIV/AIDS.

We have developed effective and safe vaccines (preventive and curative) against the HIV. We trust you would be interested in this development. You may obtain more details at our website (www.medicrest.com).

We look forward to hearing from you.
With kind regards and best wishes.

Yours sincerely,

Dr. Jeremiah Abalaka
March 21, 2000

The author did not get any response from AmFAR, implying that AmFAR was probably not interested in the author's development of safe and effective HIV vaccines.

Conclusion

The author wrote and informed relevant professional bodies, Pharmaceutical Companies and stakeholders in the HIV/AIDS scourge in his country in June 1999 about the HIV vaccines he had developed, and requested that they, in the greater interest of humanity and HIV-infected persons, take action as they deemed appropriate. In 2000, the author informed the American Foundation for AIDS Research (AmFAR) by email but received no response whatsoever, not even an acknowledgement. The first priority of the author still remained humanity and the health of the HIV-infected persons. Most of those to whom the author wrote just kept mute. It should be noted that the author did not call or give any Press Conference. Instead, he was still working hard on accumulating more scientific data on the HIV-infected persons who were taking his innovative HIV therapeutic vaccine.

Chapter XXVIII

Development of a Safe Candidate HIV Preventive Vaccine

Abstract

The author's reverse approach to HIV preventive vaccine development has proceeded well so far. But it was not possible for him to rest on his oars because he had still not achieved his target of developing an effective HIV preventive vaccine for himself. So far, he had succeeded in developing a safe and effective HIV therapeutic vaccine for those infected with HIV. There is nothing wrong in a physician making the health and life of his patient his first consideration, but the physician can only do so if he is alive and well. One of the author's guiding principles in life is to strive to love others as much as he loves himself, not to attempt to love others more than himself. The author was, and is still, not prepared to attempt to love the HIV-infected person more than himself. Having successfully developed the HIV therapeutic vaccine for those infected with HIV, the author had reached the point where he had to turn his priority or first consideration on himself. The equation of his involvement in HIV vaccine development was unbalanced at this point. There was a bonus for others who are infected with HIV but nothing for the author who developed the remedy for those who are infected with the deadly virus. It was therefore opportune for the physician to attend to himself, so to say. While turning his attention to himself, he would not abandon the HIV-infected persons seeking his remedy. He would continue to attend to them while working on how to get a safe and effective preventive vaccine for himself.

Introduction

The author has shown earlier in this book that almost all other viral infectious diseases of man are acute illnesses that run their course within a few weeks of the successful entry of the causative agent into the host. As a result, all the vaccines in use against these infectious diseases are preventive. HIV infection however is a very chronic condition that lasts for about 10 years on average before it progresses to AIDS, and a further two years before death ensues. The author's approach to HIV vaccine development had been conceived, in part at least, on the opportunistic foundation that utilized the chronicity of HIV infection. Readers may therefore wish to continuously orientate their analysis and perception of the unique features of the HIV just as the author had to do. The author was in possession of a safe and effective vaccine that cured HIV infection. The author was convinced that all he needed to do was to modify the approach that produced that vaccine for HIV preventive purposes. This is how he approached the problem.

Proceeding to the HIV Preventive Vaccine

In terms of numerical strength, the HIV load that starts HIV infection in a person is far smaller than the entire viral load in an infected person. The HIV therapeutic vaccine had been successful in eliminating the HIV in some patients despite the existence in such persons of millions of mutants of the virus, despite the presence of millions of CD4+ infected lymphocytes all of which carried the HIV provirus, despite the very high viral and proviral load in the infected person, and despite the HIV-induced immunosuppression in the infected person. In an uninfected person, the circumstances are much easier. As such, the author expected that a preventive HIV vaccine that emanates from a procedure that is similar to the one used for the therapeutic vaccine would likely be able to prime the immune system to be able to repel an HIV assault later.

The autogenous approach used for the therapeutic HIV vaccine could not be used without some essential modifications because the person who needed the preventive vaccine, unlike the HIV-infected person, is not infected with the virus. Since the author had no other sources of the deadly virus, he would still have to depend on the HIV-infected person for the raw material he would need to try and develop a candidate HIV preventive vaccine. A donor for the purpose of developing a candidate HIV preventive vaccine would need to be carefully screened to be sure he was not infected with other known pathogens such as the hepatitis viruses. The blood of such a donor would have to be compatible with the author's blood since the candidate vaccine would be taken by the author. Instead of the arbitrary dose of 20 mls of the patient's blood that the author took as a dose, perhaps the author should consider using a higher dose for the preventive vaccine.

Accordingly, the author, on March 1, 1999 took 30 mls of the peripheral venous blood of one of his blood group O+ HIV-infected patients (he is also O+) who had not started the therapeutic remedy, and used it to prepare his first candidate HIV preventive vaccine using slight modifications of the method he had been using to prepare the therapeutic vaccine. He administered that candidate HIV preventive vaccine to himself by deep intramuscular injection immediately after it was prepared. Of course, he had screened the patient and confirmed she was negative for hepatitis B surface antigen (HBsAg) and anti-hepatitis C virus (HCV) IgG antibodies.

He would give the candidate HIV therapeutic vaccine some time to hopefully prime his immune system. After that, he would proceed to assess its efficacy.

Conclusion

The author produced his first candidate HIV preventive vaccine on 1st March 1999 and administered it to himself. If it worked, he would have accomplished his target that initiated all he had gone through since the beginning of 1992. Like the autogenous HIV therapeutic vaccine that he had been using, the candidate HIV preventive vaccine that he prepared and took on March 1, 1999 was safe. He only had to wait and see if it would be efficacious also.

Chapter XXIX

Efficacy Assessment of the Author's Safe Candidate HIV Preventive Vaccine

Abstract

Even before the author received the first dose of his candidate HIV preventive vaccine, he had made up his mind about how he would proceed to assess its efficacy. He had increased his risk of acquiring HIV since he started performing the efficacy trials of his candidate autogenous HIV therapeutic vaccine; he handled on a daily basis HIV-infected blood, processed the blood till he obtained a vaccine product out of it, and then inactivated the blood to get rid of the live HIV the blood contained. He was lucky that he had not yet picked up the virus. He really needed to increase his resistance to HIV, and only a vaccine could do that for him. He would proceed as he had planned long ago, but with slight modifications. This chapter describes what some people call 'daredevil' or 'mad' approaches that the author chose. Merck's V520 HIV preventive vaccine was pompously, prematurely and unexpectedly called "the vaccine of vaccines". But when it mattered most, V520 did not just fail to protect against the wild HIV but it might have made vaccinees worse than those who got a placebo. The author delivers an important and relevant challenge for all developers of candidate HIV preventive vaccines. Find out in this chapter.

Introduction

The author found he was involved in all sorts of construction and maintenance work in the small private hospital he had just started around June 1998. He just could not avoid a cut here, a prick there or an abrasion here and there during these activities. He made up his mind that when he reached the stage of testing for the efficacy of his candidate HIV preventive vaccine, these bloody scratches, pricks, cuts and abrasions would conveniently give him the opportunity for blood to blood contact with HIV-infected blood without the need for additional painful procedures. All he needed to do was to continue to do his HIV screening frequently so that he would be able to detect whenever his body produced detectable levels of anti-HIV antibodies. Already, he was no longer scared of HIV infection because he had a reliable and safe therapeutic remedy. If he had not possessed the remedy for HIV infection, he would not have been able to proceed with his work as he did. If he ever picked up the virus in the course of his work either from the HIV-infected blood he was handling on a daily basis or from failure of his candidate HIV preventive vaccine, he would chuckle out the HIV with his therapeutic remedy and proceed. The HIV therapeutic remedy he possessed was indeed a strong pillar of courage to employ 'daredevil' or 'mad' approaches. There should be no need for field trials for any promising candidate HIV preventive vaccine. Have the developers of such candidate HIV preventive vaccines never heard of James Phipps? Let them turn themselves into James Phipps!

The Taste of the Pudding is in the Eating

As far as the author knows, the best and most reliable way to assess the efficacy of any preventive vaccine against an infectious disease is the post immunization exposure of the vaccinee to the wild or pathogenic causative agent of the disease. If such an exposure causes no disease, the efficacy of the vaccine is established; if on the other hand, such an exposure causes the disease in the vaccinee, the vaccine is not efficacious. In other words, just as the taste of the pudding is in the eating, the efficacy of any vaccine is in the ability of that vaccine to offer protection when the vaccinee is later exposed to the wild and pathogenic causative agent of the disease. Even if all laboratory experiments show the vaccine is promising, the ultimate test of its efficacy lies in its ability to protect against infection when the vaccinee is faced with the wild and pathogenic causative agent.

A month after the author took the candidate preventive vaccine, he started doing blood to blood challenge with the wild HIV. He would smear some fresh blood from various HIV infected patients over the raw wound he had. Fortunately for him, there was hardly any week that he would not get a skin wound. Most of these wounds were on his hands, so it was an easy matter for the author to smear the blood conveniently on the wounds. Every fortnight, he would do his HIV screening for even the indeterminate results, but got none. When the results continued to be negative by the end of May 1999, he was satisfied that the candidate HIV preventive vaccine was efficacious.

The author then remembered Edward Jenner and the eight-year-old James Phipps when Jenner wanted to confirm that the cowpox vaccination he did on the boy had protected the lad against smallpox. Jenner inoculated Phipps with fresh wild smallpox from a maturing smallpox skin lesion. Phipps never got the disease. Come on! Go and do thou likewise, Jeremiah.

On June 1, 1999, the climax came. The author confidently challenged himself with an intravenous injection of 2 mls of fresh whole untreated O+ blood in CPDA-1 anticoagulant taken from a confirmed HIV-1 infected patient who had not yet started taking the therapeutic vaccine and who had been screened and found negative for HBsAg and anti-HCV IgG antibodies. Like most of his HIV-infected patients then, the evidence that there was infective HIV in the blood of this patient was the assays that were routinely carried out to make sure that when the author made vaccine he used blood from an HIV-infected person. These normally consisted of the ELISA screening test used for HIV antibodies and their confirmation using Western Blot. Readers should note that the author's confidence in doing this challenge lay in the safe and effective HIV therapeutic vaccine he had developed; if the candidate HIV preventive vaccine failed, he would resort to the therapeutic vaccine to get rid of the virus before proceeding to try and conceive another type of candidate HIV preventive vaccine. As it turned out though, there was no need for him to do that.

Later in 1999, he took five more similar intravenous challenges of 2 mls each of fresh untreated HIV-1 infected blood from different O+ blood group patients on August 11, September 10, October 11, November 11 and December 10. At the time he took these five injections, PML had developed the p24 antigen assays. A day before each of these challenges, the author carried out HIV antibody screening, p24ag assay, CD4+ count, and FBC tests on his blood. The tests were all negative or normal. Since then, he has been doing these tests frequently on himself at 3-monthly intervals at the latest. All HIV parameters in his blood tested in various laboratories in Nigeria and in London have remained either negative or normal up till today.

When the author told a senior colleague recently about these challenges, he advised the author to be taking yearly boosters of the preventive vaccine in case the protection provided by the preventive vaccine he had developed lasts just 3 to 5 years. Heeding that advice, the author now takes yearly booster doses of his HIV preventive vaccine.

The author remains willing and prepared to publicly challenge himself with fresh blood group O (Rhesus D positive or negative) HIV-infected blood from any suitable person anytime anywhere to demonstrate that he is protected against HIV. In addition or in the alternative, he is willing to give his blood samples to any researchers anywhere who are interested in finding out his immune system's response when challenged with ABO compatible HIV-infected whole human blood in vitro and /or in vivo so that such researchers may proceed to try and elucidate the mechanism(s) involved. In addition, he is prepared to assist such researchers to get in touch with (some of) his HIV-infected patients that have been cured so that such patients may give them their blood samples for the same purposes, too.

Conclusion

Many HIV vaccine researchers claim that one of the problems militating against HIV vaccine development is the absence of an appropriate animal model to use, adding that there is no human being that has successfully eliminated the virus from his/her body. Such statements are not true at all. The author's immune system knows how to ward off HIV invasion. The author has dozens of patients who were confirmed HIV positive before but are now HIV negative.

Some 'experts' argue that HIV can hide for a long time in the tissues and not be detected. For the sake of argument, let us presume that the statement is correct. Human technology to date may not be able to detect such low viral loads but the human immune system does. The human immune system is so sensitively accurate that even if there is just one HIV-infected cell in the body, the immune cells recognize such a cell and mount an immune response against it. Such a person would continue to produce anti-HIV antibodies. When there is no HIV infected cell in the body, the body stops producing anti HIV antibodies. The serodeconversion to anti-HIV antibody negative status in a person previously positive for such antibodies is therefore a public announcement beyond any reasonable and unreasonable doubt that there is no single HIV-infected cell in that person's body. When the much acclaimed HAART causes persistent non-detectable levels of HIV RNA, the body continues to produce anti-HIV antibodies because the body knows it still has some HIV infected cells in the body. When such a person stops HAART, the viral load becomes detectable within a few days.

Besides, the author severally challenged himself with wild HIV nine years ago. If the author's HIV preventive vaccine has forced the virus into hiding in the author's body these past nine years and the virus can still not multiply to cause the author's immune system to respond to its presence, the author is convinced that the vaccine has done its job. After all, no one lives on this planet for ever. If the author's HIV preventive vaccine forces the virus to go into hiding for the rest of the author's life, what else would anyone expect the vaccine to do?

The author would like to throw a challenge to his critics that are at his jugular because of his efforts. The author gave his candidate HIV preventive vaccine to himself and challenged himself with the wild HIV. Let those critics who never see anything good in the efforts of others follow his footsteps.

Whenever they claim they have a promising candidate HIV preventive vaccine let them not waste time and funds looking for any volunteers for efficacy trials. Let them take their own vaccine, challenge themselves later with the wild HIV and tell us if their vaccine protected them. If they claim the vaccine had protected them, let them go further by offering themselves for public challenge with wild HIV. The author would come and witness their public challenge to confirm their claim. They should all turn themselves into James Phipps. The efficacy trials of any candidate HIV preventive vaccine would therefore be drastically reduced to just 3 months by so doing.

Let the empty noise making and false propaganda such as prematurely calling their candidate HIV vaccine "the vaccine of vaccines" stop. After all, the recent "vaccine of vaccines" did not only fail to offer protection against HIV; it might have actually made recipients of the vaccine worse than those who received a placebo! For yielding promising results in laboratory animals, Merck's V520 was described as "the vaccine of vaccines" but it failed when it mattered.

The author's HIV preventive vaccine has succeeded when it mattered most, i.e. when it protected against the wild HIV challenge. What name would they use to describe the author's vaccine then, dear reader?

Chapter XXX

Tough Rough Road Indeed to Travel

Abstract

What a tough road indeed for the author to travel! We all have different circumstances of birth, upbringing and environment. Some are born with spoons of gold, silver, bronze, iron, clay or even straw in their mouths while some are born with no type of spoon at all even in their entire environment! Some are born in countries that are super powers; some are born in developed (industrialized) but non-super power countries; some are born in countries that would soon become developed (industrialized) nations; and some are born in developing countries of different categories. In spite of this broad spectrum in the circumstances of our births, we all still hold as true and self evident that all men are 'created' equal, and that they are endowed by their 'Creator' with the brain of Homo sapiens.

The author, by the circumstances of his birth, belonged to the lowest and poorest portion of the spectrum but was fortunate enough for his illiterate peasant father to send him to school. He also had the great fortune of having a father who inculcated in him from his earliest days the importance of hard work at his studies so that he could change his social status from that of a poor peasant's son to that of a medical doctor, a surgeon for that matter. The author ignored the poor circumstances of his birth and upbringing to work hard at his studies even when engaged in manual labour activities. Fortunate enough to have had devoted and dedicated teachers, providence ensured that he would eventually qualify as a medical practitioner and surgeon.

When the dreaded, dreadful and incurable HIV/AIDS became quite widespread in his country in the late 1980s with the attendant increased risk to surgeons like the author, the author decided at the beginning of 1992 to try and tackle the HIV menace. He may probably be the only surgeon in the entire world who made such a daring decision. Since 1992, the author has been confronting one serious problem or the other. The author has been a lonely pilgrim on a really tough and dangerous road on which he has travelled since 1992, a road that became increasingly more dangerous since 1998/99 when he developed safe and effective HIV vaccines. This chapter brings to an end his account.

Introduction

This chapter will not be a recapitulation of this book. If raw, how raw was the author's approach to HIV vaccines development? When, under the circumstances in which the author found himself, one obtains the first evidence that he has developed a safe and effective HIV therapeutic vaccine, what steps should he take to ensure he accumulates further credible, confirmatory and verifiable scientific data? Are there ways forward to reduce or curtail the spread and scourge of HIV using the author's safe and effective vaccines? Was the author's journey on the perilously long, rough and tough road worth it? These are the sort of issues that would attract our attention in this last chapter of a fairly but necessarily long account.

Preparing for the Inevitable Scientific Criticisms

Informed Written Consent before Treatment for HIV Infection

In orthodox medical practice, written consents are usually required for operative procedures and /or general anaesthesia only. In other words, doctors do not obtain written consents from any patient before issuing prescriptions or getting the prescriptions supplied to the patient. The administration of drugs even by the injection route does not demand the patient's consent in writing. Written consent of the patient or the legal guardian is not required for antiretrovirals. Written consent is not obtained from patients before they are given human blood or its products. The author's HIV vaccines do not involve any operative procedure or any form of anaesthesia. However, the author decided right from the beginning of his treating HIV-infected persons in 1997 to obtain written and informed consent of the patients receiving his novel HIV vaccines for several reasons that include satisfying those critics who might wish to accuse him of using patients for dangerous purposes without their knowledge or consent. Even though written consent is not required before human beings receive prophylactic vaccines against measles, polio, tetanus, meningitis, Varicella, etc, the author decided to introduce and obtain written informed consent from those who opt for his HIV preventive vaccine. Similarly, the author decided to put into writing the information given to patients to consider before they decide whether or not to take the author's HIV vaccines. These non-mandatory steps were taken by the author just to prove to whoever might want to unnecessarily criticise him that he had such consent from the recipients.

In the early years of the author's work, this was the consent form he introduced in 1999:

'THE MANAGEMENT and STAFF OF MEDICREST SPECIALIST HOSPITAL, GWAGWALADA, ABUJA FCT.

CONSENT FOR TREATMENT FOR HIV INFECTION

I *know/have been informed that the human immunodeficiency virus (HIV) is the causative agent of the serious and deadly disease called AIDS (Acquired Immunodeficiency Syndrome), and that it is universally accepted and acknowledged that there is as yet no known cure for HIV infection. Various existing management options for HIV infection include orthodox medical antiretroviral drugs, traditional or herbal preparations, and prayer for divine healing. Dr. JOA Abalaka, Chief Medical Director i/c Medicrest Specialist Hospital, Gwagwalada, Abuja FCT, claims he has, after several years of his personal research, developed a safe and effective outpatient therapy for non-AIDS HIV infection. He has made it clear to me that like the late, terminal and advanced stages of other infections/diseases such as syphilis where cure is extremely difficult and very costly, AIDS being the advanced, late and terminal stage of HIV infection, is extremely difficult and costly to attempt to cure.

Dr. Abalaka has also emphasized that he cannot give an assurance or guarantee that his treatment will cure any particular case of HIV infection, just as he or any other human being cannot give an assurance or guarantee that any treatment will cure any other disease, not even the common malaria for which tested drugs like chloroquine sometimes fail to effect cure.

WHEREFORE,

I hereby give my free and informed consent not only for *me or my .... called (names supplied) to undergo Dr. Abalaka's innovatory treatment for HIV infection but also for Dr. Abalaka to publicise, as he deems necessary, any or all aspects of the cure.

Name (in full)
Office/Business Address
Residential Address Block
Telephone Numbers (if any:)
Office
Residence
Fax Numbers (if any):
Office
Residence

Signature Date Time

*delete as necessary or applicable'

The consent form was later updated to this:

'THE MANAGEMENT and STAFF OF MEDICREST SPECIALIST HOSPITAL, GWAGWALADA, ABUJA FCT.

Consent for Treatment for HIV Infection

I *know/have been informed that the human immunodeficiency virus (HIV) is the causative agent of the serious and deadly disease called AIDS (Acquired Immunodeficiency Syndrome), and that it is universally accepted and acknowledged that there is as yet no known cure for HIV infection. Various existing management options for HIV infection include orthodox medical antiretroviral drugs, traditional or herbal preparations, and prayer for divine healing. Dr. JOA Abalaka, Chief Medical Director i/c Medicrest Specialist Hospital, Gwagwalada, Abuja FCT, claims he has, after several years of his personal research, developed a safe and effective outpatient therapy for non-AIDS HIV infection. He has made it clear to me that like the late, terminal and advanced stages of other infections/diseases such as syphilis where cure is extremely difficult and very costly, AIDS being the advanced, late and terminal stage of HIV infection, is extremely difficult and costly to attempt to cure.

Dr. Abalaka has also emphasized that he cannot give an assurance or guarantee that his treatment will cure any particular case of HIV infection, just as he or any other human being cannot give an assurance or guarantee that any treatment will cure any other disease, not even the common malaria for which tested drugs like chloroquine sometimes fail to effect cure.

WHEREFORE,

I hereby give my free and informed consent not only for **me called.................... or *my ...., called ....* to undergo Dr. Abalaka's innovatory treatment for HIV infection but also for Dr. Abalaka and or the Hospital to publicize, as he deems necessary, any or all aspects of the cure. I also hereby agree to make **myself or the patient* available at any time Dr. Abalaka and or the Hospital may require my presence even after I have stopped taking the treatment. In addition, I agree to give evidence at any time anywhere before any court of law or investigation panel about the treatment.

Name (in full)...
Office/Business Address ....
Residential Address ....
Telephone Numbers (1) office (2) residence
(3) GSM office (4) GSM residence

Fax Numbers (1) office (2) residence

Signature............... Date......... Time...... Hospital No..................

(*delete as necessary or applicable)'

Was the Author Really Treating Human Beings or Ghosts?

Colleagues in Nigeria's Lagos University Teaching Hospital confronted the author during an International Symposium on HIV/AIDS organized by an American based NGO (FIARE) —see Chapter 33—in 2000 and asked him to be honest and tell them if he was treating humans or ghosts. In other words, they were accusing him of concocting everything. The author had prepared for such criticisms from the beginning by insisting that every patient willing to take his HIV therapeutic vaccine must produce four postcard sized photographs. Ghosts, as far as the author knows, cannot pose and take such photographs!

The reader would find samples of such photographs with a summary of the data on each patient in Figures 30-1 to 30-12. There is severe dread associated with HIV infection as the reader knows. There are really chilling but true accounts of the severe and universal stigmatization and social rejection associated with being HIV positive.

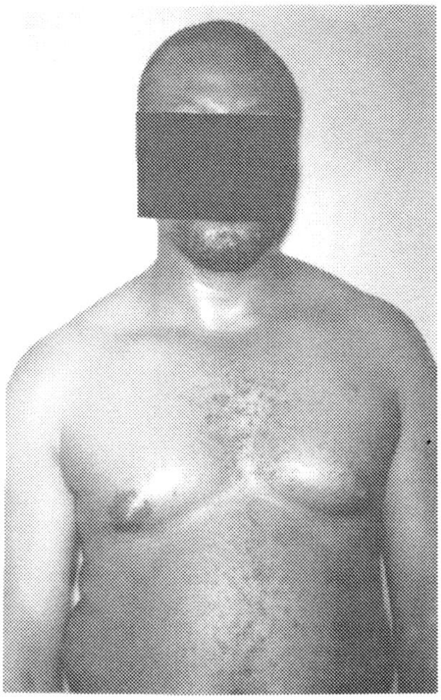

Figure 30-1. Patient AZ on 5 Oct 1999 (HN117; M29OP; SandCP240999; P24-3-240999; ST051099; SDN221099).

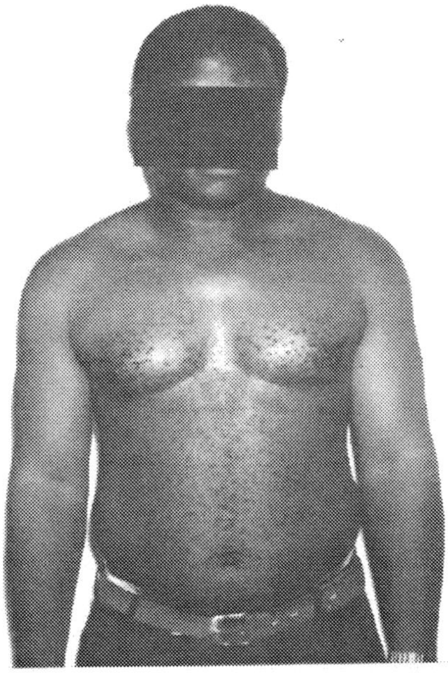

Figure 30-2. Patient BY on 13 April 2000 (HN710; M45BP; SandCP010400; P24-5-200800; WB010400-G160.120.41-P65.51.31.24.18; ST180400; SDN191200).

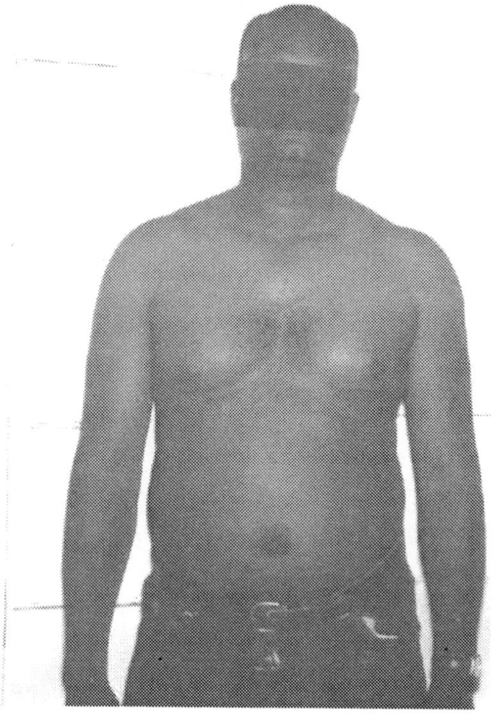

Figure 30-3. Patient CX on 26 Jun 2000 (HN1393; M34AP; WB220600-G160.120.41-P65.51.31.24.18; ST260600; SDN301000).

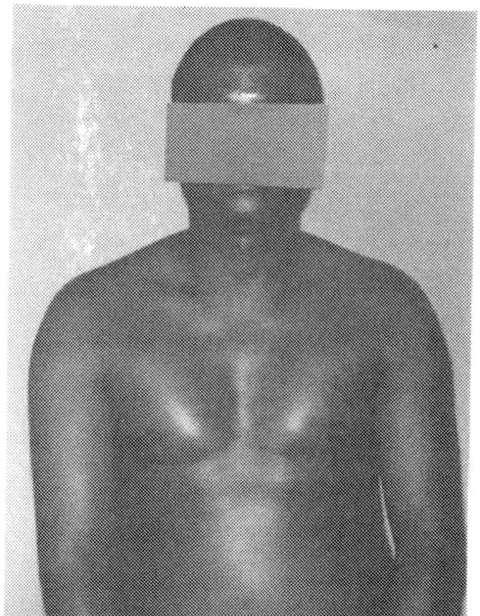

Figure 30-4. Patient DW on 18 Aug 1999 N072; M45BP; SandCP180899; ST180899; SDN170300).

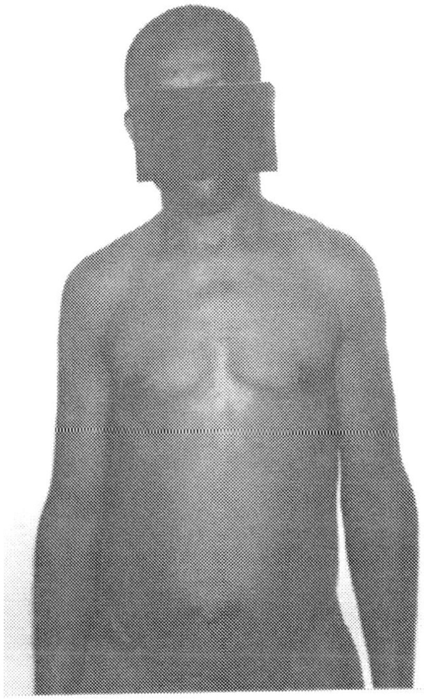

Figure 30-5. Patient EV on 24 May 2000 (HN1103; M41BP; SandCP230500; WB230500-G160.120.41-P65.51.31.24.18; ST250500; SDN191100).

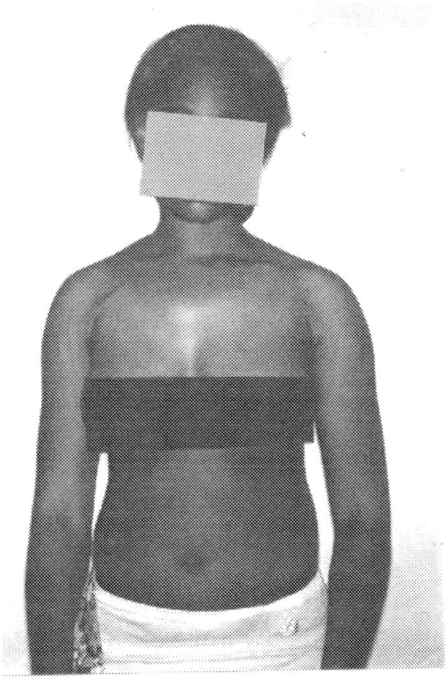

Figure 30-6. Patient FU on 17 April 2000 (HN732; F20OP; SandCP130400; WB130400-G160.120.41-P65.51.31.24.18; ST170400; SDN080101).

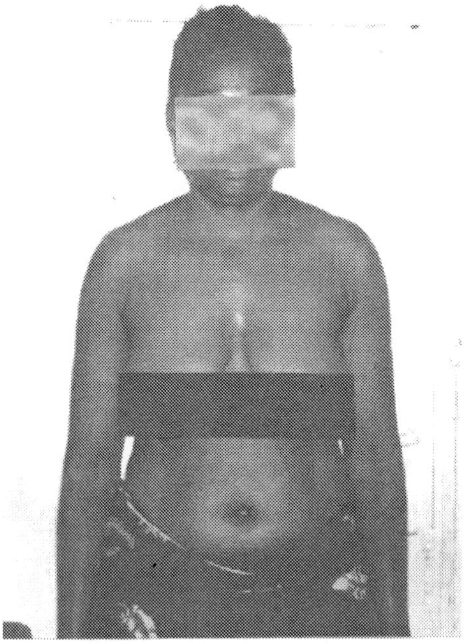

Figure 30-7. Patient GT on 26 Jun 2000 (HN1388; F42AN; SandCP240600; WB240600-G160.120.41-P65.51.31.24.18; ST260600; SDN230101).

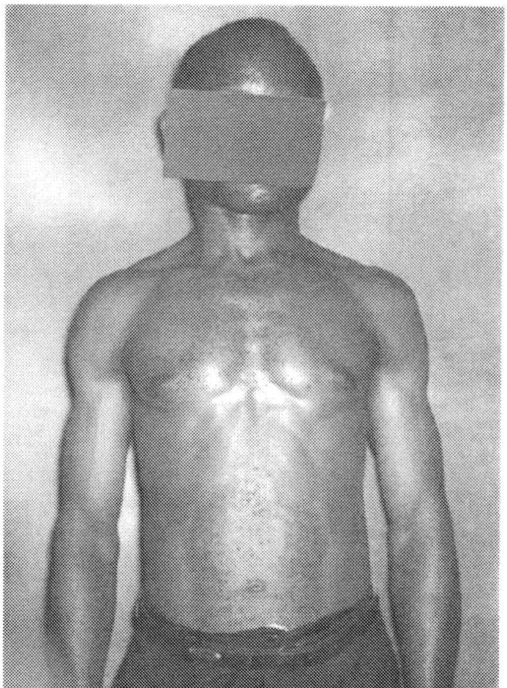

Figure 30-8. Patient HS on 16 Mar 2001 (HN3098; M44AP; SandCP171000; WB171000-G160.120.41-P65.51.31.24.18; ST230301; SDN291203; SHIVN200505.F5DLABS).

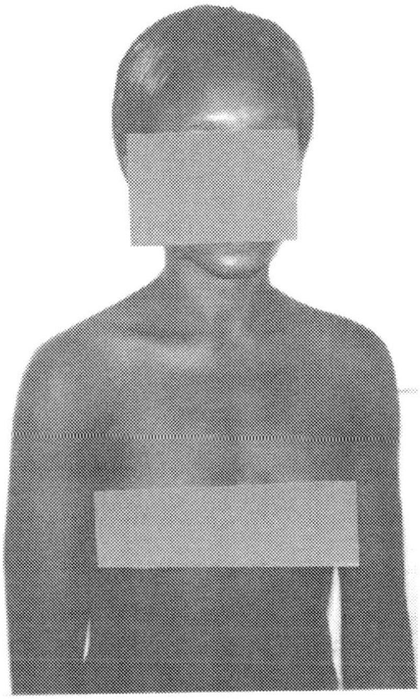

Figure 30-9. Patient IR on 22 Jun 2000 (HN1362; F20OP; SandCP210600; WB210600-G160.120.41-P65.51.31.24.18; ST200600; SDN210700).

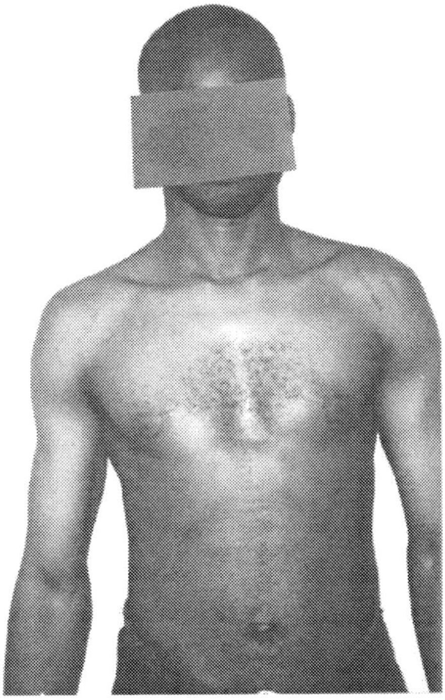

Figure 30-10. Patient JQ on 13 Mar 2000 (HN561; M24OP; SandCP070200; WB070200-G160.120.41-P65.51.31.24.18; ST130300; SDN270300)

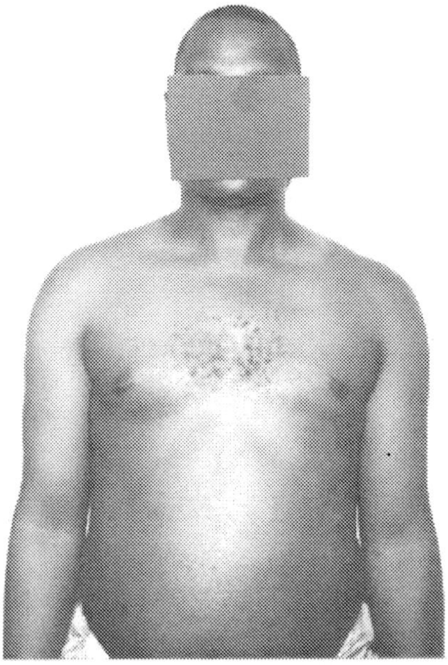

Figure 30-11. Patient KP on 17 Dec 1999 (HN221; M33AP; SandCP111299; P24-8-120500; P24-0-220500 and 170700; ST120200; SDN160600).

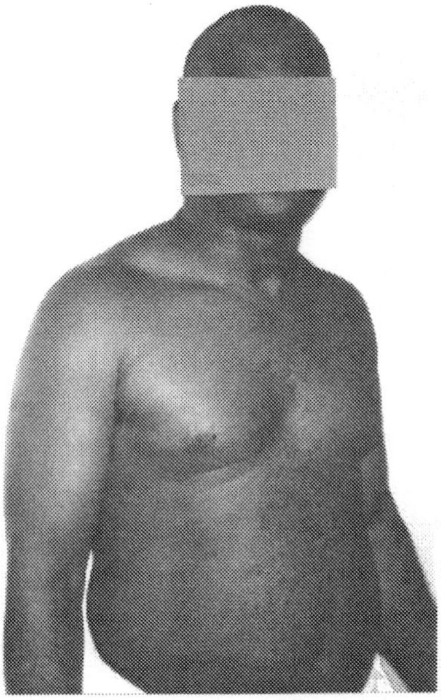

Figure 30-12. Patient LO on 22 Jun 2000 (HN1365; M43OP; SandCP130600;WB130600-G160.120.41-P65.51.31.24.18; ST220600; W64.5KG.220600; LAH280501; W74.5KG.280501).

For more than the past 20 years, it has been a crime for any HIV-positive non-US citizen to visit the USA even for one day; an HIV-positive Dutch citizen who visited the USA was found guilty of the crime and jailed for four years!

The sustained but false propaganda that HIV infection is incurable worsens the stigmatization and societal rejection. If any one should admit that he was HIV positive at any time in the past, (s)he would immediately suffer from these punishments. No one would investigate anything. Every one would just say something like this: 'Did you hear him say that he was HIV positive? There is no cure for HIV, so the man is still HIV positive!' Like an inferno, word would spread rapidly and the person's fate is sealed!

For years, the author has thrown a challenge that has not been heeded. He is still prepared to publicly inject himself intravenously with fresh compatible HIV-infected blood from any suitable HIV-infected person to show any critics that his body is capable of warding off wild HIV challenges. Many say it is unethical! What is unethical about it? The real reason for failure to accept the challenge is that it will put paid to the false propaganda about HIV. If the challenge is accepted and the efficacy of the author's HIV preventive vaccine is demonstrated publicly, that would be the end of the huge economic market for antiretrovirals and condoms, hence the challenge must be nipped in the bud with all sorts of unscientific gimmicks!

Similarly, the established knowledge of our generation is that there is no cure for HIV infection, another false propaganda. The author has battled with how to reconcile his patient's interests with the public interest about the availability of his curative HIV vaccine. The patients that have been cured do not want anyone to know that they were ever HIV infected. The author appreciates their fears. But the far more important public interest demands we should let humanity know that truly, the author has developed a safe and effective HIV therapeutic vaccine so that the millions who are infected with the virus worldwide may avail themselves of the remedy if they so wish.

In the author's still-pending 8-year-old legal battle with the Nigerian Academy of Science, many interesting episodes have occurred. After the parties had filed their pleadings, the author's Counsel was ready to start with his witnesses. In the open Court, the learned trial judge and the author's Counsel exchanged something like this:

'Mr. Okpanachi, I am not prejudiced against you and your client, but I want to remind you that even though I am a Judge, I read newspapers, listen to the radio and the television, and browse the Internet. I know like everybody else that there is no cure for HIV infection. I have seen the pleadings in this matter. Your client claims he has safe and effective HIV vaccines including the one that cures HIV infection whereas the defendants all say that there is no cure for HIV anywhere in the world. Are you sure you are not trying to waste your time, your client's time,the court's time and every body else's time with this case? Do you really want to continue with the case?'

It was obvious that the many lawyers representing the defendants were extremely happy at the development. After a few seconds of thinking about the matter, Mr. Okpanachi responded:

'My Lord, we are grateful for your concern. With the greatest respect, my Lord, we would like to continue with the case. We are grateful.'

The Court then said: 'Okay. Let us take a date for the matter to continue.'

Several months later, the author's counsel Mr. Okpanachi told the author it was crucial that the author get some of the patients who had been cured of HIV infection with his treatment to come to testify before the Court. It became a nightmare for the author. He criss-crossed the country with the residential and office addresses the patients had given him but found they were fictitious! The author had the photographs of the patients he was looking for and so he was able to get neighbours at the addresses he was given to help him locate the person he was looking for. Of course, the author did not tell them the problem. He went about with the passport photographs of the people he was searching for; he obtained such photographs by reducing a copy of the photographs in his medical records to passport size. A Good Samaritan of a neighbour came and advised the author to find his way to one Church somewhere on any Sunday morning and that he would meet the lady he was looking for and /or the husband because he knew they worshipped there regularly, but as for their residence or office, he knew nothing.

The following Sunday, the author found his way to that Church and showed the security men there the lady's passport photograph. They recognized her and told the author she was one of the choristers in the Church. They helped the author call her out. She came out in her chorister's dress!

As pleasantly as the author could muster, he greeted her generously. Her response was to tell the author that she did not know him! The author was dazed, but kept his cool. He was about to introduce himself when the lady stopped him, saying that the security man that called her out had told her about her visitor. She showed no sympathy for all the effort the author had made to locate her. The author just asked her for an appointment for him to come and discuss with her spouse with or without her. She got the author's GSM number and promised to get in touch with him later that day. She refused to give the author her own GSM number.

The next morning, the author received the following 2 text messages from her spouse:

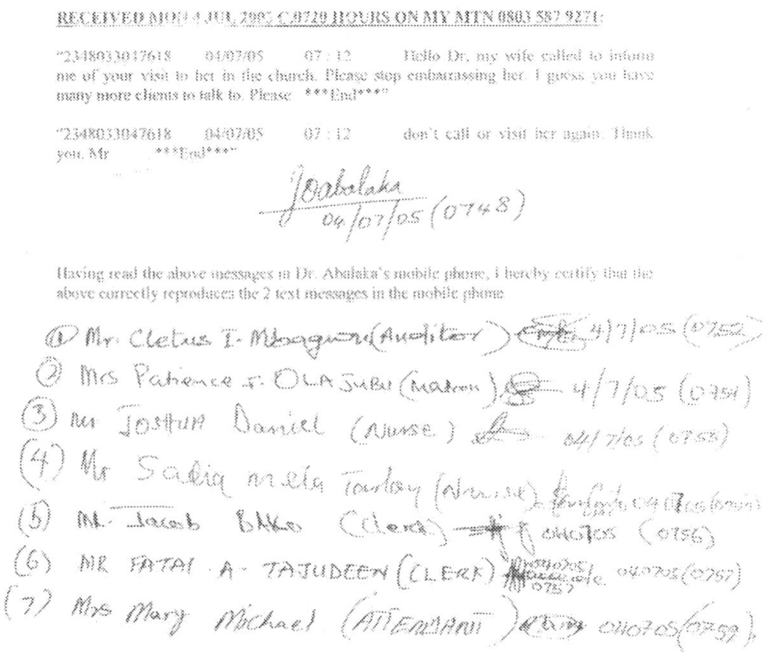
RECEIVED MON 4 JUL 2005 C.0720 HOURS ON MY MTN 0803 587 9271:

"2348033047618 04/07/05 07 : 12 Hello Dr, my wife called to inform me of your visit to her in the church. Please stop embarrassing her. I guess you have many more clients to talk to. Please ***End***"

"2348033047618 04/07/05 07 : 12 don't call or visit her again. Thank you. Mr ***End***"

JOabalaka
04/07/05 (0748)

Having read the above messages in Dr. Abalaka's mobile phone, I hereby certify that the above correctly reproduces the 2 text messages in the mobile phone

(1) Mr. Cletus I. Mbaguru (Auditor) 4/7/05 (0752)
(2) Mrs Patience F. OLAJUBU (Matron) 4/7/05 (0754)
(3) Mr JOSHUA Daniel (NURSE) 04/7/05 (0755)
(4) Mr Sadiq m. Ola Tanlay (Nurse) 04/7/05 (0755)
(5) Mr. Jacob Bako ([illegible]) 040705 (0756)
(6) MR FATAI A. TAJUDEEN (CLERK) 04/07/05 (0757)
(7) Mrs Mary Michael (ATTENDANT) 040705 (0759)

The reader can see clearly the sort of ingratitude from some patients that doctors all over the world have to bear. The lady had HIV infection. The author did not contribute in any way to her infection. She was afflicted with an incurable and fatal infection. The author developed his HIV vaccines at his expense and at the risk to his life. He treated the lady till she was cured. Right in the premises of God's House, her Church, and in chorister's dress, the lady claimed she had never known the author! She had gone beyond the limits of just fear of HIV infection. After all, she no longer had the infection. And then, see the SMS texts from her spouse. They had benefitted but they did not want to do anything that would let others benefit too. They were just ingrates of the worst order! To the stupid and selfish spouse, the author was embarrassing his wife! Yet she had signed a consent form that authorized the author to publicise any or all aspects of her treatment with him before she commenced his treatment. The spouse put his name on the SMS but the author has blotted it out so that they are not ex-communicated from their society in case someone who knows them reads this book. And the spouse is one of the senior officials of the Federal Government of Nigeria in the establishment in which he works! There are very many like this couple. If there were safe and effective HIV therapeutic and preventive vaccines, there would be a drastic reduction in the stigma, fear, dread and social excommunication of HIV and HIV-infected persons. The author's HIV vaccines readily achieve these objectives.

The HIV-infected person that has been cured of his infection by the author's vaccine would not like others to know that he was ever infected with the virus in the past. At the other end of the scale lies the public that needs solid evidence to convince it that there may be merit in the author's HIV therapeutic vaccines claim. All the HIV-infected persons that have come to the author for his HIV remedy must produce 4 copies of their photographs before commencement of therapy and after the author's confirmation of their HIV-infection. Figures 30-1 to 30-12 contain the clinical summary of each of the patients shown. Figure 30-8, for instance has the following label below the figure (photograph):

Figure 30-8: Patient HS on 16 Mar 2001
(HN3098; M44AP; SandCP171000;
WB171000-G160.120.41-P65.51.31.24.18;
ST230301; SDN291203; SHIVN200505.F5DLABS)

This is the translation. Two alphabets were chosen in a systematic manner to represent the name; the letters chosen have absolutely no relationship at all with the initials of the patient. The date the photograph was taken is indeed the real date.

HN3098 means the patient's Hospital Number was 3098.

M44AP means the patient was a male, aged 44 years when he registered at the Hospital and was blood group A Rhesus D Positive.

SandCP171000 means the patient was screened and confirmed positive for HIV on 17 Oct 2000 (first 2 digits for the day of the month, the next two digits for the month and the last 2 digits for the year).

WB171000-G160.120.41-P65.51.31.24.18 means the Western Blot result dated 17 Oct 2000 showed antibody bands for viral glycoproteins (gp) 160, 120 and 41 and for viral proteins (p) 65, 51, 31, 24 and 18 kilodaltons.

ST230301 means the patient started treatment (with the author's HIV therapeutic vaccine) on 23 Mar 2001.

SDN291203 means the patient serodeconverted to anti-HIV antibody negative on 29 December 2003.

SHIVN200505.F5DLABS means the last screening of the patient for anti-HIV antibodies was negative on 20 May 2005 and that such screening result was obtained from 5 different laboratories.

The following different shorthand information below the other figures has these meanings:

P24-5-200800 means the serum /plasma HIV P24 antigen level was 5 pg/ml on 20 Aug 2000.

W64.5KG.220600 means the patient's weight was 64.5 Kg on 22 Jun 2000. The Hospital uses the same weighing scale and the same nursing staffs to take the patients' weights in a cubicle and with standard clothing – every man's weight is taken in just his pants while ladies have their weights taken in just their pants and bras.

LAH280501 means the patient last attended the author's Hospital on 28 May 2001.

The reader should please remember that patient compliance with Hospital appointments is very poor in his country for various reasons that the author explained in earlier Chapters.

Stored Frozen Serum/Plasma Samples of Patients Undergoing the Author's HIV Therapeutic Vacciotherapy

Despite the extremely erratic, unstable and unreliable public electricity supply in the author's country (power outages may last several days or even weeks), the Chief Medical Laboratory Scientist that carries out various lab tests and assays on the author's patients agreed to be storing 1-2 ml aliquots of all the author's patients for possible independent assay by others who might wish to do so in verification of the author's claims. For several years and at much cost to the Scientist, he kept all serum/plasma samples from the author's patients before, during and after therapy. At the end, the Scientist had to stop keeping such samples when it became clear that no one was interested in carrying out any scientific verification of the author's HIV vaccines claims.

Is the Author's Approach to HIV Vaccines Development Really Raw?

Hear this, dear reader:

> One last aspect of vaccine testing to discuss is the tradition of a placebo control. In cancer chemotherapy trials, a placebo control is no longer used or considered to be ethical. Thus, "standard therapy" serves as the control group, with which an experimental group is compared. Accordingly, before testing new vaccines in the third world, at least two promising vaccines, doses and regimens should first be identified in the first world in therapeutic trials, and then compared with one another in the third world in prophylactic trials. If one vaccine and regimen is found superior to the other, it should then be used as the "standard vaccine" for comparison with an experimental vaccine in the next trial. This approach should make the idea of volunteering for a vaccine trial in the third world much more palatable and therefore decidedly more easily accomplished by first and third world scientists and physicians, working together.

Conclusions

Given the understanding of how the immune system functions, combined with the ability to rapidly and definitively test therapeutic vaccines in HIV+ volunteers, a rational and successful approach to testing therapeutic and prophylactic HIV vaccines is now within reach. However, the scientific, medical and HIV-infected communities of the first world must mobilize to perform the necessary crucial clinical research before vaccines and immunotherapies can be applied effectively worldwide as rapidly as possible.

These are the words of the American Professor, Kendall A. Smith in an article '***The HIV Vaccine***' published in 2004 in the *National Journal of Andrology* 10(1):723-8. Professor K A Smith is of the Division of Immunology, Department of Medicine, Weill Medical College, Cornell University, New York in the USA. He wrote these words several years after the author worked out his approach of developing first, an effective and safe HIV therapeutic vaccine and using that development as a springboard for the HIV preventive vaccine. Moreover, the author did not use any placebos because he considered it unethical and unnecessary for an infection that everyone says is incurable. The author believes that at the time Professor Kendall wrote his article, he was unaware of the author's approach and the results. Professor Kendall has abandoned the UNAIDS guidelines too. As far as the author knows, he has not drawn the ire of UNAIDS or his colleagues elsewhere all of whom have been condemning the author. Why have they not descended on Professor K A Smith as they have been angrily swooping on the hapless author?

And in an interview on October 6, 2008, one of the 3 winners of the2008 Nobel Prize for Medicine, Prof Luc Montagnier said, *inter alia*: "... And I appreciate that the Nobel Committee has put on the air this important disease which is not finished, and my message is that we should continue the research. And myself I'm working on a vaccine – not a preventive vaccine but on a therapeutic vaccine which is aimed at completing the antiretroviral therapy which is now given to many patients even in Africa, but which does not cure. So the idea is to eradicate the virus infection. I think this is the main step now. ..."

Good gracious! Was Luc Montagnier so elated for winning the Nobel Prize that he was talking balderdash or what? Was he inebriated? Had he gone crazy? If not, how could he be talking about an HIV therapeutic vaccine in 2008 when an internationally recognized and WHO-recognized Professor of Virology from Nigeria, Professor Tam David West wrote in August 2000 in these words:

"Abalaka's scientific (medical) adventurism can only occur in Nigeria – Nowhere else in the whole civilized world. In fact, he cannot even contemplate the saga of his so-called "HIV/AIDS vaccine" treatment." If he dares, he will be picked up and sentenced for medical recklessness. This is without prejudice to the merits (or otherwise) of his claims. It is because he has been rather reckless with the fundamentals.

Do vaccine (sic) *cure?* The answer is of course No. Even a first year microbiology undergraduate knows this.

I had argued earlier that Science is international (Never local).

Perhaps Dr. Abalaka was overzealous when he was reported to have also claimed that his vaccine also cures. This is immunology heresy. Vaccines don't cure, they prevent"

Perhaps, the author is completely out of date with the latest news from France and Sweden, two countries that are highly civilized and developed! Have the French authorities picked up Luc Montagnier and sentenced him for medical recklessness for working on a therapeutic vaccine for HIV and for bringing scientific odium on France for not knowing that vaccines dont cure, they prevent? Has Sweden withdrawn Luc Montagnier's 2008 Nobel Prize because of the immunology heresy that poured out of his lips during the interview he gave on October 6, 2008 when the Nobel Academy announced that he was one of the 3 winners of the 2008 Nobel Prize for Medicine?

Is the Long Journey Along the Perilous Rough Tough Road Worth It?

The author has had a very fulfilling pilgrimage with his self-assigned hobby of trying to develop a safe and effective HIV preventive vaccine for himself. He has achieved that target.

In addition, in the course of doing so, he succeeded first in developing a safe and effective HIV therapeutic vaccine that has cured several patients of HIV infection. Physicians like the author have kept the Physician's Oath and made the health and lives of other people their first consideration. There is that inner contentment and satisfaction in salvaging someone else from the claws of certain death as a result of disease and seeing them living normal lives thereafter. With the universal acknowledgement that HIV infection is incurable and uniformly fatal, it follows that any HIV-infected person would eventually succumb to the infection. The author has succeeded in treating some HIV-infected persons to the point that they became anti-HIV antibody negative, not temporarily but for several years that they have been followed up so far. That achievement gives the author indescribable joy and happiness. The author's HIV therapeutic vaccine has cured a number of highly placed citizens in his country including, at the time they registered with him, started his treatment and became cured, a High Court Judge and a senior military officer. The author did not envisage that his decision to delve into HIV preventive vaccine research at the end of 1991 would give such bountiful satisfying harvests that have made the long perilous journey he has undertaken on a very rough tough road really worth it.

Conclusion

Since 1981 when the first cases of AIDS were described and 1983/84 when the causative agent of AIDS, the HIV was isolated, mankind has known no peace. We have faced extraordinary times with this disease and it calls for bold and far-reaching actions to curb it. It is not the time for conventional thinking or outdated dogma but for the fresh and innovative intervention that gets to the heart of the problem, to echo Gordon Brown, the British Prime Minister. Mankind has lost many millions to the pandemic; over thirty million are still infected and the infection is spreading daily.

The author has played his part and is satisfied. He expects humanity to be allowed to reap the benefits of his efforts so that together the world can hasten the taming of the HIV/AIDS monster. Ten years have already been wasted since safe and effective HIV vaccines were developed and during that period, millions have perished. A change in our approach is long overdue in the interest of humanity everywhere.

Index

B

C

D

G

H

J

K

L

M

N

O

P

Q

R

S

T

U

V

W

X

Y

Z